The Trauma of War:
Stress and
Recovery in
Viet Nam Veterans

The Trauma of War: Stress and Recovery in Viet Nam Veterans

Edited by
Stephen M. Sonnenberg, M.D.
Arthur S. Blank, Jr., M.D.
John A. Talbott, M.D.

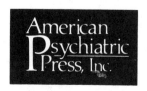

American Psychiatric Press, Inc.

1400 K Street, N.W.
Washington, DC 20005

Note: The contributors have worked to ensure that all information in this book concerning drug dosages, schedules, and routes of administration is accurate as of the time of publication and consistent with standards set by the U.S. Food and Drug Administration and the general medical community. As medical research and practice advance, however, therapeutic standards may change. For this reason and because human and mechanical errors sometimes occur, we recommend that readers follow the advice of a physician who is directly involved in their care or the care of a member of their family.

Books published by the American Psychiatric Press, Inc., represent the views and opinions of the individual authors and do not necessarily reflect the policies and opinions of the Press or the American Psychiatric Association.

Cover Design by Sam Haltom
Text Design by Richard E. Farkas
Typeset by Exspeedite
Printed by RR Donnelley & Sons Company

Library of Congress Cataloging in Publication Data

Main entry under title:

The Trauma of war: stress and recovery in Viet Nam veterans.

Includes bibliographies and index.
1. Post-traumatic stress disorder. 2. Veterans—Mental health services—United States. 3. Vietnamese Conflict, 1961–1975—Psychological aspects. I. Sonnenberg, Stephen M., 1940– . II. Blank, Arthur S., 1936– . III. Talbott, John A. [DNLM: 1. Military Psychiatry. 2. Social Adjustment. 3. Stress Disorders, Post-Traumatic—therapy. 4. Veterans—psychology. WM 184 T777]
RC552.P67T75   1985   616.85'212   85-6094
ISBN 0-88048-048-3

Contents

Dedication

Born in 1946, Eric M. was a happy child in a small American town. As a teenager, he was an accomplished student, swimmer, and photographer. He did well in college, graduating in 1968. Anticipating the draft, he enlisted in the Army in 1969 and graduated with honors from Infantry Noncommissioned Officers School. He married that same year.

In 1970 Sergeant M. was sent to Viet Nam, where he served in combat. He was awarded a Purple Heart and experienced numerous fire fights and ambushes. He later became a combat photographer, on assignment for Army publications.

On return from Viet Nam, Eric's wife, parents, and friends found him to be severely anxious and unable to resume his normal prewar life. He spoke little about his year in Viet Nam. Sometimes he awakened from nightmares. At other times he appeared to be listening vigilantly to some far-off sound that no one else could hear; he could not explain that state of mind. Occasionally there were good days, especially during a trip abroad, which he and his wife thought might clear his mind. But subsequently he remained unable to resume work, for reasons that were never clarified. Eric wanted to work and went for interviews, but he was overcome with anxiety.

In response to the stillbirth of Eric's first child, his life deteriorated strikingly. He expressed the feeling that he was biologically contaminated; he believed that was the cause of the baby's death.

Nineteen months after returning from Viet Nam, Eric agreed to psychiatric hospitalization. He entered a Veterans Administration hospital affiliated with a leading medical school. He was diagnosed as schizophrenic in the absence of any family history of significant psychopathology. Treated with phenothiazine and family and group therapy of generally high quality, his symptoms cleared after six months. He was then discharged.

Over the next three years, Eric often seemed his normal self. He and his wife had two children, he resumed working industriously, and he began studying for a masters degree. However, in early 1976, as his older child approached age three and his younger, age one, Eric became severely anxious and depressed.

He was hospitalized again, diagnosed this time as depressed, and treated as before, with the addition of antidepressant medication. He was subsequently discharged to outpatient care, in which he was treated primarily with medication.

In all, between 1972 and 1976, Eric was seen by 15 different psychiatrists, social workers, and psychologists for evaluation and treatment. Later review of the lengthy medical records revealed psychiatric evaluation and documentation of good quality and conscientious treatment efforts. However, the record includes no information regarding his tour of duty in Viet Nam. It appears that this topic was never explored during two admissions and many outpatient episodes.

In late 1976, Eric was found dead in his car in a closed garage. His death by suicide was due to carbon monoxide poisoning.

Three years after Eric's death, his wife, who had not ceased to believe that his difficulties were due to his untold experiences in Viet Nam, sought review of his case by an expert on the psychiatric effects of war. It then came to light that Eric's wife still had all of the letters that Eric wrote home from Viet Nam. They had been preserved, after having been read once and packed away in 1970 and 1971. On rereading, the following—written to his wife by Eric in Viet Nam—was revealed:

Yes, I'm back in the boonies. . . .When I picked up the bottles from the North Vietnamese base camp, I spent most of the day humping. . . .In the platoon to our flank the. . .sergeant was John Bradley—another honor graduate from my class. . . .The jungle was triple canopy. . .made it impossible to see more than 10 feet. . .constantly fighting vines and scrub brush, trees fallen from artillery—light conditions like those at twilight. . . .John Bradley, survived by his wife and child, took a direct round from a rocket-propelled grenade antitank weapon. . .a direct hit in the abdomen. . . .He like so many others never knew what hit him. . . .He was one of seven people I've seen die since I left Cu Chi. . . .

I'm back in Cu Chi. I took a shower. . .for my mind, which was disordered. I thought I should write everything I'm trying to organize, for us to disentangle our mind. . . . I owe you some explanations. . . .

Most of this month has been spent in Cambodia. . .from Cu Chi to MACV to Tay Ninh to Cambodia—Parrot's Beak—Ba Tu to War Zone

C—Kontum. . . .Guns and artillery and pain and killing and GI's and children and tortured faces. . . .The last two weeks became impossible to write around. (I'm still sorting. . .still not talking about why I'm unable to sleep.)

I can't disentangle it yet. . . .I saw three young children detonate a booby-trapped mine. . . .I was also with their father (maybe three or five years older than me) when we tried to get help even back to the aid station. . . .He was beautiful. . .pitiful. . .tortured, frantic. They were dying, the young girl and one boy died while at the aid station. The medic told me they were going to die. . .they did. The father's eyes were imploring, pleading, praying. I felt guilty, how can I say I'm not with these people. I just wanted to see what it's like. . . .And I don't like it. He can see the tears in my eyes reflected in the tears in his. . .talk about guilt.

Thus Eric wrote to his wife from Viet Nam in 1971, partway through his tour. Soon after these particular excerpts, Eric wrote that he felt his mind detach from his surroundings. For the remainder of the tour his letters did not again mention events in Viet Nam. He wrote only about returning home.

Before consulting an expert, Eric's widow had twice applied to the Veterans Administration for a determination that his death had been service-connected. She believed that his suicide had been the result of war neurosis. Her application was twice turned down.

However, in 1979, when all records were obtained and carefully reviewed, it became clear that there was no evidence for any other diagnosis than post-traumatic stress disorder. The letters from Viet Nam, along with the medical history and the statements of a number of friends and family members, were presented to the U.S. Board of Veterans Appeals in 1980. At that time, the Board determined that the cause of Eric's death was post-tramatic stress disorder. Four years after Eric's death, the board awarded his widow and children benefits due them by reason of his death having been caused by a disability connected with military duty.

Upon hearing the news of this decision by the Board in 1980, a Viet Nam veteran psychologist observed, "The system is weeping." Since 1980, there has been no river of tears, save perhaps among veterans and their families at the Viet Nam Veterans Memorial in Washington, D.C. The "system"—our institutions and the professions—appears however to be attempting to fully confront the challenge of healing the psychological wounds of the war. This attempt, yet tense and painful, is still uncertain of outcome.

Our guilt about many veterans like Sergeant M. stands in the way. However, with sufficient weeping, reparation, and clear memories, this barrier too shall be overcome. As for the weeping, we recommend our readers to their own human capacity for healing grief. As for reparation, we believe this clinical textbook provides guidance for the only true reparation from mental health professionals: good treatment for all those who need it.

As for clear remembering, this book is dedicated to the memory of Sergeant Eric M., to his widow, and to their two children. And it is dedicated to all Viet Nam veterans and their families—especially their children—who have suffered or lost their way, because of unhealed emotional wounds from the Viet Nam War, and because they could not find someone among their fellow men and women who could hear, share, understand, and ease their pain.

Foreword

 War has always had a profound effect on those who engage in combat, and psychiatric studies of the psychological effects of war are as old as the field itself. The war in Viet Nam, however, was different in many ways. First, it was the first "unpopular" war within the memory of most persons alive today. Second, it touched all elements of society because of its profoundly divisive political nature. Third, it was reported in detail by the media; recorded in detail by historians and scientists alike; and studied in detail by physicians and others in the health field, utilizing technologies never before available. And fourth, the Viet Nam War became a metaphor for American society, encapsulating within a single phrase all that connoted distrust in traditional government, limitations in the realization of the American dream, and the futility of the sacrifice of American lives for poorly understood and deeply divided values and principles.

It is no surprise, then, that the psychological effects of the Viet Nam War were also different. First, there were reports of puzzlingly low psychiatric casualty rates, originally attributed to modern methods of combat psychiatry. Second, there were widespread and disturbing reports of multiple drug abuse as well as acts of violence against both Vietnamese civilians and American officers. Third, acts of "disobedience"—refusal to take antimalarial pills, to go out on patrol, or to conform to "Mickey Mouse regulations"—seemed to reflect the zeitgeist of the war as much as the personalities of the soldiers involved. And finally, most insidious and most pervasive was the finding that despite the seemingly low psychiatric casualty rates, upon their return to "the world," many veterans exhibited significant psychiatric symptoms. These ranged from difficulty sleeping to vivid flashbacks, and are now widely recognized as comprising a syndrome heretofore acknowledged but not so codified in our nomenclature—post-traumatic stress disorder.

Our professional resistance in recognizing and treating PTSD was no different than our societal reluctance to welcome home our warriors, to reflect in literature and films our recent experience, or to openly discuss among ourselves—especially those of us who are Viet Nam veterans—our experiences, reflections, and emotional sequelae.

It has taken us a very long time as a society to begin to deal with Viet Nam; it has taken psychiatry just as long as a field to begin to deal with the war's psychological victims. This volume represents a significant milestone, for its appearance—10 years after the last American troops left Viet Nam—signals the realization that research on the psychological effects of the war has reached the point where analysis and review can lead to new insights into the effects of war itself, and specifically the Viet Nam War, on American soldiers. In addition, it is now possible to clarify what further research questions must be addressed in the immediate future to better understand the effects of war on the human psyche.

Now the critical task for all mental health professionals who are interested in this area is to translate our understanding of the psychological effects of the Viet Nam experience into effective and accessible programs for those suffering from its impact. This book, summarizing as it does our knowledge regarding specific syndromes, subgroups of the population affected, and different treatment modalities, gives us the theoretical and practical data base to transform what we have learned into action. Thousands of men and women have died and suffered as a consequence of the war in Viet Nam. It is our responsibility to use the knowledge we now have to ameliorate the plight of those who survive.

John A. Talbott, M.D.

Acknowledgments

$\mathbf{B}$etween 1979 and 1983 my work with Viet Nam Veterans was supported by two academic institutions and five foundations. Each showed foresight in recognizing that the problems of Viet Nam veterans were not over, were worthy of careful investigation, and were demanding of help. My thanks, then, to the Washington College of Law of The American University, the Howard University College of Medicine, the Eugene and Agnes E. Meyer Foundation, the Public Welfare Foundation, Inc., the Carlile Foundation, The Windom Fund, and The New World Foundation.

The definitive editing of this book took place during the academic year 1984–1985, while I served as Scholar in Residence at The Washington School of Psychiatry. My thanks to the School for supporting this project.

The original idea for this project emerged from the activities of the Committee on Federal Government Health Services of the American Psychiatric Association. The Committee and its individual members deserve much credit for the publication of this book.

Tim Clancy, the editor with whom I worked at the American Psychiatric Press, deserves the highest praise and thanks for his professionalism, technical skill, and friendship.

Peter E. Scheer was a thoughtful and helpful friend in ways too numerous to catalog. My thanks are extended to him.

In order to edit this book it was necessary to appreciate not only the foundations of psychiatry and psychology, but the evolving nature of those disciplines. John G. Sonnenberg's curiosity and penetrating questions left me ever-sensitive to that process of evolution. Additionally, it was important to appreciate the relevance of an understanding of historical events and political influences to what was far more than a psychiatric problem. Katharine L. Sonnenberg's incisive comments were invaluable in this regard. It was also essential to understand the contemporary relationship of the range of mental health disciplines and the ways helping professionals can most effectively interact. By example, and through her thoughtful observations, Dale F. Sonnenberg, A.C.S.W., provided invaluable assistance in meeting that challenge. All three Sonnenbergs were not only giving of their assistance, but generous of the time we might have otherwise spent together in easier pursuits. My sense of gratitude to them is boundless.

By their example my parents, Peggy and Leonard Sonnenberg, taught me the importance of the most fortunate in our society reaching out to the least fortunate, with concern and compassion. Those lessons served me well during this project.

Stephen M. Sonnenberg, M.D.

I am grateful to the many colleagues and friends who have contributed to the development of this book, especially Sarah Haley. In 1969, at the height of the Viet Nam War, Sarah Haley began providing psychotherapeutic treatment to Viet Nam veterans, based on creative clinical insight and brave personal initiative. Undeterred by years of skepticism and indifference, she has continued to this day to inspire many others who have now prevailed in the effort to bring enlightenment to fellow professionals, awareness to the public, and help to many veterans. Her inspiration is reflected often in this book.

I am especially grateful to the following colleagues for their support of my work: John Russell Smith, M.A., Paul Errera, M.D., D. Earl Brown, Jr., M.D., Stephen Fleck, M.D., Shad Meshad, M.S.W., and especially Ira Levine, M.D., Richard Munich, M.D., Sid Blatt, Ph.D., Charles Gardner, M.D., Victor Altshul, M.D., and the other members of our psychotherapy study group at Yale University.

Finally, and perhaps most importantly, I wish to thank my wife and principal friend in life's journey, Donna Blank.

Arthur S. Blank, Jr., M.D.

Contributors

Arthur L. Arnold, M.D.

Chief, Psychiatry Service,
Veterans Administration Medical Center,
Phoenix, Arizona; and
Lecturer in Psychiatry,
Department of Psychiatry,
University of Arizona College of Medicine

Arthur S. Blank, Jr., M.D.

National Director,
Viet Nam Veterans Outreach and Counseling Centers,
Veterans Administration; and
Lecturer in Psychiatry,
Yale University Department of Psychiatry

Ghislaine Boulanger, Ph.D.

Director, Psychology Externship Program,
The New Hope Guild Centers, New York

James Dwyer, M.S.W.

Chief, Viet Nam Veterans Liaison Unit,
Veterans Administration Medical Center,
West Los Angeles–Brentwood Division

Harry C. Holloway, M.D.

Colonel, Medical Corps, U.S.A.; and
Chairperson and Professor of Psychiatry,
F. Edward Hébert School of Medicine,
Uniformed Services University of the Health Sciences,
Bethesda, Maryland

Charles Kadushin, Ph.D.

Professor of Sociology and Psychology,
Graduate Center,
City University of New York

Lawrence C. Kolb, M.D.

Distinguished Physician in Psychiatry,
Veterans Administration Medical Center,
Albany, New York;
Professor of Psychiatry,
Albany Medical College; and
Professor Emeritus of Psychiatry,
Columbia University

Robert S. Laufer, Ph.D.

Department of Sociology,
Brooklyn College, Graduate Center,
City University of New York; and
Center for Policy Research

John O. Lipkin, M.D.

Associate Director for Psychiatry,
Mental Health and Behavioral Sciences Service,
Veterans Administration Central Office

Janet Ott, R.N., M.N.

Clinical Nurse Specialist,
National Center for Stress Recovery,
Veterans Administration Medical Center,
Brecksville, Ohio

Erwin Randolph Parson, Ph.D.

National Clinical Program Specialist,
Veterans Administration Central Office;
Former Regional Manager,
Viet Nam Veterans Readjustment Centers,
Northeastern U.S.A.,
Veterans Administration; and
Psychoanalyst in Private Practice

Bruce Pentland, M.P.A.

Social Work Associate,
Vietnam Veterans Liaison Unit,
Veterans Administration Medical Center,
West Los Angeles–Brentwood Division

Gregorio Piña, III, Ph.D.

Clinical Psychologist in Private Practice,
McAllen and Laredo, Texas

Raymond Monsour Scurfield, D.S.W.

Associate Director,
Viet Nam Veterans Outreach and Counseling Centers,
Veterans Administration

John Russell Smith, M.A.

Director, Center for Stress Recovery,
Veterans Administration Medical Center,
Brecksville, Ohio; and
Assistant Clinical Professor of Psychology,
Department of Psychiatry,
School of Medicine,
Case Western Reserve University,
Cleveland

Stephen M. Sonnenberg, M.D.

Scholar in Residence,
The Washington School of Psychiatry

John A. Talbott, M.D.

Professor of Psychiatry,
Cornell University Medical College;
Associate Medical Director,
The Payne Whitney Psychiatric Clinic,
The New York Hospital; and
President (1984–1985),
American Psychiatric Association

Robert J. Ursano, M.D.

Lieutenant Colonel, U.S. Air Force, Medical Corps; and
Associate Professor and Associate Chairman,
Department of Psychiatry,
F. Edward Hébert School of Medicine,
Uniformed Services University of Health Sciences,
Bethesda, Maryland

Candis M. Williams, Psy.D.

Clinical and Organizational Psychologist,
Denver Police Department,
Denver, Colorado

Tom Williams, Psy.D.

Director,
Post Trauma Treatment Center,
Denver, Colorado

The Trauma of War:
Stress and
Recovery in
Viet Nam Veterans

1

Introduction:
The Trauma of War

Stephen M. Sonnenberg, M.D.

1

It was a steamy July day several years ago. Stan, a Viet Nam combat hero, walked into a small clothing store. He was bedecked with his war medals and carried a fully loaded automatic rifle. He took control of the store and asked everyone in it to keep calm and take cover. He carefully explored the building, firing from time to time at the ceiling.

Several hours later, after tense negotiations with local police, Stan emerged from the store. No one had been injured or even threatened. The customers and employees told a curious story, for they believed—and they couldn't say just why—that Stan seemed protective of them during their time together.

Stan gave his lawyers and the authorities a detailed history of his life before, during, and after Viet Nam, but could not understand or explain his reason for entering the clothing store. He reported that he grew up in a home which included a large extended family. He was the only son, and his impulsive grandfather frequently beat him as a child. He observed that at such times his frightened parents stood by in silence, concerned with their own physical safety and that of his two sisters. Stan grew up with unmasked rage toward his parents for their passivity. When he reached an eligible age he enlisted in the Army and became a member of a crack combat unit in Viet Nam. He was just 18 years old.

Stan reported two vivid and horrible memories of Viet Nam, memories which haunted him in the form of powerful and frightening waking experiences, and in the form of remarkably similar dreams when he slept. First, he remembered the day when a small Vietnamese girl came running toward him and two comrades while they paused for a smoke on a country road. He saw clearly that the child held an explosive, which would detonate when she released a spring mechanism she held closed in her clenched fist. Stan called to the child, urging her to throw the bomb away. She would not or did not respond, and finally he shot and killed her when she was about 50 yards from him. When she was hit the device did detonate, and an explosion of substantial magnitude did occur. However, from that moment on he was haunted by guilty memories of what he had done.

Stan's second memory concerned an event which occurred some three weeks later. He and his platoon were caught in a Vietcong ambush, and Stan was one of three survivors. He observed his closest buddies slaughtered in cross-fire. His memories included vivid pictures of the disemboweling of these men by continued enemy fire into their dead bodies, which lay about the ambush scene. Stan recalled that a rage came over him, and—in a state of mind he could not explain, but in which he felt that he was "not really there"—he fought the enemy and almost single-handedly routed them. After the enemy had been slaughtered, he fired at their corpses, destroyed their faces with fire from his automatic weapon, and eventually had to be dragged away by his comrades. Stan added that he could not be sure, but he felt that his state of mind in the clothing store reminded him of his state of mind on that fateful day in Viet Nam. He said that his memories of the ambush were, like those involving the little girl he had killed, characterized by guilt.

Stan reported that upon his return to the United States he was still in uniform when he had an unfortunate experience with a civilian. He wanted to go to a sporting event, but he was turned away at the door because all of the tickets had been sold. Stan felt entitled to attend the event because he had sacrificed for his country in Viet Nam; he felt enraged, but he controlled his temper, muttering under his breath as he walked away. The gatekeeper noticed this, resented Stan's muttering, and challenged Stan to a fight. Stan fought this man and won; the police were called, and Stan was arrested. He was later released, but the police report which reached the Army concerning the beating Stan gave the man led to a denial of his opportunity to reenlist. Stan felt devastated.

From the day of Stan's separation from the Army to the day of his entry into the store, a period of several years, he never felt he got on track. He kept losing good jobs, such as selling real estate, even though he always did well in terms of specific employment tasks. He realized that he always felt angry at the orders he was given by supervisors, and that he never seemed able to hide this from them. He knew the firings occurred because his supervisors felt there was something distant and eerie about him, and because they were frightened by the thinly disguised rage they saw in him. Stan also reported that the same complaints were registered by his girlfriends, who also eventually rejected him because to them he seemed forever distant and uncommitted, forever somewhere else.

Stan often felt strange; in fact he often felt as though he were back at the ambush, though in reality he might have been taking a walk, talking to a friend, or watching television. At times this strange feeling blended into a sense of déjà vu, a sense he was doing something he had done before. This, too, occurred at times most notable for being unremarkable, like when he was driving a car.

Having related part of the history of Stan, a Viet Nam combat hero in trouble with the law, it is now possible to meaningfully describe post-traumatic stress disorder (PTSD) and the psychological difficulties experienced by many Viet Nam veterans (1).

Many veterans suffer from some of the symptoms of PTSD, while a smaller but still very large number have the symptoms required for the diagnosis of the condition. These veterans were exposed to conditions of extreme psychological stress. The trauma to which they were exposed was guerilla warfare, and many of those who are most substantially disturbed witnessed the mutilation of a close combat buddy or survived the ambush of their unit. Because they survived and now feel guilty for surviving when others did not, or for what they did in order to survive, they suffer emotionally.

These individuals frequently experience depression, with a full range of accompanying symptoms, such as loss of appetite. In addition to insomnia, these veterans experience nightmares of the traumatic event and in waking life can experience flashbacks. Flashbacks are altered states of consciousness in which the individual believes he or she is again experiencing the traumatic event. As dramatic as a full-blown flashback can be, it is but one point on a spectrum of more or less subtle alterations in consciousness experienced by those suffering from PTSD. Much of the psychic life of each of these individuals is devoted to reexperiencing traumatic events, and on an unconscious level these individuals strive to master their traumas by making them come out differently. The altered state of consciousness occurs in the service of this task. Since the disorder is so psychologically painful, many of these individuals sedate themselves with drugs or alcohol. Since at the core of the disorder is a fear of loss of loved ones and friends, these individuals keep distant from those around them to avoid the inevitable pain of departure and loss. Thus, they are impaired in their functioning with friends, family, and employers, and their divorce and unemployment rates are in excess of what would be predicted based on variables excluding combat service in Viet Nam.

The typical Viet Nam veteran with PTSD, or elements of the condition, is now aged in the mid-30s (slightly older in the case of women veterans) and saw Viet Nam combat at age 19½. The typical Viet Nam combat soldier was younger than the typical combat soldier of World War II or Korea and was therefore more psychologically vulnerable than those men. Viet Nam veterans will be poor and from an under-privileged racial or ethnic background in greater than expected numbers, given the size of their race or ethnic group in the population at large. Their chief presenting symptom may be poor vocational or marital adjustment or perhaps alcohol or drug abuse. They may report that their problems began immediately after combat trauma, or that there was a latency period of months to years (which resulted in the term "delayed stress reaction"), but they will consistently report some combination of the following: guilt over survival, anxiety, de-pression, nightmares, and altered states of consciousness. They may tell you that they have suffered for long years, were distrustful of the Veterans Administration, and only with the advent of the Viet Nam Veterans Outreach Center program did they consider treatment in a government facility.

Important theoretical questions about PTSD may now be consid-ered. The question of predisposition arises, since in Stan's life there were frequent episodes of psychic trauma throughout a childhood marred by the brutality of his grandfather. There is no doubt that predisposing factors must be evaluated in an individual with PTSD (2), but research findings in this book suggest that more important than premorbid personality and pathology is the nature of trauma, its immediate impact on the victim, and its subsequent intrapsychic meaning to the victim. Normal developmental factors are also rele-vant: the soldier who is a few years older than the average combatant and possesses a more integrated sense of self and purpose has greater insulation against serious trauma than does a late adolescent who is still in the process of more active maturation.

An individual's sense of self is not only a function of maturity, but also of environmental supports. It is clear that the general lack of opportunity to discuss Viet Nam with appreciative, respectful listeners back home is a factor which contributes to the development and course of PTSD in many veterans (3). This factor, too, is further discussed in this book. Finally, for minority veterans, including women, the home environment was complicated by prejudice and, as shall also be described in these pages, even less supportive of success-ful readjustment.

From a metapsychological standpoint we can see that there is much to learn about the genetics of PTSD, but clearly pretraumatic strengths and weaknesses, the trauma itself, and subsequent events and experiences are all important to an understanding of the condition.

In much of the literature on PTSD the sufferer is described as though everything relevant is conscious. Stan's case illustrates that this is not always so—he did not have any idea why he entered and took over the clothing store—and recent work by two distinguished psychiatrists suggests that to understand PTSD the nature of unconscious process in the condition must be explored. In Chapter 14, Arthur Blank describes the unconscious flashback, observed when an individual plays out a script from the past without conscious awareness of the process. In Chapter 10, Lawrence Kolb describes PTSD sufferers who are unaware of the traumas they experienced, and who can be helped by a therapy designed to restore memory and encourage abreaction.

In psychotherapy the veteran with PTSD is able to develop insight which clarifies the existence of altered states of mind, the meaning of action in terms of reworking past traumatic events, and the meaning of patterns of interpersonal behavior. In this book the full range of available therapies for PTSD will be described, including modes of assistance for special veteran groups. The following case example is intended as an introduction to the task of the psychotherapist.

Jack was referred by a lawyer in the community after he had been charged with attempted burglary. (For heuristic purposes, in this illustration issues relating to premorbid personality and childhood will be omitted.) The most striking feature of the alleged crime was the impossibility of success. Jack was not an experienced thief, in fact he had never before been in trouble with the law, and the place he allegedly attempted to burglarize had an obvious and extensive security system. Finally, Jack reported that minutes before arriving at the building, just a few blocks away, he had been stopped by the police. Why they had stopped him was unclear, but they had, and in spite of this Jack did not alter his plans. Jack was then followed by the police and arrested as he attempted to enter the building.

During initial interviews with Jack, his most impressive characteristic was that he didn't feel terribly concerned about being sent to jail. He felt that he had taken a chance and not succeeded, and now he would have to suffer the consequences. Furthermore, for several weeks he expressed disbelief regarding any of the psychodynamic explanations offered for his behavior. He remained cool, calm, distant, and unmoved.

Jack revealed that as a late adolescent he joined the Army, with the intention of going to Viet Nam to serve his country. He chose to become a medic because he wanted to help his comrades. He recalled that throughout his tour in Viet Nam he felt a great sense of responsibility to the men he treated in the field; if one died on the way to the hospital, he usually experienced remorse and guilt. He reported feeling that if he had been able to go along on the helicopter his patients would have survived.

Upon discharge Jack was distant from others and remained so by conscious design. He traveled around the country alone, avoiding interpersonal involvement. He met a woman, became somewhat close with her, and eventually lived with her. However, they staunchly maintained emotional independence of each other. As therapy progressed Jack came to feel that his style of relating to others reflected among other influences his experience of service in Viet Nam.

A few months before Jack's arrest, he had learned that his mother was dying of a degenerative disease. At first he visited her on weekends, traveling the thousand miles to her, talking with her doctor and nurses, and returning home. He became certain that only he could provide her with the supportive care she required, and he moved her to his home. Then, as his mother continued to deteriorate physically, Jack began to experience ambivalent feelings towards her. He saw her as an emotional drain, and at times wished she were dead.

Jack experienced barely perceptible confusion over his mixed feelings towards his mother, and he became minimally aware that he was feeling "down." His decision to enter the building was motivated by two conscious needs. First, he wanted money because he was concerned about how he would pay for his mother's care when her savings were depleted. Second, because he was feeling "down," he hoped that success at an adventure would give him an emotional lift, making him feel happy. At the start of therapy he was not aware that his behavior was related to a need to assert mastery at a time when he felt helpless. As his capacity for insight increased, he realized that his mother's illness had caused him to reexperience painful memories of helplessness, which in part originated in his work as a medic in Viet Nam.

Efforts to explore Jack's dream life produced information concerning two repetitive dreams. Jack reported that usually he did not dream, and that these were the only dreams he could recall. In one dream, he is going to fetch something from the garage. There, he is met by a menacing bear and feels frightened. Jack awakens just before the bear reaches him. In the other dream, Jack is sleeping on the ground in Viet Nam, and within the dream he awakens with a snake on him. He immediately associated to his hatred of snakes, said that in the dream he was frightened, and added that he actually awakened in a state of panic after waking within the dream. Efforts to develop associations to these dreams were met with thoughts of actual fears: during his childhood, living in a rural setting, Jack was afraid of attacks from animals; he really did fear snakes and had done so all his life. What was most impressive about these dreams is that in them Jack seemed to be reexperiencing something he knew and feared. Eventually, he recognized that his dream life reflected his preoccupation with real-life traumatic experiences.

Through exploration of his relationship with his dying mother, and his attemped commission of a crime which couldn't succeed, Jack learned that he had been acting symbolically in response to feelings of survivor guilt and the need for punishment to expiate guilt. Jack realized that his anxiety dreams represented an attempt to master the scars of psychic trauma, which in large measure involved combat. He recognized that his original "war crime" was that he had survived, while failing to save his friends. He saw for the first time that he had been angry at his patients for dying, and that this complicated reaction had made him feel even guiltier. Finally, Jack realized that his style of relating to others after Viet Nam was designed to shield himself from traumas in the future.

Specifically with regard to the burglary attempt, Jack came to believe it represented a complicated effort to deal with the feelings he had about past experiences, including his experiences in Viet Nam. As time passed his memory of the burglary improved. Eventually, Jack realized that during much of the burglary he was unsure of where he was; "felt" he was back in various past situations, including Viet Nam; felt very guilty; and believed that by successfully entering the locked building he would symbolically enter the hospital to help the men to whom he had ministered in the field. He also became aware of a wish during the burglary to be caught and punished.

As Jack remembered more, he became less psychically numb, more involved with his psychiatrist, and better able to struggle with painful memories of his past and how he specifically played them out in the here and now.

There is no question that psychological treatment of PTSD is effective and that this effectiveness is explained by the oldest of psychiatric principles: the process of putting painful feelings and impulses into words ameliorates psychic suffering, and the development of an understanding of the meaning of one's actions and memories and dreams has a healing effect. These truths explain the reason for the success, not only of individual psychotherapy, but of peer group counseling in the treatment of psychic trauma. In the group setting, the purposes of behavior, dreams and daydreams, and fantasies are well known to all who share the common pathway of stressful experience which leads to membership. This, too, is described in detail in this book.

From a psychodynamic perspective, both Stan and Jack illustrate that Viet Nam veterans with PTSD struggle with guilt (4): such veterans fear the loss of those close to them and fear hurting anyone with whom they develop closeness. That the condition involves the repetition compulsion, the desire to rework the past and make it come out differently, is clear. Also clear is that, since the script is already written, a different outcome is not possible.

Some of the most fascinating questions about PTSD arise with respect to the metapsychological concepts of psychic energy and structure. The psychoanalytic literature proffers the idea that psychic trauma can cause a fundamental psychobiological change (5), that is, a permanent, biologically rooted change in the way the mind works or performs the range of psychological functions. Included in this perspective is the view that psychic energy is not available as before to perform mental tasks.

These theoretical speculations about psychic energy and structure raise vital questions, which can be answered through basic and applied research. Does trauma actually alter the biological activity of the central nervous system in some potentially permanent way? If so, what is the mechanism of action? Finally, how can pharmacological or psychological intervention, or a combination of the two, return the system to proper functioning?

Those who suffer from PTSD report similar traumatic dream and waking experiences. They report altered states of consciousness and a sense that they are often "not all there." They report a vague sense that they are often doing something that they have done before. All this suggests that there may be unusual patterns to be found on the EEGs of these individuals, and that this may be an area of measurement where understanding of the biological roots of behavior can be advanced.

The relationship in traumatized individuals between dreaming and waking life, for example, clearly provides an opportunity for such investigation. From a clinical perspective an attempt to rework a past traumatic event may involve an eruption of dream life, the life of the wish, into waking life. In a psychologically traumatized man, sensory conversion reactions which represented an intrusion of the dream into waking life have previously been described (6). That formulation concerning conversion leaned heavily on the work of Levitan (7) and Lewin (8).

Altered states of consciousness in the form of flashbacks, as experienced by both Stan and Jack, may represent intrusions of dreams and traumatic memories into waking life. If this hypothesis is proved correct, it would provide an explanatory mechanism for complicated, irrational flashback activity. Another traumatized patient previously described experienced obvious hallucinations (9). While hallucinations are not described in *DSM-III* (10) as a part of the PTSD syndrome, they are recognized as occurring in traumatized individuals, sometimes as an intensification of flashbacks. Hallucinations are thought of as a dream-in-waking-life phenomenon by some who work with psychotic patients, so in fact the idea that the barrier between dreaming and waking life is disturbed by psychic trauma is compatible with a long tradition of theoretical psychodynamic formulation.

The recorded history of PTSD is almost as old as the history of humanity, sensitively reported by talented expert observers of the human condition. Not long ago the contemporary literature noted the poetically reported case of a European university student, who several hundred years ago was noted to have PTSD. The poet was Shakespeare and the student, Hamlet (11). Despite this long history of recognition of PTSD, it seemed that after Viet Nam even recent clinical experience derived from World War II and Korea was forgotten. Many psychiatrists simply did not recognize PTSD, even in veterans who showed dramatic signs of an unsuccessful attempt to reintegrate psychologically after a stressful war experience. This phenomenon indicates the difficulty all mental health professionals have in recognizing and working with problems related to stress. More than most patients with mental illness, those with PTSD arouse anxiety about the helping professional's own potential for psychopathology, as therapists recognize in themselves the capacity to act in savage ways under savage circumstances, and to suffer a protracted and agonizing stress disorder in response to that behavior.

Psychiatrists and psychotherapists can overcome anxiety and listen with empathy to those who suffer from PTSD. First, recognition of how difficult it is to do this work is necessary, and then professionals can learn that they do have the ability to bear the stress of working with this patient population. If therapists do create an environment in which veterans can tell their stories, the therapists will experience the special satisfaction of the healer who works well with the victim.

Finally, another result of working with those who suffer from PTSD is that therapists will learn much that is applicable to patients in other diagnostic categories. Victims of psychic trauma teach one to appreciate how in the lives of all people elements of reaction to stress are intermingled with elements of the more familiar neuroses and major mental disorders. While many of the situations which cause PTSD are clear-cut, it is my view that the experience of even a most horrible event as traumatic must be understood as a unique phenomenon in each patient or client. All human beings are unique, have had unique developmental experiences, and possess a singular set of psychological strengths, weaknesses, vulnerabilities, and potentials. Thus, by understanding those with PTSD, by listening carefully to their stories, much can be learned about the nature of human mental functioning, and hypotheses about psychobiology and the interplay of talking therapy and biological disorder can be generated.

Such lessons potentially advance our understanding of psychology and behavioral science and create the possibility of helping patient groups who have so far been beyond the reach of psychiatric therapy. Thus, this book has been written to serve a twofold purpose: to demonstrate the problems and needs of Viet Nam veterans suffering from the trauma of war, and to disseminate the combined experience of this book's contributors, in the spirit of aiding the advancement of psychological science and art.

REFERENCES

1. Sonnenberg SM: Statement of the American Psychiatric Association on Viet Nam Veterans Counseling Readjustment Programs (S.26, S.458, S.872), before the Senate Committee on Veterans' Affairs. Congressional Record 127(104): E3460–E3461, 1981

2. Worthington ER: Demographic and pre-service variables as predictors of post-military service adjustment, in Stress Disorders Among Viet Nam Veterans. Edited by Figley CR. New York, Brunner/Mazel, 1978

3. Figley CR (ed): Introduction, in Stress Disorders Among Viet Nam Veterans. New York, Brunner/Mazel, 1978

4. Sonnenberg SM: A disputed diagnosis of posttraumatic stress disorder: reply. Hosp Community Psychiatry 33:666, 1968

5. Winnik HZ: Contribution to symposium on psychic traumatization through social catastrophe. Int J Psychoanal 49:298–301, 1968

6. Sonnenberg SM: A hypothesis concerning the nature of sensory conversion. Paper presented to the Baltimore-DC Society for Psychoanalysis, Washington, DC, January 1974

7. Levitan H: Depersonalization and the dream. Psychoanal Q 36:157–171, 1967

8. Lewin BD: The Psychoanalysis of Elation. New York, Psychoanalytic Quarterly, 1950

9. Sonnenberg SM: A special form of survivor syndrome. Psychoanal Q 41:58–62, 1972

10. American Psychiatric Association: Diagnostic and Statistical Manual of Mental Disorders, Third Edition. Washington, DC, American Psychiatric Association, 1980

11. Sonnenberg SM: A transcultural observation of posttraumatic stress disorder. Hosp Community Psychiatry 33:58–59, 1982

2

Post-Traumatic Stress Disorder: An Old Problem with a New Name

Ghislaine Boulanger, Ph.D.

2

In this chapter I shall review the different ways in which the syndrome now called post-traumatic stress disorder has been understood by the medical profession. It has taken almost two-thirds of a century for the recognition that shell shock is a psychological rather than a physiological disorder to be officially integrated into psychiatric nosology. I shall discuss some of the factors that may have contributed to the psychiatric profession's reluctance to accept the fact that traumas that occur in adult life can have long-lasting psychological consequences, even for people who were previously without psychological problems. I shall then consider the acute and chronic phases of PTSD as they are described in the *Diagnostic and Statistical Manual of Mental Disorders*, Third Edition (1), contrasting this description with findings obtained when the list of symptoms found in *DSM-III* is subjected to a statistical program that tests the validity of a given diagnosis by determining whether the symptoms form a characteristic pattern. The chapter will conclude with a summary of the findings of a national survey of young men of the Viet Nam generation, in which Viet Nam veterans were compared with both nonveterans and non–war zone veterans on a number of social and psychological dimensions. Our findings establish the expected incidence of PTSD among those subjected to a traumatic stressor and consider its prevalence among combat veterans today. I shall also discuss the influence of a number of pre- and postservice variables in affecting the onset and maintenance of this disorder, and in so doing I shall take up the question of predisposition, which has been the source of considerable conflict in establishing this diagnosis.

The support of grant no. MH 34580-02 from the National Institute of Mental Health to Charles Kadushin, Principal Investigator, is gratefully acknowledged. NIMH is not in any way responsible for the analysis and conclusions reported in this paper.

OPPOSITION TO THE DIAGNOSIS OF PTSD

Had we returned home then, out of the suffering and strength of our experiences we might have unleashed a storm. Now if we go back we will be weary, broken, burnt out, rootless, and without hope. We will not be able to find our way any more. . . . We will be superfluous even to ourselves, we will grow older, a few will adapt themselves, some others will merely submit, and most will be bewildered; —the years will pass by and in the end we shall fall into ruin. (2, p. 254)

These are among the concluding lines of *All Quiet on the Western Front*, one of the classic novels of wartime experience. They were written of the 1914–1918 war during the course of which, as Fairbairn (3) remarked some 25 years later, "a remarkable scientific advance was undoubtedly registered by the abandonment of the term 'shell-shock' in favor of the term 'war-neurosis' " (p. 279). This change of terminology indicated a recognition of the fact that the "weary, broken, burnt out, rootless" men, whom Erich Maria Remarque described with such painful clarity, were suffering from symptoms that were essentially of psychological and not of neurological origin.

It has taken psychiatrists in the United States over 60 years to further refine this position. Those who treated combat veterans in hospitals, clinics, and their private offices after World War II, after Korea, and most recently after Viet Nam would not deny the psychological nature of the problems, but they have failed to agree on the etiology or natural course of reactions to severe trauma. In his seminal chapter on war neuroses written in 1969, Kardiner (4) commented on mental health professionals' reluctance to arrive at a consensus about post-traumatic stress reactions: "In general there is a vast store of data available. . . but it is hard to find a province of psychiatry in which there is less discipline than this one. There is practically no continuity to be found anywhere, and the literature can only be characterized as anarchic. Every author has his own frame of reference—lengthy bibliographies notwithstanding" (p. 245). It is not my purpose here to add to the anarchy by advancing yet another view, but rather to understand the reasons underlying the failure to reach a consensus until 1980.

One reason for the reluctance to build on the wealth of hard facts and empirical observations that have followed each war—indeed, each catastrophe that has overtaken a segment of the population—lies in the fact that the data challenge one of the fundamental beliefs in psychiatry and particularly in that branch of psychiatry that is influenced by psychoanalysis. The question of trauma is at the root of psychoanalysis, but the timing of the trauma is also significant, and it is this that has historically proved a stumbling block to the acceptance and appropriate treatment of traumatic neuroses. For it is commonly believed that the etiology of pathology lies not in adult but in childhood traumas. To argue that trauma in adult life can have profound and long-lasting psychological consequences even among individuals who were previously normal is to contradict this developmental theory.

Paradoxically, Freud (5) considered the "dark and dismal subject" (p. 5) of traumatic neuroses to be a separate phenomenon from neuroses whose foundations lie in childhood. In *Beyond the Pleasure Principle*, he treats the nightmares that almost always accompany traumatic neuroses as entirely separate phenomena from normal wish fulfillment dreams. He argues that nightmares that follow trauma represent the psyche's repeated attempts to master a situation that has overwhelmed the defenses. But these distinctions appear to have been overlooked by his followers, who maintain that a defense system cannot have been adequate in the first place if it was so permanently disabled by a catastrophic event. Thus the dogma of the childhood etiology of neuroses prevailed. For example, Ferenczi et al. (6) published a symposium during World War II in which they concluded that those who fall prey to war neuroses had suffered an arrest of development at the oral or anal libidinous stage, and the subsequent trauma of war forced the soldier to regress to the original state of the arrest. The British psychiatrist Fairbairn (3), who served as Visiting Psychiatrist to the Emergency Medical Service in Great Britain during World War II, puts the argument most strongly and most succinctly.

> It is rare to find a case in which evidence of preexisting psychopathological characteristics cannot be detected in the previous history (p. 257). . . . The chief predisposing factor in determining the breakdown of a soldier . . . is infantile dependence on his objects. . . . The most distinctive feature of military breakdowns is separation anxiety. (p. 79)

Such a point of view obviously precludes putting traumatic neuroses in a separate category from other neuroses. It permits, indeed encourages, the clinician to deny the significance of the trauma itself. Fairbairn, for example, made little distinction between his patients who had seen combat and those who had not. He describes one man he interviewed, a sailor whose ship was torpedoed, who had to swim for his life in order to escape the burning oil, and who was forced to drown a floundering survivor in order to prevent himself from being drowned along with him; the sailor subsequently became symptomatic. Fairbairn appears to equate this survivor's experience with the breakdown of a soldier immediately upon induction. There is a fundamental error in confusing life event stressors, such as induction into the military, with traumatic stressors. Daily environmental stimuli do influence the development of psychological and physiological symptoms (7, 8). However, one must question the implicit or explicit assumption that stressors from life events to traumatic events fall along a continuum. This is a popular claim and one that has surely obscured the recognition of traumatic stressors as producing a specific psychological reaction. The claim is made in many guises: Rabkin and Struening (9) state that studies "show a linear correspondence between the magnitude of the stressor and the extent of the disorders [that follow]" (p. 601). Helzer (10) maintains that "if stress is a significant contributor to illness, extreme events and the resulting extreme stress should show a stronger association with later outcome" (p. 1). Grinker and Spiegel (11), in their classic study of World War II combat veterans, noted,

> The psychological mechanisms under discussion in this book are those that apply to Everyman in his struggle to master his own environment. . . . The failure of adaptation of the soldier described herein mirrors Everyman's everyday failures or neurotic compromises with reality. (p. vii)

It seems almost illogical to argue that experiences such as beginning college or starting a new job, to use a couple of items from the Holmes and Rahe Life Event Scale, can be equated in type if not in magnitude with the experience of combat. But this is the argument that is being advanced by these authors. Indeed, carried to its illogical conclusion, as the examples from Fairbairn illustrate, this point of view denies the relevance of the trauma and does considerable disservice to those who have been exposed to life-threatening experiences.

One might, however, sympathize with the wish of clinicians to spare themselves the task of listening empathically to the frequently horrifying details of recent traumas by exploring their patients' pasts. Obviously, this behavior—while reducing clinicians' anxieties and enabling them to avoid confronting both their own vulnerability and the loopholes in their own theories—has serious ramifications for the treatment of stress disorders.

It is important to note that war and specifically combat are not the only causes of the psychological reaction now called PTSD. Kardiner (4) wrote, "There is no such thing as a specific neurosis of war," and the editors of *DSM-III* note that any trauma that is "generally outside the range of usual human experience" can be considered a trigger or a catalyst for developing such reactions. Indeed, at the end of the last century traumatic hysteria was called "railway hysteria" because at that time the most frequent source of catastrophes was railroad accidents. At that time, too, the question of predisposition was at issue because it was argued that if the symptoms were caused by the trauma, then the sufferers could have recourse to legal proceedings against the railroad.

One major reason this diagnosis has been so long in coming is the argument I have already mentioned, that those who fall prey to stress reactions as a result of catastrophic experiences must have been predisposed because of failures to develop sufficiently strong defenses in their formative years. Other factors that have obscured the diagnosis are the timing of the onset of symptoms, the duration of the symptoms, and finally the nature of the symptoms themselves.

Kardiner (4) commented on the fact that the symptoms of PTSD rarely present themselves during the traumatic event. "The syndromes described under war neuroses do not appear on the battlefield. All one sees are tired, exhausted, and frightened men" (p. 248). Grinker and Spiegel (11) found similarly, "Relief from combat is not a cure for war neuroses since these neuroses are not transient reactions but may even crystallize into permanent neurotic patterns if not adequately treated" (p. 212). Grinker and Spiegel noted that over 90 percent of the cases admitted to hospitals were not "casualties but casuals, recognized as needing hospital care after they returned to the United States from a full tour of duty" (p. 212).

Not only can the onset of symptoms be delayed, but once established the symptoms themselves can last indefinitely. World War II studies have documented cases of "gross stress reaction in combat" lasting five, 10, 15, 20, and even 30 years.

It is this last issue that was totally overlooked by the editors of the first two editions of the *Diagnostic and Statistical Manual of Mental Disorders* (12, 13). It is true that the editors paid lip service to the fact that in some cases individuals "without apparent underlying mental disorders could have acute reactions to overwhelming environmental stress," but they failed to define the form that these reactions might take. In 1952 in *DSM-I*, the disorder was called "gross stress reaction," and the editors pointed out that such a reaction "differs from neuroses or psychosis chiefly with respect to clinical history, reversibility of reactions, and its transient character. If the reaction persists," the editors warned, "this term is to be regarded as a temporary diagnosis to be used only until a more definitive diagnosis is established" (p. 40). In 1968, with the advent of the second edition of *DSM*, the word "stress" was dropped altogether, and the diagnosis was subsumed under the category of transient situational disturbances. The editors reiterated that "if the symptoms persist after the stress is removed, the diagnosis of another mental disorder is indicated" (p. 49).

THE SYMPTOMS OF PTSD

It is ironical that *DSM-II* was published in 1968 at the height of the Tet Offensive in Viet Nam. It is also noteworthy that, compared with the three to 10 percent psychiatric battlefield casualties in World War II and the slightly less than four percent in Korea, in Viet Nam in 1968 only one percent of the troops was evacuated for psychiatric reasons. Even as the military establishment was congratulating itself on this low incidence of psychiatric casualties and offering a number of reasons for its success (such as limited tours of duty, frequent R&R, and the new practice of treating combat soldiers quickly, near the front lines, and reintegrating them into their units as soon as possible), mental health professionals in America were beginning to see a pattern emerging among the Viet Nam veterans they treated. The pattern of symptoms, which seemed to occur independent of personality type, included intrusive recollections of traumatic events in the form of dreams, nightmares, and—occasionally—flashbacks, which are dissociative states during which the individual behaves as if he or she were reexperiencing the traumatic event. There were symptoms of excessive autonomic arousal, hyperalertness, exaggerated startle reactions, difficulty falling asleep, and the feeling of being on the verge of losing control. Hand in hand with these anxiety-related symptoms were symptoms more commonly related to depression, including a general diminished responsiveness to the world, what Robert Jay Lifton has referred to as "psychic numbing." The veteran felt detached from others, had difficulty maintaining close interpersonal relationships, lost interest in normal activities, and felt that life had lost its meaning. Often the veteran was quite unaware of the syndrome to which he or she had fallen prey and unaware of its origin in the traumatic experience of combat.

One observer, Shatan (14), argued that there were probably three reasons for the low incidence of psychiatric casualties recorded by the military. The first was the Viet Nam veteran's tendency to avoid the Veterans Administration as representative of a government that many veterans felt had betrayed them. The second concerned the delayed manifestation of the symptoms. The third concerned the failure of the American psychiatric profession to provide a suitable diagnostic framework in which these symptoms could be understood. Shatan wrote,

Post Vietnam Syndrome is not an accidental grab bag of symptoms. It bears the hallmarks of mourning, frustrated and grief impacted—frustrated and impacted because the military discourages both grief and intimacy. Without working through their unconsummated grief, it will deprive their present of meaning.

He concluded that the only way for affected veterans to find peace is to carve out a "dead place in their souls," where memories are relived forever but divorced from their emotional impact. The similarity between Shatan's observations of the Viet Nam veterans he interviewed and Remarque's description of World War I soldiers is remarkable.

Whether these symptoms form a distinct syndrome is the final bone of contention between those who deny the independent status of PTSD and those who argue that it is an exacerbation of previous pathology. It brings us full circle, for if traumatic stress reactions are the result of an ongoing character disorder or pathological reaction, then it is to be expected that the symptoms were present in some form before the trauma and further that they would take different forms depending on the nature of the original disorder. Horowitz (15), who has researched this area for over a decade, notes that the stress response syndrome may "vary across persons according to cognitive, emotional, and regulatory styles, but it can be found in some form in patients of any diagnostic or characterological category" (p. 4).

DSM-III (1) has finally given PTSD official recognition. PTSD is described as the development of characteristic symptoms following a psychologically traumatic event that is "generally outside the range of usual human experience" (p. 236). The editors go on to define an acute phase of the disorder in which the onset of symptoms occurs within six months of the trauma and lasts less than six months and a chronic or delayed phase in which symptoms either last six months or more or manifest themselves at least six months after the trauma. The editors do, however, note that "preexisting psychopathology apparently predisposes to the development of the disorder" (p. 237). The evidence upon which this statement is based is not cited.

FINDINGS

To conclude this chapter I shall examine the findings of a recent survey in which a multisite probability sample of 274 male Viet Nam veterans, two-thirds of whom had been exposed to at least moderate amounts of combat, was contrasted with 275 Viet Nam era veterans (men who were in the armed forces but not in Viet Nam) and 452 male nonveterans. This federally funded study was undertaken in 1979, and the full findings were published in April 1981 (16). I shall discuss here those findings that throw light on the questions that were raised above about the validity of the diagnosis of PTSD, the incidence of acute cases, the prevalence of chronic cases, and those factors both in the veterans' pre- and postservice experiences that may have predisposed them to the disorder. Since little difference was observed between the nonveterans and noncombat veterans (17), I shall limit myself to a comparison of those veterans who were in combat and those who were not. (For a description of the way in which combat was measured, see *Legacies of Vietnam* [16], p. 670.)

PTSD Symptoms Form a Syndrome

First, it was established that the symptoms that have so often been observed among those exposed to massive psychological trauma do indeed form a syndrome. Respondents were asked about a number of symptoms similar to those listed in *DSM-III*; these symptoms were then collapsed into seven major constructs (see Table 1). These seven constructs were subjected to a statistical program that determines whether the symptoms form characteristic patterns and whether the empirically observed patterning can be accounted for by a single underlying construct. This analytic method, called latent class analysis, could be considered a new diagnostic tool that determines statistically (rather than relying on the clinician's judgment) whether a set of symptoms are related to one another, and further determines the ways in which they have to be related. (This technique is fully explained and these data are more fully explicated in Boulanger et al. [17].) In effect, latent class analysis works like the editors of *DSM-III*, taking symptoms and determining how many must be present and in what combination in order to justify a given diagnosis. In this case, however, the relationship between the symptoms is determined on the basis of a statistical program rather than on clinical observation and judgment.

We are, then, treating the criteria—or a list of symptoms very similar to those suggested by the editors of *DSM-III*—as an hypothesis. If the symptoms cluster together and form a distinctive pattern, there is justification for the diagnosis of PTSD. If the items merely turn out to be a set of overlapping symptoms that disintegrate under the rigors of the statistical program, we could conclude that, in the long run,

Table 1. Comparison Between Stress Scale Constructs and *DSM-III* Criteria for Diagnosis of PTSD (1, pp. 237, 238)

DSM-III Criteria	Stress Scale Constructs
A. A recognizable stressor	
B. Reexperiencing the traumatic event either by:	
1. Recurrent and intrusive recollections of the event or	Intrusiveness
2. Recurrent dreams of the event or	
3. Suddenly acting or feeling as if the traumatic event occurred because of an association with an environmental or ideational stimulus.	
C. Numbing of responsiveness or involvement with external world beginning sometime after the traumatic event as shown by either:	Diminished Interest
1. Markedly diminished interest in one or more significant activities.	Detachment
2. Feeling detachment or estrangement from others.	
3. Marked constriction of affective responses.	Constriction
D. At least two of the following symptoms that were not present before the trauma:	
1. Hyperalertness or exaggerated startle response.	Hyperalert
2. Sleep disturbance.	
3. Guilt about surviving when others have not or about behavior required to achieve survival.	
4. Memory impairment or trouble concentrating.	Cognitive Dysfunction
5. Avoidance of activities that arouse recollections of the traumatic event.	
6. Intensification of symptoms by exposure to events that resemble the traumatic event.	
Associated features Among those mentioned are:	Generalized Anxiety
• Autonomic lability	
• Headaches	
• Vertigo	

stressors merely exacerbate existing pathology as the previous editions of *DSM* suggested.

Our findings indicate that PTSD is indeed a valid syndrome (17). It is characterized by distinct patterning of symptoms, although these patterns do change somewhat depending on whether the stress reaction is acute or chronic. A population can be accurately divided into three classes: those who are stressed, those who are not stressed, and those who have a number of stress symptoms that are not sufficient and not in the right combination to be considered PTSD. The slight difference in the pattern of symptoms between the acute and chronic phases reveals that in the immediate or acute reaction to traumatic stress the more subdued symptoms like loss of interest and depression are paramount. As time goes by, a chronic reaction emerges in which irritability, startle reactions, and intrusive recollections of the trauma become more pressing.

The revised criteria for PTSD, to be published in the forthcoming revision of *DSM-III* (probably in 1987), no longer distinguish between acute and chronic PTSD, nor do they allow for a latent stress reaction. Rather, it is implied that a skillful diagnostician will be able to establish that if a full-blown stress reaction eventually develops, at least some PTSD symptoms were present soon after the traumatic events. Our data suggest that the less easily detectable symptoms are the first to emerge; symptoms such as loss of interest and constricted affect are more difficult to identify. Thus, if the case is as the revision of *DSM-III* suggests, the notion of latency is a pragmatic one, based on this difficulty in clinical detection.

Since this program empirically tests the accuracy of the criteria for PTSD listed in *DSM-III*, it is worthwhile taking a closer look at the comparison between our findings and the *DSM-III* criteria. *DSM-III* asserts that everyone who has PTSD should experience intrusive thoughts or nightmares of some kind; we find that 84 percent of the chronically stressed population and 75 percent of the acutely stressed population have such thoughts. According to *DSM-III*, those with PTSD should have either diminished interest in the world, feelings of detachment, or marked constriction of affect. We find that chronically stressed individuals are more likely to have constricted affect and less likely to claim detachment or diminished interest; this order is reversed among the acutely stressed. *DSM-III* claims that at least some of the people who are stressed should be either hyperalert or have cognitive dysfunctions. We find that 90 percent of our respondents who fit into the chronically stressed class exhibit symptoms of hyper-alertness. This is true for 81 percent of the acutely stressed. Approximately 70 percent of each class have difficulty concentrating, feel confused, or have trouble remembering things. We can quibble about percentages here and there, but the fit is generally a good one and leads to the conclusion that there *is* a syndrome in which the patterning and frequency of symptoms bear a close resemblance to those detailed in *DSM-III*.

Incidence of Acute Stress Reactions and Prevalence of Chronic Stress Reactions

The scale described above was used to establish the incidence of acute stress reactions during the war and in the 12 months that followed each veteran's tour of active duty. Twenty-six percent of the men in heavy combat and 17 percent of those in average combat, compared with seven percent of the noncombat and non–war zone veterans, exhibited a sufficient number of symptoms to meet the criteria for PTSD. In 1979, between six and 16 years after the men had returned home, 36 percent of the heavy combat veterans and 24 percent of the average combat veterans, compared with 17 percent of the noncombat and non–war zone veterans, were suffering from chronic symptoms of PTSD.

We have established that acute stress reactions and chronic stress reactions are strongly related to exposure to combat. We have also found that traumatic stress reactions can develop a year or more after a veteran returned from active duty in Viet Nam. Indeed, about 10 percent of the Viet Nam veterans in our sample who were in combat did not develop a full-fledged stress reaction until more than a year after their return home.

Conditions that Interact with Chronic Stress Reactions

Next we shall consider the conditions under which stress reactions were more likely to be consolidated. Strong racial differences emerged; nonwhites (in our sample this included blacks and Chicanos) had a significantly higher proportion of stress reactions than did whites. They were more likely to develop stress reactions in response to traumatic stressors, more likely to remain stressed after the war, and more likely to develop stress reactions after the war. A number of variables were considered that might contribute to the higher incidence of stress reactions among nonwhites. It was found that college graduates tended to be less stressed than were men at other levels of educational attainment, and nonwhites were considerably underrepresented in the college graduate sample. Stable employment patterns were associated with recovery from acute stress reactions and freedom from chronic stress reactions; significantly more blacks are unstably employed both in this sample and nationally. Income of less than $10,000 a year, an income bracket into which many more nonwhite respondents fell, also interacted with exposure to combat to produce disproportionately high levels of stress reaction.

Current and past interpersonal relationships were found to play a complicated role in the development and maintenance of stress reactions. Stress symptoms generally tend to create serious interpersonal problems. Remarriage is higher among stressed veterans, who are also more likely to claim that they are dissatisfied with their current marriages.

Veterans have frequently been depicted as violent, and PTSD has been used as a successful defense in cases involving Viet Nam veterans. In this study, violent behavior was defined as having committed three or more acts of physical violence (such as being in physical fights, using dangerous weapons, or being arrested for crimes of violence) in the five years preceding data collection. Our data show that although combat veterans were no more likely than controls to have violent dispositions before the war, at the time of the study—between 10 and 16 years after their return from the military—combat veterans committed significantly more acts of physical violence. Furthermore, there is a strong association between PTSD and violence. Respondents with PTSD are three times more likely to be violent than those without the disorder (18).

Predisposition to PTSD

Now we turn to the question of predisposition that has been at the center of so many debates on this topic. Given the difficulty of assigning diagnoses retrospectively to our respondents, we created a measure of the amount of objective stress to which they were subjected during their formative years, for example, the deaths of significant others, separations or divorce, poverty, unemployment, or crowding in the family home. We combined these indications of family distress with "symptom" behaviors that are known to be associated with poor adult adjustment, such as getting into trouble with the authorities, knowing other children who did, or being truant from school frequently. Our respondents were divided into men from very stable families, men from average families, and those from very unstable families.

We found that men from unusually stable family backgrounds have a higher stressor tolerance than men from average families. The former tended to develop stress reactions only in response to heavy combat; the latter reacted more often under relatively low levels of combat. Men from unusually unstable families tended to show traumatic stress reactions not simply to combat but also to the stressors of everyday life. These findings can be interpreted to mean that every man has his breaking point, the breaking point being contingent not only on the severity of the stressor but also on the level of stability that existed in the respondent's family of origin.

Individuals at Risk to Develop Chronic Stress Reactions

When all of these findings are weighed together rather than considered independently of one another, as they have been so far, it is possible to assemble the portrait of an individual who is most at risk for developing a stress reaction and remaining stressed. (These data are excerpted from Boulanger [19], pp. 189–210.)

Parenthetically, it should be noted that although Viet Nam was rumored to be a war that was fought by blacks and the lower classes, and that men who went to Viet Nam were predisposed to psychiatric disorders in the first place, Martin and Boulanger (20) report that race, class, and predisposition can be ruled out as determining the amount of combat to which a man was exposed. Thus, we can assert that combat is a determining variable in the development of PTSD, not a mask for the effects of race, class, or predisposition.

Combat has a strong effect on the development of postwar stress reactions. Coming from an unstable family in which one or both parents were absent from the home, for example, or where poverty and uncertainty were a way of life, also had a direct effect on the development of acute stress reactions.

The presence of a chronic stress disorder is more strongly associated with having developed an acute stress disorder during or immediately after the war and with marital dissatisfaction and employment stability than it is with race, parental class, the amount of time that has elapsed since the war, or with educational achievement. Race and class do, however, have indirect effects, for if a respondent was either nonwhite or lower class or both, he was more likely to have come from an unstable home. This alone was sufficient to lead to a postwar stress reaction, but this was even more likely if the man had to bear arms in Viet Nam. As a result of this postwar stress reaction, the respondent was likely to be dissatisfied with his marriage and unstably employed at the time our data were collected, making the determination of causality highly complex. His employment and marital predicaments, coupled with the acute postwar stress reaction and the residual effects of his unstable early life, were likely to result in an ongoing stress reaction.

CONCLUSION

In this chapter we have suggested reasons why the diagnosis of PTSD has been so controversial. Among these reasons is the fact that before 1980, when the American Psychiatric Association adopted the diagnosis officially, those who continued to show the psychological effects of a traumatic stressor after the stressor had been removed were considered to be suffering from another mental disorder. Evidence from a recent survey of Viet Nam veterans has been presented to show that a distinct syndrome of stress response symptoms can be elicited by exposure to a traumatic stressor. In some cases this syndrome can manifest itself more than a year after the stressor has been terminated. Although individuals from unstable families of origin are more likely to manifest the symptoms of PTSD than are those from very stable families, if the stressor is sufficiently intense, even those from stable families can develop the syndrome.

REFERENCES

1. American Psychiatric Association: Diagnostic and Statistical Manual of Mental Disorders, Third Edition. Washington, DC, American Psychiatric Association, 1980

2. Remarque EM: All Quiet on the Western Front. Boston, Little, Brown & Co, 1929

3. Fairbairn WRD: Psychoanalytic Studies of the Personality. London, Routledge, Kegan Paul, 1952

4. Kardiner A: Traumatic neuroses of war, in American Handbook of Psychiatry. Edited by Arieti S. New York, Basic Books, 1969

5. Freud S: Beyond the Pleasure Principle. New York, W.W. Norton, 1961

6. Ferenczi S, Abraham K, Simmel E, et al: Psychoanalysis and the War Neuroses. New York, International Psychoanalytic Press, 1921

7. Selye H: The Stress of Life. New York, McGraw-Hill, 1956

8. Dohrenwend BS, Dohrenwend BP (eds): Stressful Life Events. New York, John Wiley & Sons, 1974

9. Rabkin JG, Struening EL: Life events, stress, and illness. Science 194:1013–1020, 1976

10. Helzer JE: Methodological issues in the interpretation of the consequences of extreme situations, in Stressful Life Events and Their Contexts. Edited by Dohrenwend BS, Dohrenwend BP. New York, Neale Watson, 1981

11. Grinker R, Spiegel JP: Men Under Stress. Philadelphia, Blakiston, 1945

12. American Psychiatric Association: Diagnostic and Statistical Manual of Mental Disorders. Washington, DC, American Psychiatric Association, 1952

13. American Psychiatric Association: Diagnostic and Statistical Manual of Mental Disorders, Second Edition. Washington, DC, American Psychiatric Association, 1968

14. Shatan CF: The grief of soldiers—Viet Nam combat veterans' self help movement. Am J Orthopsychiatry 43:640–653, 1973

15. Horowitz MJ: Stress Response Syndromes. New York, Jason Aronson, 1976

16. Kadushin C, Boulanger G, Martin J: Legacies of Vietnam, Vol IV: Long-Term Stress Reactions: Some Causes, Consequences, and Naturally Occurring Support Systems. Washington, DC, U.S. Government Printing Office, 1981

17. Boulanger G, Kadushin C, Rindskopf D, et al: Post-traumatic stress disorder: a valid diagnosis? in Vietnam Veterans: Facts and Fictions of Their Psychological Adjustment. Edited by Boulanger G, Kadushin C. New Jersey, Lawrence Erlbaum, 1985

18. Boulanger G: The violent veteran, in Vietnam Veterans: Facts and Fictions of Their Psychological Adjustment. Edited by Boulanger G, Kadushin C. New Jersey, Lawrence Erlbaum, 1985

19. Boulanger G: Conditions Affecting the Appearance and Maintenance of Traumatic Stress Reactions Among Vietnam Veterans. Doctoral Dissertation, Columbia University, New York, 1981

20. Martin R, Boulanger G: Who went to war? in Vietnam Veterans: Facts and Fictions of Their Psychological Adjustment. Edited by Boulanger G, Kadushin C. New Jersey, Lawrence Erlbaum, 1985

3

War Trauma and Human Development: The Viet Nam Experience

Robert S. Laufer, Ph.D.

3

During the past decade, following presentations, lectures, and classes on the effects of the Viet Nam War on its soldiers, listeners often ask if it is possible to argue that the war was a positive experience for some. One can approach the question on two levels. First, the answer is no. The destruction of other human beings, their possessions, and their environment and exposure to death or mutilation, all of which are intrinsic to war, can hardly be described as a positive experience. One can then rephrase the question: Do some soldiers make something positive out of the maelstrom of war? The answer is yes. For veterans who do make something positive out of the war years, the effort to come to terms with the experience of war is usually difficult. It may be haunted by memories which echo Brecht's lament, "We who sought to transform the world could not ourselves be kind." It remains to be said that making something positive out of the Viet Nam War does not represent the achievement of the majority of Viet Nam veterans (1).

The reader might ask, "Why do you focus on the negative side of the experience of those who survived the Viet Nam War?" This country has assumed an obligation to America's war veterans to facilitate healing the physical and psychological wounds of war. This responsibility exists after every war, not just Viet Nam. Healing is based on knowledge of the damage inflicted by war; acquiring an understand-

The findings presented in this paper are part of the Viet Nam Veterans and Controls Study. Funding for this study has been provided by NIMH grant R01 MH26832-06 and Veterans Administration Contracts V101(134)P-610 and V101(134)P-130. I wish to express my appreciation for the support of this study to both the National Institute of Mental Health and the Veterans Administration. The author is solely responsible for the findings and conclusions in this chapter.

I want to thank my colleagues Ellen Frey-Wouters, Mark Gallops, and Elizabeth Brett for their careful reading and helpful suggestions with prior drafts of this chapter.

ing of the effects of war requires that we focus on the human destruction caused by war.

Many decry the accumulating evidence on the destructive effect of the Viet Nam War on the majority of those exposed to it, claiming that this encourages Viet Nam veterans to feel injured by the war. We feel, to the contrary, that such research, by identifying the source of their troubles, has helped Viet Nam veterans recognize that their problems do not necessarily reflect personal failures. To the extent that this has happened, the subterranean forces in the lives of these veterans have been exposed to light. Insight is the first step in healing individual trauma; support for the recognition of individual travail is the essential step for our society to acquire an awareness of the legacy of Viet Nam.

For those of us fortunate enough not to have been engulfed by the experience of the war, the fantasy that a nation can put a war behind it is a fallacy from which we need liberation. Our choices are to be hurtled blindly into the next abyss because we refuse to recognize the living legacy of war, the survivors, or instead to come to terms with the world we have created by understanding the human costs of Viet Nam. Although there may well be times when that ultimate sacrifice is necessary for the survival of the society, there is no sense in which war in itself is positive for the psychological development and maturation of individual soldiers. In the aftermath of any war, it behooves us to recognize the profound price paid by the soldier-survivors.

BACKGROUND, WAR STRESS, AND OUTCOMES

How does war stress affect the lives of Viet Nam veterans? The literature has been growing steadily over the last 15 years. It can be divided into six areas of study, including the following:

1. Difficulties in readjustment to civilian life problems among Viet Nam veterans;
2. Differences between Viet Nam veterans and veterans of other wars;
3. The relationship of predispositional factors to adjustment problems among Viet Nam veterans;
4. Combat or in-country experiences as factors producing post-war adjustment problems;
5. Strategies for treating disturbed Viet Nam veterans; and
6. The social and political alienation among Viet Nam veterans.

Our discussion will concentrate on the literature in the first four categories.

Prior to 1975 the primary concern in the literature involved alerting mental health professionals to the evidence that readjustment to civilian life was proving more difficult for Viet Nam veterans than the optimistic expectations of military psychiatrists suggested (2–6). Concurrently, many clinicians were pointing out that Viet Nam veterans appeared different from the veterans of other wars (7–10).

The twin notions that Viet Nam veterans were different from veterans of other wars and that they were having significant difficulties in readjusting to civilian life generated a range of studies. Two points of view developed. Some researchers concluded that there were few, if any, differences in post-service adjustment between Viet Nam veterans and their peers who did not go to Viet Nam or serve in the military, and that those differences which did exist could be explained by predispositional factors. Other researchers found that it was combat exposure and service in Viet Nam which made the difference in readjustment to civilian life and subsequently had a substantial negative effect on veterans' mental health.

Over the last 12 years seven major studies provide the data which form the basis of our present knowledge. Each of these studies had a relatively large sample of Viet Nam veterans (11–21). Five of the studies used a control group in their research (11, 13–16, 18–21). In addition, five of the studies utilized some systematic sampling strategy (11, 13, 18–21). Only the study by Borus (11) was conducted with men who were still in military service. All of the other studies were conducted with veterans, men who had left the military.

The Borus study reported that Viet Nam veterans were not different from their peers in the military who did not go to Viet Nam. Unfortunately, Borus did not study the effects of combat exposure. The studies by Robins et al. (13, 15) are of special interest because they include a follow-up of a subset of veterans which was conducted two years after the initial interview. During the second interview a nonveteran control group was added to the study. Thus, Robins et al. interviewed Viet Nam veterans one year and three years after they were released from the military. These studies concluded that drug and alcohol problems were part of an unfolding disposition toward deviant behavior, usually evident before the men entered the service. When they compared veterans and nonveterans with respect to psychological adjustment in their second and third years after Viet Nam, they found no differences, regardless of whether they controlled for preservice adjustment.

Research by Nace et al. (16) provided support for both the hypotheses that Viet Nam service is related to postservice adjustment problems and that certain postservice problems (criminality and narcotic use) are accounted for "primarily by preservice experience." This study also reported that there was a diverse group of adjustment indicators, including psychological depression and alcohol use, which were found to be strongly related to service in Viet Nam. The range of postservice problems among Viet Nam veterans may have been one of the most important findings of Nace and his colleagues. Unfortunately, it did not receive the attention it deserved.

Subsequent studies by Wilson (17) and Harris (18) provided evidence that the combat experience was the critical factor in postservice adjustment. However, the Wilson study was self-selected and lacked a control group, while the Harris study contented itself with a cross-tabular analysis of the data. Consequently, the consistency of the findings was to some extent undercut by the limitations of the design and analysis.

The major study supporting the thesis of postwar adjustment problems among Viet Nam veterans was *Legacies of Vietnam* (22). This was the only study which approximates a general population sample and both Viet Nam era veteran and nonveteran control groups. It employed a threat-to-life measure of combat (20), examined a broad range of social and psychological indicators of adjustment (20, 22, 23), and controlled for the influence of predispositional factors. The study found that exposure to combat significantly exacerbated the problems of readjustment to civilian life (20, 22). Specifically, it reported that combat veterans were reluctant to reach out to their peers and family after leaving the military, and that exposure to combat is associated with alcohol consumption, postservice arrests, medical problems, angry feelings, and symptoms of post-traumatic stress disorder (PTSD) for those veterans who served after 1968. (There was no relationship between stress symptoms and combat for the pre-1968 group.) The study also found support for the Nace theory that a broad range of problems are associated with combat exposure; that is, men who exhibited certain kinds of problems were substantially more likely than their peers to have other problems (20). Finally, Rothbart (22) found that it was service in Viet Nam rather than combat which was the best predictor of educational and occupational problems.

The most recent study, done by Card (21), has substantially confirmed the findings of *Legacies of Vietnam*.

INTERPRETING THE FINDINGS

How can we interpret the results to date? There are two plausible interpretations of the disparate findings over the last decade or so of research on the effects of the Viet Nam War. One way of reading the findings is that manifestations of war stress delay making their appearance for some years after men leave the military. The persistent finding of combat-related social and psychological problems in the most recent studies strongly suggests this line of reasoning. Our research shows that among combat veterans less than half of the current stress symptoms developed during the war or in the first year after leaving the military (24). The pattern of arrests found in *Legacies of Vietnam* (20) suggests that a relatively small proportion of the total postservice arrests occur during the first two years after leaving the military. The Veterans Administration reports that only in the late 1970s did they begin to notice a substantial increase in Viet Nam veterans seeking treatment for alcohol problems. A plausible explanation of the delayed expression of the effects of the war is that they gradually unfold in the process of developing interpersonal relations and in the pursuit of educational or occupational goals.

The building of the early adult life course structure is the central task young veterans face after leaving the military. The early period after release from service begins this process. It takes time for plans and relationships to develop and to go awry. This suggests that the period after release from military service represents a time of heightened expectations and planning, which serves to insulate some veterans from the trauma of their war experience.

Another interpretation of the findings is that we are confronted by several measurement problems. The conceptualization of the problem of Viet Nam veteran postservice adjustment has evolved over the years. As the conception of readjustment has changed, so too have approaches to the measurement of predisposition, war stress, and outcomes. There are four dimensions of the measurement central to the field of Viet Nam veteran research: 1) predisposition, 2) the war experience, 3) symptomological and behavior outcomes, and 4) patterns of life course development after service. (This last dimension of the effects of war has yet to be systematically examined.)

The Measurement of Predisposition

The measurement of predisposition varies across these studies. The findings of Robins et al. (13, 15) are the most important basis for arguing that controlling for predispositional factors eliminates the apparent effect of combat, although it is important to note that the Robins combat measure has its limitations. They argue that when one controls the effects of their Youthful Liability Scale (a measure of preservice delinquency), the effects of combat on postservice behavior are no longer significant. Thus, they conclude that post–Viet Nam problems were continuing a preservice pattern.

In *Legacies of Vietnam* (22) and in subsequent analysis of the *Legacies* data, the predisposition hypothesis was carefully tested. In *Legacies*, Laufer et al. (20) controlled for demographic and family characteristics as well as preservice arrest history and found that on postservice arrests and drug and alcohol use these predispositional factors did not diminish the effects of combat. Kadushin et al. (23) compared men from advantaged and disadvantaged backgrounds and found there was a combat threshold which led to elevated symptomatology on the PTSD scale. Rothbart did a careful analysis of educational and occupational careers using the Institute for Social Research job history protocol and found that service in Viet Nam had the effect of diminishing educational and occupational attainment, even after controlling for preservice educational and occupational histories (22).

Finally, in our most recent analysis (24, 25), my research group constructed indicators of preservice delinquency which include truancy, family problems, and other difficulties, such as juvenile fights, trouble with the law, or drug and drinking problems. Our findings indicate that these predispositions do have an independent effect, but they do not suppress the effects of the war experience. We are led to conclude that although preservice delinquency does influence subsequent reports of symptomatology and behavior, the stress of war also has a significant and substantial long-term influence on the lives of Viet Nam veterans.

Our findings suggest that the more fruitful line of future inquiry is to explore the combined effects of predispositional factors and war stress. The findings of Nace et al. (16) and Laufer et al. (20) that Viet Nam veterans exhibit a broad range of disruptive symptoms and behavioral problems indicate that the form of disruption resulting from the war experience may be linked to predispositional factors.

The Measurement of War Stress

The most glaring failure of research on Viet Nam veterans has been that war experience has been conceptualized unidimensionally. Researchers have limited themselves to measuring a single dimension of war stress—combat exposure. They have ignored other dimensions, such as the arbitrary use of violence and the effects of the moral climate of the war. For this reason, we need to expand the conceptualization and measurement of war experience.

As Figley (26) noted, a great deal of the early research on the effects of war stress neglected even to differentiate Viet Nam veterans who were exposed to combat from those who were not (11, 12, 27–31). Except for Strayer and Ellerhorn's study, which uses four categories of combat (4), the studies prior to 1979 that did take account of combat all tend to use two-category or three-category, interval level, measures of combat exposure (14, 16, 17, 26, 32–34).

It wasn't until *Working Papers: The Psychosocial Adjustment of Vietnam Era Veterans to Civilian Life* (19) and *Legacies of Vietnam: Post-War Trauma* (20) that the combat experience was conceptualized as a continuum of life-threatening experiences which could lead to qualitatively different outcomes. Subsequent research has adopted this approach to the measurement of the combat experience (17, 18, 35–38).

A great deal of literature on the Viet Nam War and the experiences of Viet Nam veterans has focused on the unique character of the conflict. The Viet Nam War was novel to the American experience because it was primarily a guerilla war. There were no clear boundaries to demarcate friends and foe, or the zone of safety from danger. There was no front line. The soldier in a guerilla war was continuously faced with the threat of death, injury, or violence. Despite the extensive discussion of the ramifications of this situation on the soldier's experience, few attempts have been made to empirically define the dimensions of war stress in this context.

My colleagues and I hypothesized that the degree of exposure to the threat of death, injury, or violence was central to the experience of combat in Viet Nam. We concluded that operationalization of the Viet Nam experience should reflect the character of the war experience. In *Legacies of Vietnam* we constructed a scale of combat exposure which did not only focus on direct military confrontations with the enemy but rather took into account an array of experiences which indicated whether the veteran was exposed to a serious threat to life or limb.

Conceptualization of War Stress

The above studies are consistent in their reliance on a single measure of war stress—combat or war experience. This assumes either that all experiences associated with war can be subsumed under the "combat" label—that is, the only relevant stress associated with war is the combat experience—or that all activities related to soldiering in war are perceived by the soldier as part of the combat experience (35, 39).

From a theoretical perspective it seems unlikely that either of these assumptions is correct. In all wars soldiers engage in violence which leads to the killing or severe injury of enemy combatants and comrades and the threat to one's own life. This is the essence of the combat experience. (Precisely who enemy combatants are may differ depending on the kind of war we are discussing. Although civilians may suffer death or injury during military engagements, their deaths are still considered part of the combat experience when such attacks include the threat to life of the soldier. Conceptually, we accept only those situations where the personal safety of the soldier is directly threatened as part of the combat experience.)

Warfare generates other behaviors and situations in which soldiers' lives are clearly no longer in jeopardy, but in which life is taken or human beings are systematically or intentionally injured or killed; this is what is meant by the abusive use of violence. There are situations in which the anger, fear, or anxiety associated with the combat experience leads military units and individual soldiers to strike out. Abusive violence is clearly part of the war experience of the veteran population which we do not think should be grouped together under the rubric of combat. The class of actions we are concerned with includes situations in which combatants who are no longer armed, usually prisoners of war, are deliberately mistreated; women are raped; women, children, or other civilians are killed or mistreated; whole communities are severely disrupted or destroyed; and the dead are mutilated. It seems evident to us that single measures of war stress, like "combat exposure," will fail to pick up those aspects of the experience which may be a source of indelible troubling memories. The experience of abusive violence is associated with combat exposure, but it also constitutes a distinctive domain of war stress which independently influences the lives of soldiers and veterans.

The differentiation of etiology is especially important since it appears that as a rule combat does not have a generalized disabling effect (16, 20), but instead seems to disrupt veterans' lives in different ways. Some men get into trouble with the law or substance abuse while others report elevated rates of psychiatric symptoms. Aside from the severely psychologically disabled, in whom we would find more of an overlap between social and psychological disorder, disruption over the life course resulting from war stress will most likely require services able to help veterans cope with specific problems. In order to diagnose and treat those veterans, we need to know as precisely as possible the relationship between the dimensions of war stress and symptomatology or life event crises.

EMPIRICAL EVIDENCE FOR A MULTIDIMENSIONAL APPROACH TO WAR STRESS

There is some evidence that noncombat war experiences continue to disturb the lives of Viet Nam veterans long after they have left the military. Foy et al. (35) created a Viet Nam Experience Scale which included participation in the killing of civilians. Their findings suggest that a significant number of their respondents diagnosable as suffering from PTSD were involved in the killing of civilians. The conceptual point that violence against civilians in war is significantly implicated in postservice symptomatology is important. However, in our judgment it would have been more useful to determine whether or not exposure to this kind of abusive violence plays a distinctive role in postservice symptomatology rather than incorporate this indicator into another unidimensional scale of combat exposure.

Data from the Viet Nam Veterans and Controls Study also covered exposure to and participation in abusive violence. In the last year my colleagues and I investigated this issue in some depth. From a reading of our transcript material, it was evident that abusive treatment of civilians and prisoners of war was a recurrent theme in the troubling memories, nightmares, and flashbacks of our respondents. In order to explore the effects of exposure to or participation in abusive violence, we needed to determine whether we could meaningfully differentiate our combat scale from other aspects of war trauma.

DIFFERENTIATING COMBAT FROM
ABUSIVE VIOLENCE IN WAR TRAUMA

In addition to the pervasive and ubiquitous character of threat to life in the context of a guerilla war, there is the prevalence of abusive violence. The insights provided by an intensive review of our transcripts as to the importance of this feature of war experience was emphasized by our finding that one-third ($N = 112$) of our sample of Viet Nam veterans was exposed to some episode of abusive violence and one-tenth ($N = 31$) participated in these episodes. Exposure to abusive violence is moderately associated with the level of physical threat (combat) faced by the serviceman. Comparing the group of those who were exposed to abusive violence with those not exposed to abusive violence, the average score of the former group on the combat scale was significantly higher (8.4 vs. 4.7; the combat scale ranged from No Combat [0] to Heaviest Combat [13]). However, there was little difference in the average combat score between those who only witnessed abusive violence and those who participated in it (8.4 vs. 8.5).

Previous studies have often maintained that the subjective perception of combat and the war experience is important. We too were aware that subjective perceptions of the experience of war might significantly affect postwar behavior or symptoms. In this regard we carefully examined the effects of 1) perception of threat to life, 2) the extent to which Viet Nam veterans felt that their survival was the key element in their war experience, 3) the salience of physical discomfort during the period they served in Viet Nam, and 4) their response to abusive violence, that is, distancing themselves from it or recognizing its cruelty. None of these variables systematically predicted postservice problems. The absence of effects attributable to these indicators led us to the conclusion that subjective perceptions of war stress are relatively poor predictors of subsequent problems in civilian life. Our research suggests that the effort to specify war stressors should concentrate on indicators of behavior and actual experience.

These findings in the measurement of war stress (23) have led us to believe that there are at least three dimensions of war trauma relevant to predicting subsequent symptomatology and behavioral problems: 1) exposure to life-threatening situations, 2) exposure to abusive violence, and 3) participation in episodes of abusive violence.

The importance of this multidimensional approach to conceptualizing and operationalizing war stress cannot be overstated, particularly as it relates to the Viet Nam conflict. Veterans clearly articulate the ambiguity of their situation and its consequences. The inability to distinguish friend from enemy and civilian from combatant created a milieu which encouraged the military and the individual soldier to justify a personal broadening of the "rules of war." The level of exposure to abusive violence we find in our data suggests it was a relatively common feature of the Viet Nam veteran's war experience.

INDICATORS OF PSYCHIATRIC SYMPTOMATOLOGY AND PSYCHOLOGICAL WELL-BEING

Studies of postwar adjustment among Viet Nam veterans use different indicators of psychological adjustment. The confusion—or more precisely, the lack of clarity—on the psychological effects of war stress is partly a result of the different measures employed by the several studies, partly from the contradictory results reported, and partly due to unresolved issues raised by the contrasting behavior of scales which purport to measure postwar sequelae and those which measure generalized mental states.

The study by Robins et al. (15) reports no difference between veterans and nonveterans with respect to psychological adjustment. (The Robins measure of adjustment is a general psychological adjustment scale.) The PTSD Scale (40) was unavailable to Robins et al. because the diagnostic category did not exist when they conducted their study. Whether a particular instrument is the best measure of stress disorder remains in question (41). However, the measurement of stress is clearly important (38, 41, 42). The failure to measure this aspect of postservice psychological disruption is a major problem in comparing the findings of the Robins study with subsequent studies concerned with readjustment problems among Viet Nam veterans.

MEASURES OF ADJUSTMENT

A number of instruments have been used to assess patterns of psychiatric symptoms among Viet Nam veterans. We utilized two in our study: 1) the PTSD Scale (40), which is a single additive scale of stress symptoms often mentioned in the professional literature on PTSD, and 2) the Psychiatric Epidemiology Research Instrument (PERI) (43), which consists of a number of scales tapping general psychiatric symptomatology. We used 11 of these scales: 1) demoralization, 2) feelings of guilt, 3) feelings of anger, 4) active expression of hostility, 5) perceived hostility of others, 6) somatic problems, 7) lack of mastery, 8) suicidal thoughts, 9) distrust, 10) sex problems, and 11) repression of anger. It is important to note that these scales do not measure psychiatric disorder, rather they tap general patterns of symptoms which indicate the presence of psychological tensions of different types.

The findings in *Legacies of Vietnam* (22) pointed to an association between combat and the PTSD Scale for Viet Nam veterans who served after 1968; however, except for the angry feelings scale, combat effects did not appear on any of the PERI scales. The lack of consistent findings in the effects of combat on the PTSD Scale and almost all of the PERI scales places a heavy burden on the concept of stress disorder as the primary psychological disruption associated with war stress.

The more general issues of psychosocial development were to some extent addressed by the *Legacies* study (20, 22). Like *The Forgotten Warrior* (17) and *Myths and Realities* (18), the *Legacies* findings suggested that though some Viet Nam veterans turned the crisis of combat to their advantage, combat did have a generally negative effect on psychosocial development.

In summary, the available findings suggest that combat exposure does have a negative effect on psychological well-being, principally as measured by the PTSD Scale of the *Legacies* study, and that it also has an effect on psychosocial development. However, the existing stress measures cannot as yet be reliably differentiated from anxiety and other psychiatric anxiety indicators that do not show the predicted effects of combat.

A MULTIDIMENSIONAL APPROACH TO WAR TRAUMA AND POSTWAR ADJUSTMENT

If we are to understand the effects of war trauma, it is necessary to explore why the PTSD Scale in *Legacies of Vietnam* showed the effects of combat in the post-1968 group, while the PERI scales seemed to be immune to these effects. We explored two lines of analysis: 1) the war stress model in *Legacies* was misspecified, and 2) the approach to PTSD used in *Legacies* was too general.

Our first working hypothesis was that over time the generalized threat to life measure (combat) contributed most strongly to specific postwar sequelae, while the more intense experiences of exposure to and participation in abusive violence was more likely to contribute to general psychiatric symptomatology as measured by the PERI scales (23). Our findings support the above hypothesis. Including the exposure and participation measures in the model of war stress, we found a systematic relationship between five PERI scales (demoralization, guilt, angry feelings, perceived hostility of others, and active expression of hostility) and exposure and participation. In addition we also found a relationship between participation and drug use (marijuana and heroin) (25). However, the effects of exposure to and participation in abusive violence did not follow a simple additive pattern: exposure leads to more symptoms than combat, and participation leads to more symptoms than exposure. Instead we found that blacks and whites responded differently to the stress of war. Whites exposed to abusive violence and blacks who participated in abusive violence both showed more symptoms on the PERI scales. White participants, however, scored markedly lower on the five PERI scales. After careful analysis of a broad range of measures which tapped attitudes toward the Vietnamese and conduct of the war, we concluded that the postwar effects were related to meanings attributed to these experiences in Viet Nam, that is, the social context of the white participants was more supportive and less likely to challenge the moral basis of this behavior than that of the black participants (23). Drug use among participants, however, did not vary by race.

The second hypothesis we explored was that the *DSM-III* formulation of PTSD reflected in the PTSD Scale (40) used in *Legacies* was composed of discrete dimensions which were differentially related to war stress. We identified four dimensions of PTSD (intrusive imagery, hyperarousal, numbing, and cognitive disruption) from the *DSM-III* PTSD diagnosis (44). The most important modification in the *DSM-III* formulation we made was to differentiate criterion D (a miscellany of symptoms) into two dimensions (hyperarousal and cognitive disruption). The analysis showed that combat and exposure to abusive violence were both associated with intrusive imagery in the 12 months preceding the interview, that combat elevated hyperarousal scores, and that neither combat nor exposure was significantly contributing to symptoms of numbing or cognitive disruption. Participation in abusive violence contributed to significantly higher levels of numbing and cognitive disruption, as well as hyperarousal, but was not related to intrusive imagery. Again, we found some important differences between black and white participants. Black participants' scores on the cognitive disruption scale accounted for all of the effect on that dimension. Black participants also reported high rates of intrusive imagery. However, both black and white participants had significantly higher rates of numbing symptoms.

In summary our findings demonstrate that war stressors do have an effect across a broad range of psychiatric and behavioral indicators of postwar problems. Further, our data indicate that there is no substantive reason to focus on PTSD as the single disorder related to war stress in Viet Nam. PTSD is clearly a major element in post–Viet Nam psychiatric symptomatology, but an exclusive focus on this outcome does not adequately serve the needs of Viet Nam veterans. Our analysis also suggests that PTSD symptomatology varies as a result of the types of war stress the veterans experienced. These findings indicate a complex relationship between the stress of war and the process of postwar development. The last part of this chapter is an analysis of the developmental process at work in coping with the war experience in early adulthood.

A CONCEPTUAL APPROACH TO WAR TRAUMA

The problem which confronts us is to conceptualize the relationship between war stress and the developmental tasks of the early adult years and then to develop a model of how the interaction between war stress and early adult development influences the rest of the life course. The model of human development proposed is primarily concerned with the process of adaptation to life through the interaction of psychosocial maturation and social history (45).

We generally send young men (18 to 24 years of age) to fight our wars. Obviously, some portion of the officer corps and a group of the noncommissioned career soldiers who lead armies are older. However, the brunt of battle is carried by young men who would be busy building their lives were it not for the call to arms. Many of these young men deemed old enough to die for their country would be too young to buy a drink in a bar in many states. If these men were civilians they would be going to school and would likely be dependent on their families for financial support, living at home or at a college or university subject to parental or in loco parentis regulation of their lives, or beginning their occupational careers. Our armies rely on young men who are only recently adolescents, who in most circumstances would be labeled preadults or youths.

The task for people at this age, except for the intrusion of war, is to develop in their late teens and early 20s a stable identity, to complete school, to enter the occupational world, and—within the norms of their communities—to find spouses, that is, to establish early adult life structures. There is abundant literature (45–51) which indicates that this process is complex, time consuming, and fraught with peril even under the best of circumstances. To paraphrase Keniston (48), this period involves the process of establishing a sense of self and a relationship between the self and society.

It is a confusing, often tumultuous period in the development of the individual. Under the right social conditions, it can be a period of social as well as personal rebellion (52). This is a time when young men explore their options and exhibit a sense of immortality, recklessness, and commitment. It is, most of all, a time for experimentation, of slowly crystallizing beliefs, ideologies, and commitments.

The dominant characteristic of the young men we send to war is that they are only partly formed—they are still in the process of becoming. The ego defenses are maturing, ideas about the world are likewise being developed, and social identity too is at a formative stage. The young soldier, prior to his entry into war, can be described as a cauldron of emotions, ideas, and themes waiting to be forged. War is a force which turns the emotional and moral world young men grew up in on its head. For example, the archtypical foundation of civil society, the injunction "Thou shalt not kill," is waived in war.

A Viet Nam veteran from Los Angeles describes his initiation into the rites of passage of a warrior as follows.

> We were on a search and rescue mission and we were . . . uh . . . told not to take prisoners and we took about seven prisoners and . . . uh . . . this one individual had been in Viet Nam before . . . and he said he could get everything out of them and he wouldn't have to hurt them here . . . and we couldn't understand what he meant. Well, it ended up all seven of these people died of natural causes—they all had heart attacks.

Vaillant's work on ego development (45) offers us a productive point of departure for interpreting the consequences for the development of young adults through their immersion in warfare, because he so explicitly focuses on the contribution of specific types of ego mechanisms to "healthy" adult functioning. Vaillant elaborates a hierarchy of ego mechanisms which, he argues, contribute to effective social functioning. He uses labels such as mature, neurotic, and immature to characterize specific ego mechanisms to emphasize that mental health (self-actualization) is enhanced by developing mature ego mechanisms, and that the ego styles also contribute to more satisfying social relations and careers.

The moral order of warfare presents a radically altered social order, which requires individuals to significantly restructure their ego mechanisms. The "mature" ego mechanisms of everyday life for the management of interpersonal relations and intrapsychic stress are likely to prove ineffective. In general the skills necessary for survival in war are largely uncorrelated with those learned in civil society.

A white veteran from Chicago who served as an officer reflects on the pressures and tensions which work on soldiers in combat and their consequences over time.

> The kind of tactics that the Vietcong and the NVA [North Vietnamese Army] used to . . . uh . . . kill Americans, maim Americans with the mines, the pungi sticks, and the booby traps . . . and . . . uh . . . uh . . . the kind of type warfare because of that type of thing when men would see their friends injured and killed and maimed and because of mines, booby traps, and the like and . . . uh . . . see their arms blown off and their legs blown off it would—it was the kind of thing that I think had . . . uh . . . worked on their minds and made their killing of the enemy when they had the chance and the opportunity much easier and less . . . less impersonal. And I think where troops did mutilate the dead and the soldiers or where they shot and killed the enemy soldiers when they didn't have to and they shot them when they were defenseless or whatever or when they burned the villages or whatever, I don't really feel, knowing the troops—and knowing how they were thinking at the time, that they found any kind of. . .uh. . .anything but gratification in it and no conscience.

The mature defense mechanisms of civil society, suppression, altruism, humor, or sublimation may not necessarily be as effective in the warfare society. Indeed, a reasonable argument can be made that if preoccupation with survival so characteristic of soldiers is one of the dominant values of men at war, then such neurotic or immature defenses as repression, displacement, dissociation, reaction formation, acting out, and projection may well prove effective, that is, they serve as mature mechanisms, because they enhance the chances of survival.

If survival is the prime concern of the soldier, the solidarity of the unit in which the soldier fights comes a close second because the functioning of the group is instrumental to individual survival (53). Protection of the group and its solidarity in the environment of war involves aggression and violence against all those who threaten it.

In civil society group protection is also important, but within strictly defined boundaries. In war, although there are supposed to be some boundaries, they are more often observed in the breach than in routine. Certainly there is ample evidence that, forced to choose between the safety of the unit and civilian's rights or those of prisoners of war, soldiers are prone to protect themselves first; more importantly, their behavior was likely to be supported by their peers and superiors.

Warfare by definition involves projection and displacement of aggressive impulses outward against the "enemy." The dehumanization of the enemy is characteristic of warfare:

> I mean killing a gook was nothing really. It didn't bother me at all. Could have butchered them like nothing really. I really had no feelings. As far as the kids in the village or something, we would not really touch them unless something happened. I guess it would not have fazed me. . . .You got a wounded gook and he is wounded bad and you put him out of his misery. As far as just shooting them, to me it was like shooting a deer or something like that . . . really no feeling about the job.

Release of aggression through what we normally label immature or neurotic defenses is accompanied by anxiety reduction in the soldier. The connection which appears to develop is that acting out against the enemy provides a psychic release from fear. The soldier learns to connect anxiety reduction with acting out; he is encouraged to feel this is a "mature" response because the sources of tension can be categorized in terms which make acting out acceptable.

A veteran from Chicago illustrates the fundamental tendency among soldiers in Viet Nam to adopt an attitude which legitimizes random violence and impulse release to enhance their stature and exercise power over civilians.

> It was not so much direct combat action against civilians as it was riding roughshod over the population. They were there in some respects to lick our boots and, by god, if they were not going to lick our boots then we were going to stomp on them. That was probably a general attitude of many people I was involved with. I can remember shooting dogs and

cats and water buffalo and other animals: farm animals, pigs, chickens, goats. We would be half drunk riding down the road in a jeep and we would see this civilian obviously working in a rice paddy, six or eight hundred yards away. You would pick up your rifle and take a couple of pot shots at him just to scare the shit out of him. That was the type of a situation. I can remember doing that.

The above examples of how the hierarchy of ego mechanisms of civil society are inverted in the normative order of warfare raises important questions about the transition to civilian life for soldiers. The problems are especially acute for young men in the process of identity formation. If we assume that the process of maturational development proceeds in all societies, then we must ask, "How is identity formation affected by entry in a society of war during late adolescence and youth?" And we need to ask, "How are the serial transitions from civil society to war and back to civil society in a period of three to four years experienced in terms of perception of the self?"

In Viet Nam the tour of duty for most soldiers was only 12 months. Thus, the individual barely settled comfortably into his violent soldier's identity before he was pulled back out again. It is often argued that the limited duration of the war experience makes the subsequent transition easier. An alternative explanation seems perhaps more plausible. The rapid transition to civilian life leaves the individual traumatized because the moral order into which he entered during the war continues to exert tremendous power over his values.

A veteran from Chicago poignantly explains the difficulty of reentry into society after being in an environment which breaks the boundaries of civilian society.

I think a rehabilitation program where they teach a person how to live around civilian people again . . . is a good one. Teach them how to be a human being with human rights, even though he probably knows; but, people do forget when their mind is in an uproar. Kind of analyze him to see if he is capable of handling civilian life, instead of just letting him go on his own.

The transition to civilian life is likely in its early stages to lead to generalized anxiety accompanied by intense feelings of confusion. Indeed, our data suggest that the sense of disorientation often described in the early postservice period is likely to result from the feeling that there is a concentrated attack by significant others on the most strongly valued elements of identity constructed in the crucible of war. The transition from war to no war involves unlearning a whole host of reactions and patterns of behavior which are essential for survival in war but frightening and disturbing to or perceived as peculiar by civilians.

As two veterans from Brooklyn vividly illustrate, the war continues to play a role in their lives after their return home, which often leads to bizarre behavior and exaggerated fears about the hostility of the environment.

I would not come out of the house—not unless it was night and I was going to see my fiancée. [How long did this last?] Oh, about a couple of months. Then, finally, I went looking for jobs. . . .

[When you came out, what kind of person were you?] Oh, a little shaky. See, like, the cars come by and they could blow their horn and it would frighten me. . . . You could speak to somebody and they would not speak, like they did not know you. I would get mad. [What was important to you?] I don't even know. [You said that you had psychological problems. What kind of problems?] I got a nervous problem, a communication problem; I cannot explain things.

For a significant proportion of soldiers, the return home is also accompanied by identity diffusion. The problem the soldier faces after the experience of war is to resocialize himself and to cope with the experience in which his self-image must be reworked if he is to survive in civil society.

A veteran from South Bend explains the need he felt to be resocialized into civil society and emphasized the problem of accepting the norms of society after being in war.

[I was] totally confused in terms of right and wrong. I don't think my ambitions were as strong. And I had a lot of hate feelings which I really can't explain. It was just hate and mistrust.

A veteran from Westchester emphasizes the loss of direction and identity diffusion which resulted from his wartime experiences.

I had no ambition, no outlook on life. I did not care. I did not want to work. I did not want to do anything. . . . Hanging out and doing nothing. Sleeping all day and staying out at night. . . . We smoked and we drank. This went on for five years now.

And veterans must discover or rediscover the capacity for empathy and intimacy which too often withers under the stress of war.

Veterans from South Bend and Los Angeles both testify to the effect war had on their relationships with others, which made it much more difficult to respond to the needs of significant others in their environment.

More hardened. Much more hardened. [What do you think was responsible for the change?] Being in a place where you have the constant knowledge that you can be killed at any time, I suppose.

I was a much more changed person. . . . I had . . . uh . . .more . . . uh . . . I had a completely different outlook on life. I had seen how people take advantage of other people and . . . I would say I had a more violent temper. . . . I . . . just couldn't handle things.

Furthermore, as John Wilson points out (17), the premature encounter with mortality contributes to psychologically accelerated aging, which interferes with the need to build a life structure in early adulthood.

The consequences of the traumatic encounter with death and dying is evident in the response of a veteran from Los Angeles to the question, "What did you do when you returned home?"

Bumming around—collected unemployment. Started drinking pretty heavy. . . . [Had you changed?] Oh yes, I just did not care anymore. I thought I was dead, you know? For quite a while I could not believe I came back. . . . But then I started to make a go . . . like I had a second life—a second chance—so I said I wanted to do better now.

From the preceding discussion we hypothesize that at the stage of life of most soldiers in Viet Nam, exposure to war constituted a major interference with the maturational process. The interference may be conceptualized as a trauma which involves the general inversion of the young adult's moral order, the freezing of his social development (interpersonal and career), and the stunting of his emotional development (empathy), all of which occurs because it is necessary for fulfilling the soldier's role and is related to the premature encounter with mortality.

We need to see the effects of war stress on the developmental process in terms of a decisive trauma which requires the development of extraordinary adaptations which are singularly useful in a uniquely limited setting. When the individual leaves that setting, these limited adaptive styles are profoundly ineffective in "normal" human settings. The transition from warrior to civilian-veteran encompasses the psychological problems of reorganizing ego defenses and identity.

The veteran of war faces one problem all veterans encounter: catching up on the early adult tasks of career development. However, there is also the added burden of readaptation to the civil society and the incorporation of the war experience into an integrated identity that morally connects the early stages of development to the "warrior" and postwar self. The problem can be seen as the difficulty in answering the question, "Who am I?" after learning more than one wants to about the question, "What am I capable of?" To put the issue somewhat differently, the image of the self the adolescent grew into is irrevocably shattered by the experience of war. The problem is to find a postwar self-image which acknowledges the capacities of the self learned in war without being swamped.

The developmental transition described requires an extended moratorium after leaving the military. There is, as described below by a veteran from the Northeast, a need to be alone.

> [I] kept pretty much to myself. Unless there was another guy that was there, then you could always talk about it. I was reluctant to get involved, I guess.

The ability to cope with the life course tasks of early adulthood for veterans exposed to war stress depends then on the capacity to undertake a major reorganization of adaptive ego mechanisms. The process of adaptation to the second preadult stage for Viet Nam veterans becomes a life-long factor in their development. In projecting the effects of war stress through the life course, we need to account for the direct effects of war experience on mental health, quality of life, and physical well-being, but there is also the need to account for the indirect effect through the life course structure built out of and during the period of adaptation to civilian life. We should expect to find that decisions about school, job, marriage, and children made during the period of adaptation will reflect tensions and unresolved conflicts associated with war stress.

As this veteran from Chicago shows, the war could also profoundly change the direction of men's lives.

> I was psychologically wounded, not mentally disturbed to any great degree, at least I did not realize the degree that I had. [You had given up on the plans to become a surgeon?] To go into medicine, yes . . . it takes many years before you can get yourself in a position to go back to school. I just could not adjust to the lies and deceptions in school, so I just put it aside.

The basis for subsequent disruptive expressions of war stress are thus laid down during the period of adaptation and early adult life course development. To the extent that important components of war trauma are repressed, unresolved, or ignored, they become key candidates for later eruptions. Unfortunately, late-appearing symptoms or deviant behavior are not necessarily going to be intuitively identified as war related. Thus, identifying the etiology of later adult life crises among war veterans involves a complicated analysis of the effects of war stress on the different stages of the life cycle.

We cannot as yet provide answers to all of our questions. If we are ever to get an answer, we will have to follow the fate of Viet Nam veterans as they age. After 12 years of research on Viet Nam veterans, we have to face the hard reality that our work has only begun.

REFERENCES

1. Egendorf A, Remez A, Farley J: Legacies of Viet Nam, Vol 5: Dealing with the War. Washington, DC, US Government Printing Office, 1981

2. Bourne PG: The Viet Nam veteran: psychosocial casualties. Psychiatry in Medicine 3:23–27, 1972

3. Lifton RJ: Home from the War: Viet Nam Veterans, Neither Victims nor Executioners. New York, Simon & Schuster, 1973

4. Strayer R, Ellerhorn L: Viet Nam veterans: a study exploring adjustment patterns and attitudes. Journal of Social Issues 31:81–94, 1975

5. Fendrich JM: Todays veteran. Paper presented at the 16th Annual Veterans Administration Conference, Perry Point, Md, V.A. Hospital, 1971

6. Stenger CA: Perspectives on the post–Viet Nam syndrome. Newsletter for Research in Mental Health 16:1–4, 1974

7. Shatan CF: Soldiers in mourning—Viet Nam veterans self-help groups: the post–Viet Nam syndrome. Am J Orthopsychiatry 42:300–301, 1972

8. Shatan CF: The grief of soldiers: Viet Nam combat veterans self-help movement. Am J Orthopsychiatry 43:649–653, 1973

9. Haley SA: When the patient reports atrocities. Arch Gen Psychiatry 30:191–196, 1974

10. Peck CP: The Viet Nam veteran. Newsletter for Research in Psychology 13:11–14, 1971

11. Borus JF: Reentry, II: making it back in the States. Am J Psychiatry 130:850–854, 1973

12. Borus JF: Incidence of maladjustment in Viet Nam returnees. Arch Gen Psychiatry 30:554–557, 1974

13. Robins LN: The Vietnam Drug User Returns. Special Action Office Monograph, Series A, No. 2. Washington, DC, US Government Printing Office, 1974

14. Robins LN, Helzer JE: Drug abuse among Viet Nam veterans—three years later. Medical World News 27:44–49, 1975

15. Robins LN, Hesselbrock M, Wish E, et al: Polydrug and alcohol use by veterans and nonveterans. Current Alcohol 4:239–256, 1979

16. Nace E, O'Brien CP, Mintz J, et al: Adjustment among Vietnam drug

users two years post-service, in Stress Disorders Among Vietnam Veterans. Edited by Figley CR. New York, Brunner/Mazel, 1978

17. Wilson JP: Identity, Ideology, and Crisis: The Viet Nam Veteran in Transition, Part I. Unpublished monograph, Cleveland State University, 1977

18. Harris L: Myths and Realities: A Study of Attitudes Toward Viet Nam Era Veterans. Washington, DC, US Government Printing Office, 1980

19. Egendorf A, Kadushin C, Laufer RS, et al: Working Papers: The Psychosocial Adjustment of Vietnam Era Veterans to Civilian Life. Washington, DC, Veterans Administration, 1979

20. Laufer RS, Yager T, Frey-Wouters E, et al: Legacies of Viet Nam, Vol III: Post-War Trauma, Social and Psychological Problems of the Viet Nam Veteran in the Aftermath of the Viet Nam War. Washington, DC, US Government Printing Office, 1981

21. Card JJ: Lives After Viet Nam. Lexington, Mass, Lexington Books, 1983

22. Egendorf A, Kadushin C, Laufer RS, et al: Legacies of Viet Nam: Comparative Adjustment of Veterans and Their Peers. Washington, DC, US Government Printing Office, 1981

23. Kadushin C, Boulanger G, Martin J: Long-term stress reactions: some causes, consequences, and naturally occurring support systems, in Legacies of Vietnam, Vol. IV: Comparative Adjustment of Vietnam Veterans and Their Peers. Washington, DC, US Government Printing Office, 1981

24. Laufer RS, Gallops MS, Frey-Wouters E: War stress and trauma: the Viet Nam experience. J Health Soc Behav 25:65–85, 1984

25. Yager T, Laufer RS, Gallops MS: Some problems associated with war experience in men of the Viet Nam generation. Arch Gen Psychiatry 4:327–333, 1984

26. Figley CR (ed): Stress Disorders Among Viet Nam Veterans. New York, Brunner/Mazel, 1978

27. Huffman RE: Which soldiers break down: a survey of 610 psychiatric patients in Viet Nam. Bull Menninger Clin 34: 343–351, 1970

28. Enzie RF, Sawyer RN, Montgomery AF: Manifest anxiety of Viet Nam returnees and undergraduates. Psychol Rep 33:446, 1973

29. Worthington RE: The Viet Nam era veteran, anomie and adjustment. Milit Med 14:169–170, 1976

30. Worthington RE: Demographic and pre-service variables as predictors of post-military service adjustment, in Stress Disorders Among Viet Nam Veterans. Edited by Figley CR. New York, Brunner/Mazel, 1978

31. Panzarella RF, Mantell DM, Bridenbaugh RH: Psychiatric syndromes, self-concepts, and Viet Nam veterans, in Stress Disorders Among Viet Nam Veterans. Edited by Figley CR. New York, Brunner/Mazel 1978.

32. Helzer JE, Robins LN, Wish E, et al: Depression in Vietnam veterans and civilian controls. Am J Psychiatry 136:526–529, 1979

33. Helzer JE: Methodological issues in the interpretation of the consequences of extreme situations. Unpublished paper, Washington University School of Medicine, 1980

34. DeFazio VJ: The Viet Nam era veteran: psychological problems. J Contemp Psychother 7:9–15, 1975

35. Foy DW, Sipprelle RC, Rueger DB, et al: Etiology of post-traumatic stress disorder in Vietnam veterans: analysis of premilitary, military, and combat exposure influences. J Consult Clin Psychol 52:79–87, 1984

36. Polk K, Alder C, Cordray S, et al: Cohort Careers and the Vietnam Experience (final report). Bethesda, Md, National Institute of Mental Health, 1982

37. Hough R, Gongla P: Delayed Stress Disorders in Hispanic Veterans (study in progress). Brentwood, Calif, V.A. Medical Center 1982

38. Brett E, Mungine W: Imagery and post-traumatic stress disorder in Viet Nam veterans (unpublished manuscript). West Haven, Conn, V.A. Medical Center, 1983

39. Wilson J, Krauss GE: Viet Nam Era Stress Inventory: Forgotten Warrior Research Project (unpublished). Cleveland State University, 1980

40. Boulanger G, Kadushin C, Martin J: Legacies of Viet Nam, Vol IV: Long-Term Stress Reactions. Washington, DC, US Government Printing Office, 1981

41. Hough RL, Gongla P, Scurfield RM: Natural history of post-traumatic stress disorder. Paper presented at the Annual Meeting of the American Psychological Association, Annaheim, Calif, August 1983

42. Horowitz M, Solomon GF: A prediction of delayed stress response syndromes in Vietnam veterans. Journal of Social Issues 31:67–80, 1975

43. Dohrenwend BP, Shrout PE, Egri G, et al: Nonspecific psychological distress and other dimensions of psychopathology. Arch Gen Psychiatry 37:1229–1236, 1980

44. Laufer RS, Brett E, Gallops M: Dimensions of post-traumatic stress among Viet Nam veterans. Paper presented at the Annual Meeting of the American Psychiatric Association. New York, 1983

45. Vaillant G: Adaptation to Life. Boston, Little Brown & Co, 1977

46. Adelson J: The political imagination of the young adolescent. Daedalus 100:1013–1050, 1971

47. Erikson E: Identity, Youth and Crisis. New York, W.W. Norton Co, 1968

48. Keniston K: Youth and Dissent. New York, Harcourt, Brace & World, 1972

49. Hogan DP: Transitions and Social Change. New York, Academic Press, 1981

50. Elder GH: Children of the Great Depression. Chicago, University of Chicago Press, 1974

51. Winsborough HH: The transition from schoolboy to adulthood (working paper 76–13). Madison, University of Wisconsin Center for Demography and Ecology, 1976

52. Laufer RS, Bengston VL: Generations, aging and social stratification: on the development of generational units. Journal of Social Issues 30:181–205, 1974

53. Moskos CC: The American Enlisted Man. New York, Russell Sage, 1970

4

Social Networks, Helping Networks, and Viet Nam Veterans

Charles Kadushin, Ph.D.

4

Two of the more common behavioral science terms that have recently entered the English language are *social support* and *network*. The latter has even been turned into a verb so that one "networks." Both social support and networks are held to be a good thing: the more one has of each the better. Networks, the skein of relations between people, are often held to be equivalent to social support. Networking may be regarded as the social intervention of choice in the 1980s, since it is cheap, voluntary, and effective and is potentially appealing to interest groups across the political spectrum.

In this chapter I will examine the effects of social support and networking for Viet Nam veterans. It is important to note that the conditions under which social support of one kind or another is effective need to be carefully examined. First, one can have too much of a good thing so that support feels oppressive; second, the effects of support are not necessarily additive, but one type of support may substitute for another—for example, if one's wife is supportive, then one may not also need support from friends; third, not all friends are the same—different kinds of friends may perform different functions; and fourth, the effects of networking and social support may be conditional on some characteristics of the larger social environment—for example, networks may work out differently in larger cities as compared with smaller towns. I will draw on work reported in Kadushin (1, 2) and Kadushin et al. (3).

A vast recent literature has focused on social support as one of the structures which may alleviate the effects of everyday life stressors as

The support of grant no. MH 34580-02 from the National Institute of Mental Health to Charles Kadushin, Principal Investigator, is gratefully acknowledged. NIMH is not in any way responsible for the analysis and conclusions reported in this paper.

well as the impact of traumatic stressors such as the war in Viet Nam (for reviews see Gottlieb [4], Husaini [5], and Biegel and Naparstek [6]). Since the referents of the term social support are extremely broad and mean different things to different writers, the concept *interpersonal environment* is introduced to help sort out the many conditional relationships prevalent in networks and support systems. By interpersonal environment I mean simply the sum of all persons who are known to and have some direct relationship to a given focal person (7). There are between 500 and 2,000 or more persons in a typical interpersonal environment (8)—a greater number than most of us imagine. In studying interpersonal environments one must necessarily concentrate on a small subset of relationships which are relevant to particular sets of problems or interactions. We can then ask what it is about these interpersonal relationships that may or may not be supportive to Viet Nam veterans.

There are three fundamental attributes of the interpersonal environment:

1. The structure of the interpersonal environment, that is, the pattern of relations between the members;
2. The type of persons in the environment and their presence or availability—whether they are friends, lovers, kin, Viet Nam veterans, and the like;
3. The specific actions taken by these relevant others—whether these individuals encourage, act as confidants, talk with the focal person, and so on.

The interpersonal environment can impact in three ways on mental health: 1) stressful situations may be prevented or encouraged; 2) immunities or sensitivities to stressors may be developed; and 3) stress reactions themselves may be intensified or alleviated. In our case, the stressors are combat experiences in Viet Nam, events that occurred before our measurement of either stress reaction or the characteristics of the interpersonal environment. The first effect, the prevention of stress, is largely ruled out in the present discussion, although it is possible that some of our measurements of reactions to stress are sensitive to everyday life stress or to traumatic stressors that have occurred after veterans returned from combat. Perhaps we are dealing with immunization effects, but most likely we are dealing with the alleviation of existing stress reactions or what are often called "buffered" effects, because social support serves as a buffer between a stressor and reaction to stress (for a discussion of some complexities of the buffering effect, see Thoits [9]).

THE DATA: *LEGACIES OF VIET NAM*

This study of the interpersonal environment of Viet Nam veterans comes from a larger study commissioned by the United States Congress to evaluate the current status of Viet Nam veterans (as described in Kadushin et al. [10]). Included in the present analysis are 274 Viet Nam veterans and 275 Viet Nam era veterans (men who were in the armed forces during the period of the Viet Nam war but who did not serve in Southeast Asia) between the ages of 24 and 37 who were interviewed in 1979, in Chicago, South Bend, rural Indiana, Atlanta, rural Georgia, Columbus, Georgia, and Los Angeles County. In our discussion of the effects of marital support versus the support of available friends, we necessarily include only married men but broaden our base to cover nonveterans and men interviewed two years earlier in Brooklyn, New York, Westchester County, New York, and Bridgeport, Connecticut, for a total of 919 men (for details of the sample design, see Kadushin et al. [10]).

In this study we asked our respondents for the names of persons who found them their current job (if anyone), who was their partner or spouse, who their best friends were (up to four), and—if none of these individuals was a Viet Nam veteran—for up to four names of Viet Nam veteran friends. For the purposes of this research, these persons constitute the interpersonal environment of the respondent. (We also asked about friends a man had when he registered for the draft, and friends he made in the service or during an equivalent time if he was not a veteran, but these data are not reported here.) Our respondents then gave us some data on each of the persons in their interpersonal environment—how they got to know them, their occupation, whom they turned to for help with serious personal problems, and so on. We know whether the respondent talked about Viet Nam with each of these others; who, if anyone, among the four best friends was a Viet Nam veteran; and who in the current interpersonal environment knew whom. For wives or partners we also know whether they agreed with the respondent on making important decisions, how often they disagree in general, how affectionate and comfortable they are with their spouse, and how satisfied they are with their marriage.

WIVES AND FRIENDS: WHO IS MORE SUPPORTIVE?

Let us begin with the difference between two types of persons in the interpersonal environment: the spouse on the one hand and friends who were not also spouses or females living with the veteran on the other hand. This analysis draws upon work by Martin (11, 12). Spouses are presumably always available whereas friends may or may not be; we will want to know who is more effective in helping Viet Nam veterans and under what conditions. Effectiveness is measured in terms of levels of psychological demoralization (13), a construct which includes such symptoms as poor self-esteem, feelings of hopelessness and helplessness, a sense of dread, sadness, anxiety, confused thinking, and psychophysiological problems. It is important that while demoralization is one of the consequences of combat, it is also a consequence of other stressors. Given the literature, we should not be surprised if we find that men who have supportive spouses and available friends are less demoralized. Two critical questions are at issue, however.

- Are spouse support and/or available friendship especially ameliorative of the effects of combat, or do these supports also help with the effects of the stressors of everyday life?
- Are spouse support and friend availability additive or functionally alternative? That is, a man may feel twice as good if he has both an available friend and a supportive wife, or the one may be useful only if the other is not.

In order to answer these questions we must check for some possible confounding factors. Stress, in the form of combat, might alter one's ability to form attachments and hence might affect our two indicators of social support. This is not the case, however, since neither spouse support nor friend availability is related to the experience of combat, at least for this sample. Moreover, it is perfectly possible for spouse support and friend availability to be functional alternatives, since they are not related to one another. It should be obvious that our analysis has to be confined to married men, since we are comparing the effects of spouse support and friendship.

In brief, here is what Martin found. First, spouse support is effective in reducing levels of demoralization both for those men who have experienced combat and for those who have not. This suggests that spouse support is helpful in reducing the effects of life event stress as well as the traumatic stress of combat, a finding well anticipated by the literature.

It is also true, however, that spouse support is even more helpful for men exposed to combat. Since combat occurred before current levels of spouse support, it does seem that spouse support has an amelioration effect as well as possible direct effects which immunize one from the stresses of everyday life.

Third, peer or friend availability is only helpful for those married men who are not supported by their wives, and then only for men who have experienced combat. That is, friend availability is a functional alternative to spouse support and acts to ameliorate the negative consequences of combat. The important consequence of this finding is that structural availability of friends has special meaning for combat veterans, an effect which we will now examine more closely.

Several aspects of the interpersonal environment and friendship can further be specified.

- What is the social structure of friendship? Specifically, are the friends a "gang" in the sense that most of the friends know one another, or are they simply an aggregate of people unconnected to one another that the respondent just happens to know?
- Further, what are the effects of the size of the place in which a veteran lives? Is living in a smaller city or in the country and being surrounded by a gang of friends more supportive than when living in a metropolis? What kinds of friends are especially useful in anonymous big city environments?
- What difference does it make if a veteran's friends are themselves Viet Nam veterans?
- Finally, does it matter what a man does with his friends? Specifically, does it matter whether he talked with them about Viet Nam or not?

In considering these effects of friendship, we will be especially concerned with two kinds of outcomes.

- Can friends ameliorate the psychological consequences of combat? While demoralization reflects the general emotional "temperature" of an individual, there is a special set of symptoms which is known to be the consequence of combat for some individuals and which is called post-traumatic stress disorder (see Chapter 2). The interpersonal environment of veterans may have a special impact on these symptoms, especially if the environment includes other veterans and if the subject of Viet Nam has come up in conversation.
- If a veteran indeed has many of the symptoms of PTSD, he may have sought professional help for these symptoms. To what extent, then, are his friends a substitute for such professional help? Is it possible that under some circumstances talking with one's friends is more effective in alleviating PTSD symptoms than seeing a professional?

We should expect that the conditions under which one kind of friend is helpful and another kind less helpful will vary. We believe it is important to pay attention to these "it depends" conditions, because too many blanket statements have been made about peer groups and veterans. What works in one situation may in fact not work in another or might even be harmful.

Let us now look at the effects of the interpersonal environment on PTSD symptoms and consider the matter of social structure in that connection. There is a myth that in traditional village societies—those in which everybody knows everybody else—norms are firmly established, violations are noted and corrected, everybody knows where he or she stands in the community, and help for problems is readily forthcoming. This kind of clarity may prevent stressors from occurring in the first place, may make the stressors seem less severe, or may help to alleviate problems if they do occur. The latter is, of course, the factor that might be operating in our study.

A reasonable indicator that a person is surrounded with an interpersonal environment which duplicates the conditions of traditional societies is the degree of social density in the environment. If everyone knows everyone else, then social density is high. We constructed an index of density from data on up to nine persons in the interpersonal environments of each man in our sample. The index is simply the proportion of persons reported to know one another, divided by the number of possible relations.

We no longer live in traditional societies, however. The situation in large cities today is further complicated by the fact that people may belong to a number of different social circles. Within each circle people may know one another and be supportive, but there may be few connections between one circle and another. A respondent may be the sole point of contact between the members of the various circles in his interpersonal environment. So we should expect that social density will have different consequences in large cities as compared with smaller ones, which is indeed the case. High density is associated with lower levels of PTSD symptoms in smaller cities, but there is no relationship between density and PTSD in larger ones.

Thus we have our first "it depends." The structure of the interpersonal environment, in this case the social density of the environment, affects men who do not live in metropolitan areas. Density is of no help elsewhere.

The second "it depends" has to do with the effect of the presence of a circle of Viet Nam veterans. There has been much discussion of the effects of peer groups on veterans. For example, the Veterans Administration's Vet Centers are based on the notion that peer counseling is useful. In terms of the natural situation of Viet Nam veterans, if a man lives in an interpersonal environment in which there are a substantial number of Viet Nam veterans whom he calls his good friends, then he can be said to have a set of friends who understand him and his problems. This may lead to his being able to overcome PTSD symptoms. To operationalize this idea, we said that if one-third or more of a man's good friends were Viet Nam veterans (more than the average), then we would assume that he was a "member" of a circle of Viet Nam veterans. Such a circle in metropolitan areas was indeed associated with reduced levels of PTSD symptoms on the scale described in Boulanger et al. (14). But there is also a tendency for men with veteran friends in smaller cities to be worse off than men without such friends.

For all the reasons that social support might be effective, a circle of veterans should be associated with reduced levels of PTSD symptoms. Whatever the problem is, talking about the problem, knowing others who have been through the same experiences, and knowing others who have problems like one's own all seem to be helpful in wide varieties of informal support and self-help groups (15). But why should such a circle, under some circumstances, make things worse? The answer has to do with the motivation to acquire a circle of veteran friends. In large cities, whether or not one has Viet Nam veteran friends is largely a matter of accident. In smaller towns and perhaps among men with parental supports in larger cities, a veteran with problems seeks out others like himself. The men with problems reinforce one another and perhaps become "professional veterans." A cosmopolitan circle of Viet Nam veterans, on the other hand, contains veterans with many interests other than being a veteran. This kind of circle can be helpful to the veteran with problems. This interpretation of our data has obvious practical implications for treatment to which we shall return.

FRIENDS AND PROFESSIONALS: WHO IS MORE HELPFUL?

Thus far we have shown the effects of the social structure of the interpersonal environment and of the presence in the environment of certain types of people on the prevalence of PTSD symptoms. No one has actually done anything, however. Suppose these others in the interpersonal environment talk with our respondent about Viet Nam, or at least listen to him? Having someone to talk with about Viet Nam is supposed to be very important to veterans. Our data suggest that talking to just anyone is not particularly useful, however, and is not associated with lower probabilities of PTSD symptoms. Talking with a Viet Nam veteran, however, is quite a different matter. Just about all of the veterans in our sample report talking with friends who are Viet Nam veterans about Viet Nam, as one might expect. So the findings for talking about Viet Nam with a good friend who is a Viet Nam veteran are identical to those already reported about having a circle of veteran friends: such talk is especially helpful for veterans in large cities whose parents are not available. Nonetheless, talking about Viet Nam with nonveteran friends is not altogether without consequences and this brings us to some rather astounding findings.

We now need to consider not PTSD symptoms per se, but the likelihood of consulting professional help for mental problems. In the second set of data which were collected from the Midwest, the South, and the West—the data which contained the PTSD scale—we asked an extensive series of questions about help seeking. These questions were used to determine whether a veteran sought help for his problems. Because of an error in data collection, we seriously underreported mental health professionals in this study and can safely report only on visits to professionals generally. With this caveat, let us briefly review some findings on respondents seeking professional help for mental problems.

First, there are essentially none of the usual demographic correlates of help seeking for mental problems in this sample. Class, education, city size, income, region, marital status, etc. are not important factors. Veterans do have facilities to go to, apparently, if they wish. Second, help seeking is obviously strongly related to stress reaction, not only because of the way the questions were asked but also because the more PTSD symptoms a veteran had, the more likely he was to seek help. Our third finding is particularly important. If we look only at men who reported PTSD symptoms during or in the year after the war and who are combat veterans, then men who subsequently sought help for these symptoms are more likely than other men to have symptoms today. At the very least, there is no evidence in our data that seeing a professional who is not specially trained in work with Viet Nam veterans reduces the level of symptoms. However, this is not the case for veterans who talked to Viet Nam veteran friends. Men who reported symptoms during or a year after the war were less likely to report them today if, in the meantime, they had talked with veteran friends.

All of this information, while very important, is merely background to our discussion of the effects of the interpersonal environment on seeking help for mental problems. If veterans talk with good friends who are Viet Nam veterans, then this makes little difference in their likelihood of seeking professional help for mental problems. In fact, they are less likely to seek help, especially in large cities. But the more nonveteran good friends a combat veteran has talked with about Viet Nam, the more likely he is to seek professional help.

We interpret these findings to mean that veterans, who are aware that consulting most professionals about PTSD symptoms is not very helpful, are not especially likely to tell their friends they need professional help if they do talk about their problems. On the other hand, nonveterans do believe in the efficacy of professionals, make no distinctions for PTSD symptoms, and tend to refer to professionals veterans who talk a lot about Viet Nam. Once more, the effects of the interpersonal environment depend on which persons within the environment one is talking about. Talk is not necessarily support.

CONCLUSION

Although these data were collected before the Veterans Administration established Vet Centers, and although they refer only to naturally existing networks, there are some obvious practical implications to this analysis of networks and support systems. First, professionals in their usual guise may not be helpful to veterans with PTSD symptoms. Second, the community itself in smaller cities, if it is cohesive, can be helpful. Spouses also, if they so desire, are effective under any and all circumstances, although men with unhelpful spouses are worse off than men who are not married. All of these forces can and should be better mobilized. Third, well-meaning friends may not be very useful and possibly can even be harmful to men with PTSD symptoms. Veteran circles too may backfire, although under the right circumstances, talking to other veterans is quite effective. Friends can be especially important if spouses are not supportive. Finally, if one tries through professional intervention to match the results of beneficial natural networks, then much thought must be given to the way one constructs such circles. Poorly formed "support" groups may not be helpful and may even make things worse.

REFERENCES

1. Kadushin C: Mental health and the interpersonal environment: a reexamination of some effects of social structure on mental health. Am Sociol Rev 48:188–198, 1983

2. Kadushin C: The interpersonal environment and Viet Nam veterans. Paper presented at the Annual Meeting of the American Psychological Association, Washington, DC, 1982

3. Kadushin C, Boulanger G, Martin JL: Effects of professional and informal help on Viet Nam vets. Paper presented at the Annual Meeting of the American Association of Public Health, Montreal, 1982

4. Gottlieb BH: Social Networks and Social Support in Community Mental Health. Beverly Hills, Calif, Sage Publications, 1981

5. Husaini BA (special ed): Stress and psychiatric symptoms: personality and social support as buffers, in Community Psychology, vol 10. Brandon, Vt, Clinical Psychology Publishing Co, 1982

6. Biegel DE, Naparstek AJ (eds): Community Support Systems and Mental Health: Practice, Policy, and Research. New York, Springer Publishing Co, 1982

7. Rossi PW: Research strategy in measuring peer group influence, in College Peer Groups. Edited by Newcomb TM, Wilson EK. Chicago, Aldine, 1966

8. Poole IDS, Kochen M: Contacts and influence. Social Networks 1:5–52, 1978

9. Thoits PA: Conceptual, methodological, and theoretical problems in studying social support as a buffer against life stress. J Health Soc Behav 23:145–159, 1981

10. Kadushin C, Boulanger G, Martin JL: Legacies of Viet Nam, Vol IV: Long-Term Stress Reactions: Some Causes, Consequences, and Naturally Occurring Support Systems. Washington, DC, U.S. Government Printing Office, 1981

11. Martin JL: The effects of social support on psychological distress among Viet Nam veterans and their peers. Paper presented at the Annual Meeting of the American Psychological Association, Washington, DC, 1982

12. Martin JL: The effects of partner support and peer support on psychological demoralization: a comparative analysis of young adult men and their Viet Nam veteran peers. Unpublished doctoral dissertation, Department of Psychology, The City University of New York, 1981

13. Dohrenwend BP, Shrout PE, Egri G, et al: Measures of nonspecific psychological distress and other dimensions of psychopathology in the general population. Arch Gen Psychiatry 37:1229–1236, 1980

14. Boulanger G, Kadushin C, Rindskop D, et al: Post-traumatic stress disorder: a valid diagnosis? Paper presented at the Annual Meeting of the American Psychological Association, Washington, DC, 1982

15. Gartner A, Riessman R: Self Help in Human Services. San Francisco, Jossey-Bass, 1977

5

Irrational Reactions to Post-Traumatic Stress Disorder and Viet Nam Veterans

Arthur S. Blank, Jr., M.D.

5

When . . . correspondent Jonathan Schell was touring Quang Ngai Province in late summer of 1967. . . a GI who was driving him around in a jeep suddenly turned and said, "You wouldn't believe the things that go on in this war."

"What things?" Schell asked.

"You wouldn't believe it."

"What kind of things, then?"

"You wouldn't believe it, so I'm not going to tell you," the GI said, shaking his head no. "No one's ever going to find out about some things, and after this war is over, and we've all gone home, no one is ever going to know." (1)

A psychiatric commentary in 1984, which sought to persuade the reader of the insignificance of post-traumatic stress disorder in the Viet Nam veteran population and of the inconsequential role of war experiences in producing such a condition, began with this interesting generalization: "History has shown war veterans to be a problem for society" (2).

In this chapter I will discuss how, following the Viet Nam War, society was a problem for war veterans. I will further present selected examples of the irrational reactions which have intruded into psychiatric diagnosis and treatment of Viet Nam veterans. One purpose of this chapter is to minimize such reactions in professional practice in the future.

The conviction of the GI in Quang Ngai Province in 1967 portrayed above—that there would be no listener for him to tell about his

---

The views expressed in this chapter are solely those of the author and do not necessarily represent those of the Veterans Administration or the publisher.

experiences—in fact came true in many postwar encounters of veterans with mental health professionals. A second purpose of this chapter is to accelerate the decline, now well underway, of such noncommunication.

As Shakespeare, among others, might have expected (see *Henry IV, Part I* [act 2, scene 3, lines 38–65] for Hotspur's wife's comments about her husband's war stress manifestations [3]), between the years 1964 and 1975 perhaps several hundred thousand men and women returned from the Southeast Asia war zone bearing the psychological impact of traumatic stress. In many cases, this proved sufficient to, sooner or later, produce diagnosable PTSD. It is possible that epidemiologic study will establish that the percentage of individuals affected (out of over 3.5 million persons who served in the war) was 20 to 25 percent. Estimates of the fraction of veterans affected at a clinical level are highly conjectural. At present such estimates can be based only on inferences drawn from two nationwide surveys on non–treatment seeking populations (4, 5). Harder epidemiologic data will be produced by the Veterans Administration's National Viet Nam Veterans Readjustment Study, to be reported in late 1986.

An affected percentage of 20 to 25 percent would be modest, all things considered. The war was highly confused in its purposes. The public and the troops themselves were sharply divided as to whether the cause was just or unjust. From 1970 on, especially, military morale was significantly impaired. Therefore, many observers have expected that the adverse psychological consequences among veterans would be even more widespread than is apparently the case.

However, what might have been a significant but manageable need by some veterans for debriefing, counseling, and psychotherapeutic services deteriorated into a major public health problem. Ultimately, by the end of the 1970s, this involved significant human tragedy among veterans and their families.

This situation occurred because of a pervasive repudiation of the Viet Nam experience by much of the general public, so that most veterans were discouraged from talking to friends or family members —to any extent—about their war experiences. This general repudiation of veterans and their experiences was at times accompanied by extraordinary hostility. This is vividly crystallized in the following account of what happened to one veteran when he returned to college from Viet Nam:

> In the fall of 1968, as I stopped at a traffic light on my walk to class across the campus of the University of Denver, a man stepped up to me and said, "Hi."

Without waiting for my reply to his greeting, he pointed to the hook sticking out of my left sleeve. "Get that in Viet Nam?"

I said, "Yeah, up near Tam Ky in I Corps."

"Serves you right."

As the man walked away, I stood rooted, too confused with hurt, shame, and anger to react. (6)

This veteran is now the distinguished director of prosthetics of the Veterans Administration.

Generalized public hostility toward Viet Nam veterans, from both persons who supported and persons who opposed the war, was directed against both veterans who supported and veterans who opposed the war. This will not be discussed further here. My goal is to carefully note that the irrational reactions of mental health professionals, which will now be reviewed, occurred in and were strongly influenced by a much larger societal reaction.

Prior to 1980, professional repudiation of and hostility toward Viet Nam veterans, and toward the clinical reality of PTSD, was sufficiently common as to produce remarkable nationwide professional phenomena. These profession-wide features will be briefly reviewed before the focus is shifted to specific types of frequently observed irrational reactions which affect individual clinicians.

KEY TRENDS BEFORE 1980

Nondiagnosis

In 1968, the American Psychiatric Association removed the diagnosis, "gross stress reaction," from its *Diagnostic and Statistical Manual of Mental Disorders (DSM)*. This diagnosis in the first edition of *DSM* had specifically referred to combat by way of example. Although it had inaccurately specified that the condition could only be temporary, it conveyed at least a glimpse of stress disorder. As the return of troops from Viet Nam was reaching a crescendo, the psychiatric profession's official diagnostic guide backed away from stress disorder even further, and the condition vanished into the interstices of "adjustment reaction of adult life."

Thus for 12 years, 1968 through 1980, most American psychiatrists and other mental health professionals based their encounters with Viet Nam veteran patients on the official view that no such thing as PTSD existed. By contrast, the full-blown appearance in *DSM-III* in 1980 of the richly detailed diagnostic category of PTSD is all the more striking. These dramatic shifts from *DSM-I* to *DSM-III* suggest the hypothesis that—as part of a highly complex social and intellectual phenomenon—irrational influences have deeply affected the recognition and appreciation of this diagnosis by organized psychiatry.

The nonavailability of accurate guidance about diagnosis during the period 1968 through 1980 produced clinical situations which were dysfunctional and bizarre. For example, in a retrospective review of all Viet Nam veteran cases seen at one V.A. mental hygiene clinic between 1964 and 1972, I discovered 11 undiagnosed cases of traumatic war neurosis with unmistakable classical manifestations. At the same facility, between 1972 and 1980, 64 previously undiagnosed cases emerged from the normal clinical operations of the outpatient clinic and the general psychiatric wards. In 1980 the phenomenon of initial non-diagnosis stopped in that facility. Similar surveys with similar results have been conducted (7).

Since 1980, the previously widespread pattern of nondiagnosis has been thoroughly documented in the veteran population seen at the Veterans Administration's Vet Centers and V.A. mental hygiene clinics, in community mental health centers, and in the offices of private therapists. Currently, cases with a history of diagnosis missed prior to 1980 are routinely noted and taken for granted.

Perhaps the most extraordinary example of this phenomenon I know is related below:

Sam K. returned from a 12-month combat tour with the Army in 1968. At a stateside Army post he was jumpy and irritable and had flashbacks of combat and severe insomnia. All symptoms sharply worsened when he was assigned the duty of acting as a Vietcong in mock Vietnamese village training exercises for new recruits. A psychiatrist evaluated Sam, diagnosed traumatic war neurosis, and recommended that he be immediately relieved from this duty, which continuously provoked intrusive recall of war events. The recommendation was ignored by command. Sam then went AWOL. When he later returned, he was intensely symptomatic. He was diagnosed as acutely schizophrenic by other psychiatrists. For the next year, he was a patient at a succession of Army, then V.A. hospitals. He was repeatedly diagnosed as schizophrenic; he finally received a medical discharge and a 100 percent service-connected disability pension (for schizophrenia).

For the next 12 years, Sam lived a nomadic life. He married, divorced, and drifted. Much of the time he was asymptomatic, but now and again he experienced an intensification of symptoms in response to major events which reminded him of Viet Nam (for example, the end of the war in 1975). For each of these exacerbations he was admitted to a V.A. or private hospital, rediagnosed as schizophrenic, treated with phenothiazines, and given no stress disorder–specific treatment. At all admissions, his tour in Viet Nam was totally ignored.

At the end of these 12 years, Sam was arrested for a minor crime during which he had unconsciously repeated in detail a critical traumatic event which he had experienced in Viet Nam. The true nature of the situation was first unearthed upon forensic evaluation. The evaluators obtained all records from all hospitalizations (including Army, V.A., and private sector hospitals) and reviewed them. There was no documentation of schizophrenia anywhere in the record—including that of the Army medical board—but rather a listing of severe PTSD symptoms with a labeling of them as representing schizophrenia. No details of Sam's experiences in Viet Nam were recorded anywhere in the record. Furthermore, extensive interviewing by two expert clinicians revealed no evidence of schizophrenia, past or present. It was noted that Sam's postwar history had included a period of one year spent living in an African jungle in an isolated base camp situation; in this way, this veteran had dramatically recreated his life in Viet Nam.

PTSD-specific treatment was arranged for the veteran, his service-connected disability diagnosis was converted to PTSD, and he has been free of any recurrence of his severe symptoms for the past three years.

Nontreatment

Prior to 1980, it was generally impossible for Viet Nam veterans with PTSD to obtain specific treatment from mental health professionals, whether in the Veterans Administration or in the private sector. Nondiagnosis was of course one principal reason. I am one of approximately 25 clinicians—out of several thousand—who have been identified as having regularly provided specific psychological treatment for stress disorder in Viet Nam veterans, within the Veterans Administration system, during the 1970s. Those clinicians who carried out this work during that period uniformly report skeptical and occasionally hostile reactions, from otherwise close colleagues, concerning the existence of PTSD, the validity of Viet Nam veterans' complaints, and any key role for combat experiences in the production of the disorder.

At least two specialized units for the treatment of Viet Nam veterans with PTSD were established in V.A. hospitals during the 1970s. Both were closed, accompanied by hostility directed at the staff from colleagues. The few private sector clinicians who correctly diagnosed and treated PTSD in Viet Nam veterans during the 1970s report similar skepticism or hostility from colleagues as a standard feature of their work.

Effects

Although the widespread occurrence of nondiagnosis and nontreatment prior to 1980 is now well documented clinically in Vet Centers and V.A. Medical Centers, what is not yet clear is the resulting human cost.

Expert clinicians who have understood and treated PTSD since

1970 are all able to account for some suicides, other extremely unto-ward events, and numbers of seriously impaired lives because of nondiagnosis and nontreatment. There has been an understandable reluctance to report those cases in the professional literature, because of the possibility of lawsuits or other adverse reactions.

A Specialized National Treatment Program: Opposition and Support

Two events then occurred, essentially simultaneously, in late 1979. The American Psychiatric Association adopted the current diagnosis of PTSD, and the Veterans Administration, upon the direction of Congress, established a nationwide system of specialized counseling centers (Vet Centers) for a wide range of readjustment problems in Viet Nam veterans, including PTSD.

This chapter's survey of society- and profession-wide avoidance of PTSD, and of the latest generation of war veterans, would be incomplete unless it were noted that the formation of the Vet Centers came only after the Veterans Administration, the veterans organizations, and the House of Representatives had opposed for 10 years the Senate's legislation to do so. In the end, all parties acceded in 1979 to the support of the public, new Viet Nam veteran leadership in the veterans organizations, some mental health professionals, and the first Viet Nam veteran chief of the Veterans Administration, Max Cleland.

This new psychological services structure to treat Viet Nam veterans was created largely because of the incapacity of traditional treatment facilities in the Veterans Administration, in state systems, and in the private sector to provide the needed assistance. To a considerable degree, this incapacity was in turn based primarily on the hostility and avoidance described in this chapter. It is also true that some Viet Nam veterans were alienated and mistrusted the Veterans Administration, as has been widely publicized. This situation provided an additional barrier to treatment. However, the alienation and mistrust of veterans may have been less a primary phenomenon, and more one that was secondary to the nonresponsiveness of mental health professionals, than has heretofore been appreciated or publicized.

Two other aspects of this story are worth noting: 1) A civilian federal psychological services structure for reactions to wartime trauma in veterans has never before existed in the United States; it is unprecedented. 2) This structure has recently been duplicated by the Australian Ministry of Veterans' Affairs, which opened nine Viet Nam veteran counseling centers in 1983 (8).

PRINCIPAL MANIFESTATIONS OF
IRRATIONAL REACTIONS TO PTSD

I shall now review 16 attitudinal or behavioral reactions to Viet Nam veterans and to PTSD that have been seen among clinicians and clinical researchers. You will note that some of these reactions could be manifested toward veterans of other wars, or toward survivors of other types of traumatic stress, such as rape, kidnap, and natural disasters. Sorting out generic and Viet Nam War–specific elements in the following discussion is a vital task, awaiting future research; it will not be attemped here.

The following is a catalog of negative or problematic phenomena, with the purpose of identifying certain reactions not previously described in the literature. It is important to note that considerable diagnostic, therapeutic, and research efforts are presently underway in this field which are both effective and free of the phenomena described here. The purpose of this chapter is to shed light on the problematic reactions, with the hope that these may be avoided in the future.

Several types of reactions are commonly associated with the actual avoidance of diagnostic or therapeutic work with veterans. Others more often occur in the context of a clinician's attempts to provide useful diagnostic and therapeutic assistance. These two broad categories will be considered separately. An additional interesting feature is the appearance of various irrational reactions in the field of clinical research, from which some examples will be drawn.

ACTIONS ASSOCIATED WITH AVOIDANCE
OF VETERAN PATIENTS

Denial of the Validity of the PTSD Construct

Several key milestones support the contemporary consensus on the existence and nature of PTSD:

- Early psychoanalytic findings concerning traumatic war neurosis (9);
- Demonstration of chronic cases by Abram Kardiner in the 1930s and 1940s (10);

- Confirmation of chronic cases by Archibald and Tuddenham after World War II (11);
- Clarification of the generic PTSD phenomenon by Horowitz during the 1970s (12);
- Formulation of the diagnosis of PTSD in *DSM-III* in 1980 (13); and
- The awarding by the Veterans Administration of service-connected disability ratings for PTSD to over 9,000 veterans of the Korean and Viet Nam Wars, and World War II, since 1980.

Nonetheless, one still finds clinicians and researchers who openly deny the existence of PTSD. In the clinical sphere, such wholesale denial—common prior to 1980 and usually accompanied by the provision of another diagnosis (14)—is now on the wane. However, it may appear from time to time in a striking fashion, as in the following examples taken from reviewers' comments on proposals submitted to a research funding organization.

It is premature to expend thousands of dollars and research energy looking for the etiology or biological correlations of PTSD when the syndrome has yet to be clinically validated.

Investigation and clinical acumen has [sic] yet to accord that such a phenomenon [PTSD] exists.

Another example is the following from a clinical context:

At a conference of senior psychiatrists, a clinician in charge of a large psychiatric inpatient and outpatient service reported his belief that some substantial number of cases of "so-called PTSD" in Viet Nam veterans, particularly those with flashbacks, were probably in actuality a syndrome of perceptual and imagery derangement caused by the excessive smoking of marijuana in Viet Nam during the war.

Denial of Diagnosis Workability

The consensus in psychiatry, as of 1985, is that the clinical construct of PTSD is valid. Wholesale denial of the existence of the disorder is now less common, and negative attitudes about the diagnosis are now more commonly expressed in one of the following attenuated ways:

- Assertion that the diagnosis is "circular," because *DSM-III* requires demonstration of a traumatic stressor; this is usually accompanied by the assertion that it is hard to define a traumatic stressor;

- The claim that there is poor diagnostic agreement when two or more clinicians evaluate the same case;
- Fear about misuse of the diagnosis in criminal cases and compensation cases; and
- The claim that the condition is easily faked by veterans, resulting in incorrect diagnosis.

As an example of the first type of attenuated wholesale denial, at a major research conference in 1984 a nationally known psychiatric researcher asked, with evident disbelief, "What is a trauma anyway? How can you define a traumatic stressor? It is impossible to define." This view is usually accompanied by the assertion that the diagnosis of PTSD is somehow defective because it is circular—that is, that the stressor is defined as traumatic because it produces a traumatic stress reaction.

This view, that a stressor cannot be defined and that it should not be included in the diagnosis, expresses a nihilism which does not spring from clinical reality, scientifically apprehended. In fact, the events of life which qualify as traumatic stressors are usually clearly definable and limited, on the basis of current data, to combat, wartime or concentration camp imprisonment, torture, severe vehicular or air crashes, overwhelming natural disasters, rape, devastating collapse of buildings or other structures, severe fires, assaults, and being kidnapped or taken hostage.

Indeed there is an element of degree involved—as is the case for most aspects of human behavior, as well as psychiatric diagnosis. But for most clinicians and researchers that fact does not interfere with determining what is a traumatic stressor and what isn't. Defining a traumatic stressor is no more difficult than many other situations which commonly require clinical judgment from mental health workers and researchers.

The environmental traumatic stressor of course interacts with the individual mind and brain to produce stress reactions and PTSD. The characteristics of the individual thus heavily influence the stress disorder. This complex and somewhat undefined interaction, however, does nothing to diminish the impact, on normal individuals, of such stressors as those listed above.

The second form which denial of workability takes is the contention that the PTSD diagnosis is tenuous and unreliable when compared to other diagnoses.

Various reviewers wrote, in evaluating proposals for funding of research on PTSD:

Treatment outcome studies . . . are premature when the clinical characterization of the PTSD is so inadequate, imprecise, and probably not specific. Given the likely imprecise nature of diagnosis, . . .

If one is to accept the validity (never demonstrated) of *DSM-III* criteria for this disorder. . .

It is also [our] feeling . . . that PTSD has been so poorly characterized clinically that it may be premature to conduct treatment studies with PTSD at this time.

In fact, existing research on the reliability of the PTSD diagnosis indicates a quite acceptable degree of correlation between diagnosticians (15).

Some clinicians and clinical researchers have expressed their fear that a Pandora's Box has been opened through the utilization of the PTSD diagnosis as a criminal defense. This fear is usually expressed only with reference to Viet Nam veterans. In my experience, equivalent concern over the use of a PTSD defense by criminal defendants who are victims of rape, natural disasters, concentration camps, or torture, is not voiced.

In fact, this defense has been used in a significant number of cases since 1980, and the results are apparently well within the boundaries of controversy typical for the forensic use of any psychiatric defense. One recent comprehensive legal review commented the following:

Because PTSD is a relatively new way of describing and explaining client behavior in litigation, *and because none of the cases in which it has been used successfully by the defense at trial have reached appellate level*, the "case law" on PTSD is necessarily limited to cases in which defendants were unable to present the defense in a convincing manner. The cases, however, make it clear that PTSD is recognized as a proper subject for expert testimony in at least twenty-one states and five federal districts. In addition, a number of majority and dissenting opinions have taken trial judges and attorneys to task for failing to take PTSD seriously in both sentencing and trial. In one appellate case, in which PTSD was implicated, the Supreme Court of Minnesota rejected an appellate argument based upon PTSD because counsel had failed to properly raise the issue at trial. This disposition, however, should not be read as a rejection of PTSD. Rather, it is an indication that, like other factors influencing client behavior, PTSD must be properly presented at trial. It re-emphasizes the premise of this article, that attorneys must properly present PTSD, in order to adequately represent those veteran clients exhibiting symptoms of PTSD. (16; emphasis added)

With regard to compensation, the Pandora's Box concern has eased since 1981, when it was feared that compensation for PTSD in Viet Nam veterans was a social danger.

> At a regional meeting of V.A. Chiefs of Psychiatry, several senior clinicians expressed the opinion that so many disability ratings for PTSD might be awarded as to cause a serious drain on the Veterans Administration's budget and perhaps on the U.S. Treasury itself. (Some of their colleagues, of course, disagreed.)

Since the institution of the PTSD diagnosis in 1980, sometimes it has been claimed that the disorder is easily faked by Viet Nam veterans, resulting in incorrect diagnosis. Although not commonly raised as an issue with rape victims or survivors of major civilian disasters, the concern about fabrication itself is legitimate. There is a long tradition of such concern based on the role of secondary gain when compensation is available.

However, the claim of *easy* fabrication is another matter and is unique. The following excerpt from a review of a research proposal exemplifies such unusual concern:

> The [Principal Investigator] points out that the diagnosis of PTSD lacks evidence of reliability and validity and that the clinical diagnosis is based on self-report data which can easily be exaggerated or faked.

Indeed, the creation of factitious PTSD by a Viet Nam veteran is certainly no easier than the factitious creation of any psychiatric condition. In fact, it is possible that fakery may be unusually difficult on the part of a Viet Nam veteran, because a very long clinical course must be fabricated. The clinical picture requires a 10- to 20-year story, the details must fit together well, and memories must relate to long-ago traumas in a dynamically sound fashion.

Irrational Insistence on the Primacy of Predisposition

This particular reaction to PTSD must be understood against the background of the rise and fall of the predisposition theory of war stress reactions. The predisposition theory is the view that pretrauma personality characteristics—defects, flaws, and weaknesses—are the primary or most influential variable in the production of the condition. This view has its roots in the early writings of European analysts, who observed traumatized soldiers during and after World War I and interpreted their findings in terms of the early theories of psychoanalysis (9). This work emphasized—quite naturally, in light of what was being discovered by psychoanalysis at the time—reverberations of war trauma with early childhood memories and conflicts. In part because of a resulting *post hoc, ergo propter hoc* fallacy, this led to significant enthusiasm, among American psychiatrists at the time of World War II, for predicting which soldiers would break down in combat on the basis of psychiatric history and examination.

By 1944, a massive screening program by Selective Service psychiatrists had resulted in the rejection of about one million men from military duty for psychiatric reasons. However, by about the same time during the war, it was noted that about one million men had been discharged for psychiatric or personality reasons. An Army Inspector General recommended that the screening program be abandoned as ineffective, since about a million men had been psychiatrically screened out, but about a million had been discharged anyway for psychiatric or personality reasons. The program was abandoned, and never since has the military attempted a general psychological screening program for vulnerability to war stress based on the notion of predisposition (17).

In the early 1950s, Eli Ginsberg, on behalf of the Conservation of Human Resources Project at Columbia University, formally inquired of a number of the psychiatrists who had participated in the screening program as to their retrospective views of the lessons learned. Ginsberg's report reflects the conviction that predisposition had not been established as the major factor in the production of war neurosis (18).

Later during the 1950s, the principles of modern military psychiatry were established. These included the view that acute stress reaction to combat is influenced by multiple factors, including the following:

- The nature, quantity, and timing of the trauma;
- Combat unit cohesion and morale;
- Combat effectiveness;
- Personality factors;
- The short- and long-term post-trauma environment of the stressed individual; and
- Conveying expectancy of recovery to the affected soldier.

A similar multicausal view with respect to chronic PTSD has been supported by the bulk of research during the post–Viet Nam War period. One feature of this research has been careful control for the degree and kind of combat trauma experienced by various subgroups. Two examples which indicate the leading role of the multicausal view are described below.

1) Frye (19) surveyed a 1969 Ft. Benning Officers Candidates School graduating class, many of whom went to Viet Nam. In this

group of well-educated and well-functioning officer veterans, the five factors which significantly distinguished those with PTSD from those without PTSD were the following:

- Negative perception of family helpfulness upon return to the United States and less talking to family members about Viet Nam;
- Higher level of combat in Viet Nam;
- An external locus of control;
- A more immediate discharge from active duty after the war; and
- A more positive attitude toward the Viet Nam War before entering the service.

2) The second example, a major nationwide survey by Card (20) of a group of 1963 high school graduates, compared those who had gone to Viet Nam with those who had not. It failed to find any preservice predictors of postwar stress-related symptoms. It is important that this is the only large-scale study on stress disorder in Viet Nam veterans to date which has been able to utilize prospectively obtained data.

Because of these developments, and also because of common clinical experience, the predisposition theory (as defined above) has no standing at all among expert clinicians who treat significant numbers of war veterans, nor does it have a standing among those treating stress disorder in rape victims or survivors of civilian disasters.

Thus has the predisposition theory risen and fallen over the past 65 years, whereas the multicausal view has coalesced in research and clinical work over the past two decades. However, especially among clinicians with little or no experience in treating war veterans, one continues to find the belief that PTSD is primarily the result of premilitary personality defects. Sometimes this view is buttressed by clinical researchers with case material in which personality factors are indeed apparently more influential. The fallacy lies in drawing epidemiologic conclusions from small and nonrepresentative numbers of cases.

Perhaps what is most significant is that this view of the primacy of predisposition involves a failure on the part of both clinicians and researchers to evaluate premilitary, military, and postmilitary variables and influences carefully and without bias. At this time the predisposition theory is an instance of blaming the victim.

The Comorbidity Theory

The fading of the predisposition theory, and the emergence of the multicausal view, have been recently followed by a new phenomenon:

the view that PTSD is usually accompanied by other psychiatric disorders. This view may lead to either dismissal of the condition as an epiphenomenon or attributing it, along with other concomitant psychopathology, to more general underlying mental dysfunction. One study by Sierles et al. (21) has reported on 25 Viet Nam veterans hospitalized for PTSD and found that 21 showed one or more additional diagnoses. However, the study was flawed in that consistent methods were not used in making the various diagnoses, and some diagnoses were based on interviews by two of the authors with no independent raters. Furthermore, in 12 of the cases, the "other" diagnosis was either drug dependence or alcoholism. The treatment of Viet Nam veterans with PTSD has revealed that substance abuse is sometimes a secondary manifestation of PTSD; this study shows no effort at all to determine whether the substance abuse was primary or secondary to PTSD.

More recently a communication to the *American Journal of Psychiatry* (22) reported that, in 31 outpatients with PTSD, a certain number had other psychiatric disorders, although the writer does not specify how many. Like the previous study, this report too was flawed. The "other" disorders included alcoholism, multiple drug abuse, depression, sociopathy, and caffeinism, yet the communication does not mention that substance abuse may be secondary to stress disorder, depression may be an associated feature (23), and sociopathy may be a misdiagnosis when PTSD is present in Viet Nam veterans. The communication reflects no effort to consider those questions, which are well known to clinicians and researchers in this field; this again raises a question of objectivity.

The emergence of the comorbidity theory, as a recent addition to the series of unscientific reactions to the phenomenon of PTSD, is strikingly crystallized in the following sweeping statement from a recent commentary by Van Putten:

> Judging from veterans now in treatment, *most patients with PTSD* have coexisting psychiatric disorders. . . . (2; emphasis added)

Clearly, the point is precisely that one cannot make such a judgment from patients in treatment, because these subjects represent a unique subgroup of the universe of veterans with PTSD. Van Putten bases his unjustified generalization on the previously discussed flawed study by Sierles (21) on hospitalized patients, and also on yet another paper by Escobar et al. (24), which purports to show extensive co-occurrence of other psychiatric disorders in PTSD patients. However, Escobar's report has the following major defects:

- Again, the entire sample is treatment-seeking. Accurate epidemiologic conclusions cannot be drawn from a treatment-seeking sample.
- All of the sample was from a particular ethnic-cultural group, which constrains the ability to generalize.
- Many of the supposed second *DSM-III* diagnoses either were possibly secondary to PTSD (e.g., alcoholism or drug dependence) or may represent PTSD symptoms (e.g., depression or social phobia) registering as a false-positive diagnosis of those disorders. Most importantly, no clinical investigation which might untangle these diagnostic issues is noted in the report.
- Forty percent of the sample met the *DSM-III* criteria for antisocial personality on the Diagnostic Interview Schedule (DIS). Some of these cases may represent a factitious antisocial personality DIS pattern secondary to PTSD and the Viet Nam War experience. If this is not the case with a large number of subjects in this study, then the sample would appear to be skewed, since no such correlation of antisocial behavior and stress symptoms has appeared in nationwide non-treatment-seeking samples of Viet Nam veterans (5, 20).

In summary, Van Putten's claim that "most patients with PTSD have co-existing psychiatric disorder . . ." relies on a study of 25 hospitalized veterans and another study of 41 treatment-seeking Mexican American veterans with a supposed 40 percent rate of diagnosis for antisocial personality. Both studies completely lack differential analysis of symptoms known to be secondary to or associated with PTSD. Neither study supports any epidemiologic conclusions.

Although the relation between PTSD and other psychiatric disorders is an extremely important topic for investigation, the foregoing examples illustrate how this approach may be affected by nonobjective attitudes.

Generalized Professional Paralysis

Fear, confusion, and other irrational reactions in professionals confronted with Viet Nam veteran patients may manifest themselves as a general inhibition of professional functioning. When this occurs, a therapist or a ward staff take no action or provide no treatment, and the patient remains unusually suspended for a long period of time.

It was finally determined that an inpatient, misdiagnosed as schizophrenic for years, was suffering from severe PTSD with psychotic-level symptomatology. Following correct diagnosis, the patient remained on the psychiatric ward for several weeks with no change in treatment until finally the patient's family asked the ward staff what was going to be done. Only after the family's intervention did the staff begin to make changes and formulate plans.

A veteran under extreme pressure from undiagnosed PTSD symptoms created a serious hostage and barricade incident. A senior police official, who was a Viet Nam veteran, resolved the situation. The patient remained in jail and pretrial confinement for one year. The prosecutor, defense attorney, and the various psychologists or psychiatrists who saw him (though they had the correct diagnosis in mind) were all unable to formulate clear recommendations to the judge as to how to proceed. An expert consultant finally obtained a more in-depth history, sorted out the diagnostic picture (a hysterical conversion symptom had been misdiagnosed as migraine), and made recommendations at a sentencing hearing for a treatment program. This was accepted by the court and has worked well to date, after three years of follow-up.

Generalized Hostility and Contempt Toward Viet Nam Veterans

During the postwar period, clinicians treating Viet Nam veterans have noted numerous and striking episodes of intense hostility or contempt for veteran patients from otherwise well-functioning fellow professionals. This has not been an easy topic to address, either in the literature or in daily professional work, for it is understandably accompanied by significant feelings of shame or guilt in hostile or contemptuous clinicians.

A veteran patient with severe, chronic, and painful PTSD symptoms—and also a possibly unrelated sexual problem—was being interviewed in front of a group of professionals at a case conference in the department of psychiatry of a distinguished university. Halfway through the interview, which was being conducted delicately and which was going well, a physician member in the audience, who was aware of the veteran's sexual problem, suddenly interrupted and said to the patient, "You haven't told him about your sexual thing. Don't you think that should be discussed?" The interview was derailed.

A scientific reviewer of a research proposal recommended against the researcher's plan to pay a small fee to both Viet Nam veteran and civilian control subjects. The reviewer wrote that the civilian controls should be paid, but the Viet Nam veterans should not. "The payment to subjects is not justified. Given their symptoms, PTSD patients [the Viet Nam veterans] should be highly motivated to find out what's wrong with them. Some payment to normals is reasonable."

An experienced psychiatrist was evaluating a veteran patient, who had severe PTSD symptoms and repeatedly expressed fears of losing control. There was no history of violence, except of course in combat. The patient was desperate for help and terrified of what harm he might cause others. After one evaluation session, the psychiatrist and the patient by chance encountered each other informally in the waiting room. The psychiatrist jokingly commented that he hoped the patient would not take him hostage in the waiting room. The patient did not return to the psychiatrist. Subsequently, the patient was given a psychotropic drug by another psychiatrist for insomnia and, influenced by the marked disinhibiting effects of the drug, created a barricade incident when overcome by war flashbacks. This was peacefully negotiated by police who were more familiar with PTSD than was either psychiatrist, and successful treatment was the ultimate outcome. The patient went on to help the police department improve its procedures for handling other similar situations.

Hostility Toward Professionals Who Treat Viet Nam Veterans

Professional hostility toward colleagues who treat Viet Nam veterans has been observed by experts since the early 1970s. Particularly since 1980, this phenomenon is fading somewhat, as clinical understanding of the problems in Viet Nam veterans has grown. However, it is still occasionally manifested in striking ways.

The clinical psychologist director of a Viet Nam veterans counseling center had successfully completed part of his clinical training on the Psychology Service of the supporting V.A. hospital, to the documented satisfaction of his supervisors. Now fully qualified, the Vet Center director's V.A. career appointment was nonetheless blocked by the Psychology Service Chief, who admitted he wanted no Vet Center psychologists to hold career appointments. The appointment was finally awarded on orders from V.A. headquarters.

This hostility at times extends to whole groups of persons and programs which provide effective counseling services to veterans.

In late 1984, a senior V.A. medical official, fortunately reflecting a minority opinion among his associates, stated that the Veterans Administration's Viet Nam veteran counseling centers should not have been created. He said they were harmful to the Veterans Administration because they unfairly compete for funds.

It is interesting that by the time this judgment was expressed the Centers had seen over 325,000 people at much less than the cost per visit of regular psychiatric clinics, had three times been endorsed by unanimously passed legislation in Congress, and were strongly supported by veterans and the public.

Instances of such hostility encountered by mental health workers who treat Viet Nam veterans are understandable in that the work indeed deals with the dark side of life—war—and with one of the darkest periods in the history of our nation in this century. At times, it seems to both the therapist and his or her associates that there is no end to the death, mutilation, and ethical and political conflict which such patients bring to the fore. Underlying revulsion and anxiety about such matters is one factor creating this hostility.

REACTIONS ASSOCIATED WITH NONAVOIDANCE OF VETERAN PATIENTS

The following reactions are seen among clinicians who do provide treatment to Viet Nam veterans, who accept the validity of the clinical construct of PTSD, who regard the diagnosis as workable, and who strive to avoid hostility or contempt for veteran patients.

Normal Reactions of Mental Health Professionals to War, Violent Death, and Horror

PTSD is produced by contact between the individual and the darkest and most violent forces of human nature. War, murder, rape, floods, etc. take the victim over the edge of life into a serious confrontation with death or uncontrolled violence. Some individuals are thereby transformed and become, at some level, bearers of the traumatic experience. The therapist with whom they come into contact is thus inevitably exposed to the war, rape, flood, etc.

As details of the events of war and the actions and feelings of the combatant come forth in treatment, normally there are produced in the listener such reactions as punishing or retaliatory wishes, sadistic impulses, fear and anxiety about the former warrior's violence, and existential fear of death accompanied by a deepened sense of one's own vulnerability. These reactions may also be accompanied by feelings of helplessness, concern, sympathy, and strong empathic reactions.

These nearly universal reactions to material about the violence and death of war, unlike other emotional manifestations mentioned in this chapter, have already received some attention in the literature (see Haley [25, 26], Lifton [27], and Margolin [28]).

Superficial Praising or Reassurance by Mental Health Professionals

During the 1980s our society generally has begun to swing away from disavowal and repudiation of the Viet Nam War experience and of its veterans, toward a more reflective position about the war and a more accepting and understanding rapport with the approximately

3.5 million Americans who participated in it. Many citizens, including mental health professionals, now have regrets, specifically about hostile attitudes and nontherapeutic receptions which some returning veterans encountered.

As a result, one reaction now seen in diagnostic and treatment situations consists of explicit expressions of support, respect, praise, and reassurance from therapists. Early in an evaluation or a treatment —long before the veteran's combat experiences have been delineated and long before his or her therapeutic needs have been established— the clinician may respond, on the basis of personal discomfort or guilt, with superficial reassurance or praise. Although a veteran's reaction to this may at first be positive, ultimately such expressions are experienced as rejection or repudiation. They should be scrupulously avoided if evaluation is to be accurate or treatment is to be successful. What is required of the clinician is respect in the form of provision of one's best skills.

Excessive Self-Disclosure by Mental Health Professionals

Treatment during the past decade has shown the need by some, though not all, veteran patients for an unusual kind of self-disclosure on the part of the therapist (29). Certain attitudes and fears found in these patients, based on the character of the war and the indifferent or hostile reception after the war, may require the therapist to reveal his or her attitudes about the war and its veterans. This may be needed to develop sufficient therapeutic trust as a prerequisite for any treatment relationship to occur. Also, in the case of therapists who were of draft age during the Viet Nam era, the patient may require some information about the therapist's status during the war: whether the therapist served in the military and went to Viet Nam. With many patients, it just does not do for the therapist to act as though he or she had no actual connection to an historical experience which profoundly affected most citizens. Some patients indeed must learn—if there is to be any possibility of therapy—the crucial details of how the therapist dealt with the draft, the possibility of service in Viet Nam, or where he or she stood on the war.

However, as an irrational manifestation, such transparency may be overdone in reaction to treating a Viet Nam veteran. The therapist may be unduly self-revealing in a way which does not contribute to the working alliance, and which is driven largely by personal reactions to the patient (for a clinical example, see Chapter 8, p. 180). Finding the right amount of therapist self-revelation for a patient, especially concerning Viet Nam–related matters, is one of the most difficult and complex technical issues in treating this patient group. Many therapists can benefit from consulting with colleagues about choices that have to be made about what to reveal.

Overindulgence by Mental Health Professionals

A related reaction manifests as withholding of needed limit-setting on patient behavior, which Margolin has called "acting-out giving" (28).

A patient repeatedly mentioned his fear of losing control and shooting someone with his rifle. His relationship with weapons was highly influenced by perseverations from the war. The therapist made no suggestions about removing the weapon from the veteran's easy access, until finally the patient shot it off, narrowly missing a family member. The police intervened, and the patient's clinical state markedly worsened. Later he revealed his wish that the therapist would have asked him, or would have told him, to get rid of the weapon.

A psychiatric ward, specializing in the treatment of PTSD, lacked sophisticated and consistently applied controls on abusive acting-out patient behavior. Finally, such behavior deteriorated to the point of frequent drinking and marijuana smoking; disregarding of various rules; three suicides of current or former patients in a one-year period; and, ultimately, nationwide publicity about the foundering state of the ward.

It is axiomatic that such staff behavior may derive, in addition to the usual sources, from unresolved guilt about prior hostility toward Viet Nam veterans. Conflict-laden features of the staff member's own relationship to the Viet Nam War may also contribute.

It may be especially difficult to distinguish such emotionally motivated lack of structure from flexibility about time and scheduling sometimes necessary for individuals recovering from PTSD. Intensity of catharsis or the pressure of newly unlocked memories, for example, sometimes mandate ad hoc hours or sessions lasting longer than scheduled. Conversely, at times, patients may need to interrupt treatment for several weeks or months in order to fully digest and master what has been recalled and felt in therapy. In general, there is an inner timetable of recovery from PTSD based on internal processes of binding of aggression, mastery, integration, and unfolding of meaning. Sometimes the schedule of these processes cannot adhere to an appointment book or a ward schedule. On the other hand, provision of structure and organization in a therapeutic context may be critical to the needed development of new internal structures in the veteran.

Abrupt Dismissal or Abandonment of Patients

Expert clinicians are all too familiar with occasional cases of veterans with PTSD who commit suicide, instigate violence, or deteriorate clinically in some other way, following precipitous discharge from a psychiatric ward or hasty termination of outpatient psychotherapy. Of course these situations occur with other types of patients as well; they may not result only from therapist reactions which are specific to PTSD or the Viet Nam experience. Sometimes the dismissal does appear to be a specific reaction, as in the following example:

The patient, a corporate executive, was in analysis with a senior training analyst. The treatment focused on what was thought to be typical obsessional difficulties. The patient began to talk about his experiences as a combat infantryman in Viet Nam. Almost immediately, the analyst reacted by contacting a clinician whom he knew to be an expert on PTSD in Viet Nam veterans, requesting a consultation. When the patient arrived for the "consultation," he indicated that his analyst told him that the task would be to "work out" the Viet Nam experiences with the consultant, and that when that was completed, he could return to the analysis. Of course, after the veteran's war experiences were "worked out," the veteran had no desire to return to the original analyst.

Avoidance of the Military History

Perhaps the most remarkable and dramatic irrational professional reaction to Viet Nam veterans is the failure to obtain a military history in an otherwise complete psychiatric workup. By 1980, this phenomenon had become so well known in the Veterans Administration medical system that the appearance of a thick psychiatric file of a Viet Nam veteran with multiple psychiatric visits or admissions, but no military history ever having been obtained, attained nearly pathognomonic status—for PTSD.

A case was presented at psychiatric grand rounds with excellent detail and formulation, but with no material at all about the patient's tour of duty in Viet Nam. The diagnosis presented was borderline personality disorder, notwithstanding excellent functioning for three years in the military. A visiting consultant asked about the missing Viet Nam military history, to which the senior psychiatrist on the patient's unit responded by asserting that the individual had not been in combat, but rather in the "rear" support forces, and that his job had been "merely" to direct artillery strikes. Therefore, concluded the psychiatrist, there was no war trauma present and no need to pursue the details of the year in Viet Nam. Indeed, the military history was not further pursued. Sometime later the patient killed himself.

Similar cases seen in treatment suggest the hypothesis for this case that unresolved guilt over the damage done by the artillery shelling, for which the veteran felt responsible, may have played a crucial role in his difficulties. Also, guerilla attacks occurred in many "rear" areas during the war and have led to PTSD in some veterans.

A patient had several admissions for alcoholism over a number of years. The military history was never obtained. Nonetheless, the psychiatric record revealed multiple notations that the patient had hallucinated, while he was in delerium tremens, "Asians" and persons who were disemboweled or torn to pieces. The material of these hallucinations was referred to in the record as "primitive" and "psychotic." The only reference to Viet Nam in the records of several admissions was that the patient had not been "in combat." However, investigation revealed that the patient operated a heavy gun on a ship shelling Viet Nam, and he was consciously aware that his hallucinations, plus preoccupations during normal states of awareness, were his imaginative constructions of the effects of the shelling on the people in Vietnamese towns and villages. He further indicated that his constructions had been based on accounts of destruction from fellow veterans who had been in extensive combat on the ground. Indeed, his alcoholism had concealed severe underlying PTSD with intense guilty preoccupation about various war events. There was no family history of alcoholism and no alcoholism prior to Viet Nam. The alcoholism was secondary to PTSD and represented the patient's desperate attempt to quiet the undiagnosed war still raging within himself.

Another patient was referred to an expert consultant after having been seen at length by a senior psychiatrist for severe unrelenting insomnia. The psychiatrist considered the problem to be due to PTSD, and treatment had been active and apparently appropriate. During the consultant's workup, when the history reached the point of the veteran's tour of duty in Viet Nam, the patient informed the consultant that he could not discuss Viet Nam, and in fact he had never done so during the treatment with the referring psychiatrist. With considerable care, the consultant ultimately enabled a discussion of the war experiences. The patient decided that he wished to continue with the consultant.

Intrusion of the Therapist's Unresolved Traumatic Experiences

If the therapist has experienced extreme trauma during childhood or adult life, the impact of which is still unresolved, this may impair the assistance he or she can provide.

A therapist, a Viet Nam veteran, conducted group therapy for veterans with PTSD. The group was open-ended and included many patients over a three-year period. Most patients did well clinically. Analysis of the process in supervision revealed that the therapist made hardly any effective interventions directly in response to specific memories of the patients about Viet Nam; all such interventions came from other members of the group. Also, the therapist reported being diffusely anxious after most group meetings. Five years later, the therapist experienced an acute upsurge of PTSD symptoms accompanied by recall of repressed memories of war experiences, for which he engaged in psychotherapy. Subsequently, he was able to respond to other veterans' traumatic memories with indicated interventions.

An analyst was treating a veteran patient. Apropos of some expressed anger from the patient, the analyst warned him not to "throw out the baby with the bath water." Later, apropos of nothing, the analyst told the patient that he (the patient) thought that he was "superior" to the analyst ("superior" in the sense of a superior person).

Both comments stimulated free-floating anxiety in the veteran patient, could not be further clarified, and were forgotten. Six months later, intense and previously repressed painful memories about war-damaged Vietnamese babies and children emerged in the patient.

Subsequently, the veteran learned that the analyst, who was Jewish and a native of Germany, had seldom been able to discuss his own experiences in connection with the Holocaust. After extensive review of this episode in a later treatment, the hypothesis was strongly supported that the analyst had been unconsciously experiencing the Viet Nam veteran patient as a Nazi ("You think you are superior to me") murderer ("Be careful not to throw out the baby with the bath water"). This reaction had been in response to a telegraphing, in the patient's associations, of the imminent uncovering of the veteran's repressed memories of harm to babies and children in Viet Nam, which was caused by soldiers of the analyst's adopted country, to which he had fled to escape the Nazis.

A Viet Nam veteran patient experienced severe PTSD symptoms accompanied by intense grief with long episodes of sobbing. He saw for consultation a distinguished senior clinician who was renowned for his publications on empathy and treatment technique. The patient presented his problems and Viet Nam experiences in considerable detail. The consultant's first response was to heatedly ask, "Are you sure you can tolerate your grief? It can be very intense and difficult. I know a great deal about that." The psychiatrist went on to inform the patient that he had lost all of his family members in the Holocaust, and that the grief had been overwhelming and painful for years.

While the psychiatrist did not explicitly discourage the patient from further visits, the veteran interpreted the message as a warning that the psychiatrist would not be comfortable in dealing with another war/holocaust.

Intrusion of the Mental Health Professional's Unresolved Viet Nam War Experiences

To be carefully distinguished from such extreme traumas in the mental health professional's personal history is the history of his or her own encounter with the Viet Nam War, which may intrude into the clinical context.

> *For some years, the director of a psychiatric inpatient service had experienced skepticism about the steadily increasing numbers of veterans with PTSD admitted to his service. Such admissions increased further following the opening of a Vet Center (V.A. Viet Nam Veterans Counseling Center) in his community in 1980. At that time, the director startled his staff in a clinical conference by informing them that these new veteran cases had brought him to the following realization.*
>
> *During his tour stateside during the war, as a military psychiatrist, he had often been assigned the duty of visiting the families of servicemen to inform them that their husbands, or sons, had been killed in Viet Nam. He was one of two officers assigned for this mission, but since he was the psychiatrically knowledgeable of the two, when there was a strong reaction, the other officer sometimes left him to handle the situation alone.*
>
> *The psychiatrist, recalling these experiences with his staff in 1980, said that he had shut off this encounter with the reality of the Viet Nam War for years, and that it had not come up in his psychoanalysis, which had been completed years before. He said further to his staff that he now understood the view that many mental health professionals had unresolved Viet Nam histories, since he himself was experiencing significant, long-shut-off feelings about these memories. He also indicated that he now felt less inclined to avoid thinking about Viet Nam veterans' cases than he had previously.*

> *During a session, a clinical psychologist responded to a veteran patient's expression of strong antiwar views, not with interpretation or an investigative response, but by directly stating his own passionately held similar views about the war. The psychologist still felt angry and frustrated about American activities in Viet Nam. The response, however, had the effect of shutting off further therapeutic exploration of the veteran's feelings about his Viet Nam experiences, which in fact remained shut off for the rest of the otherwise largely successful treatment.*

And a final example:

> *During the treatment of a veteran patient, the psychiatrist, in response to a flood of material about Viet Nam, angrily and explicitly denounced the more vigorous antiwar protestors of the wartime period, stating that they were unpatriotic, gave aid and comfort to the enemy, etc. As it happened, however, the patient agreed with those whom the psychiatrist denounced. The veteran considered himself and the antiwar protestors all to be quite patriotic. Feeling assaulted, the veteran terminated the treatment not long after. The psychiatrist was profusely apologetic for his outburst. Later it was determined that the psychiatrist, unlike the patient, had gone to significant trouble to avoid military duty during the war.*

The Poor Soldier Theory

Although long ago abandoned by military psychiatry as regards acute breakdown in combat, occasionally civilian clinicians or researchers put forth the view that soldiers who do well in combat, who perform and respond the way a good soldier should, do not develop stress reactions. The view that PTSD is correlated with, or caused by, poor combat adaptation is the latest in an evolving series of views which sees the veteran affected by stress as a poor soldier. In its pre–19th century version, this series saw combat breakdown as due to cowardice. For example, the *Report of the Committee of Enquiry into Shell Shock* of the British War Office (1922) described the pre–19th century view:

> No doubt there were men who, from one cause or another, broke down in every campaign . . . but such breakdowns, when they are recorded, are not very sympathetically treated, and unless a man had proved himself of good courage earlier in action, are dismissed as not differing greatly from cowardice. Of course, numbers of men went out of their minds in the old campaigns as they still do. (quoted in reference 30)

Recently, Hendin and Haas (31) studied 10 cases of veterans who were exposed to intense combat but did not develop PTSD. Other than referring to the study as an "introductory analysis," the authors state no limits on the generalizability of observations on 10 cases to a population of over 3.5 million persons. They list 13 characteristics of the 10 non-PTSD cases, which can be summarized and paraphrased as follows:

- Showed calmness under pressure and place value on staying calm;
- Showed intellectual control;
- Showed acceptance of fear;
- Had a lack of excessively violent or guilt-arousing behavior (e.g., atrocities);
- Saw impulsiveness as a threat in combat;
- Felt one's skill as a soldier would ensure survival;
- Strove to find purpose in the situation in Viet Nam;
- Tolerated the lack of purpose in the war;
- Saw the war in more rational terms;
- Did not obey silly or dangerous orders;
- Did not like being violent;
- Did not dehumanize the enemy; and
- Have little or no survival guilt, due to low intensity of buddy relationships.

The authors summarize these findings under the rubric of "good combat adaptation," which they claim provides a "systematic form of protection" against PTSD. Apparently the authors relied solely on the veterans' reports in determining how they had actually behaved in the war.

It is useful, in order to clarify the implications of this report, to list the apparent opposites of the characteristics of these authors' "good combat adaptation." In other words, the following are the putative characteristics of veterans *with* PTSD, derived from the views of Hendin and Haas:

- Showed excitement under pressure and do not value calmness;
- Had a lack of intellectual control;
- Repudiated fear in combat;
- Were excessively violent and engaged in guilt-arousing behavior (e.g., atrocities);
- Did not see impulsiveness as a threat in combat;
- Did not feel one's skill as a soldier would ensure survival;
- Did not strive to find a purpose in the war in Viet Nam;
- Could not tolerate experienced lack of purpose;
- Saw the war in less rational terms;
- Obeyed silly or dangerous orders;
- Liked being violent;
- Dehumanized the enemy; and
- Have survival guilt, due to [over] involvement with buddies.

Although these authors formally eschew the predisposition theory, it appears that the "good combat adaptation" view is the "poor soldier theory" and represents the belief that those who have what it takes to do well in war do not sustain lasting emotional wounds. The Hendin and Haas report presents the predisposition theory in a new disguise and conveys a generally derogatory view of Viet Nam veterans with PTSD. This derogatory view is not supported by most clinicians who have diagnosed and treated veterans. Rather, they have found that PTSD affects veterans with all kinds of combat performance impartially—including a great many with medals for heroism, distinguished military careers, and overall outstanding performance.

CONCLUSION

This chapter has cataloged irrational reactions on the part of clinicians and researchers to veterans of the Viet Nam War and the concept of PTSD, reactions which have impaired treatment and research. Although such reactions will continue to occur, they can be anticipated and ameliorated by both patients and therapists, particularly when cast in an objective light. This chapter has considered the topic on the phenomenological level, as a first step in a study of irrational, nonobjective manifestations specific to this group of patients. Two further steps which can be hoped for in future study are a clarification of the feelings and impulses underlying these phenomena and a consideration of the role played by the patients and their specific difficulties in evoking the reactions identified.

REFERENCES

1. Hersh SM: My Lai Four: A Report on the Massacre and Its Aftermath. New York, Random House, 1970

2. Van Putten T, Jager J: Post-traumatic stress disorder. Arch Gen Psychiatry 41:411–413, 1984

3. Shakespeare W: Henry IV, Part I, in The Yale Shakespeare. New Haven, Conn, Yale University Press, 1954

4. Louis Harris and Associates: A Study of Attitudes Towards Viet Nam Era Veterans. Washington, DC, Louis Harris & Associates, 1980

5. Egendorf A, Kadushin C, Laufer R, et al: Legacies of Viet Nam. Washington, DC, U.S. Government Printing Office, 1981

6. Downs F: The Killing Zone: My Life in the Viet Nam War. New York, W.W. Norton & Co, 1978

7. Haley S: Treatment implications of post-combat stress response syndromes for mental health professionals, in Stress Disorders Among Viet Nam Veterans. Edited by Figley CR. New York, Brunner/Mazel, 1978

8. Evaluation Report: Viet Nam Veterans' Counseling Service Part I (mimeo). Sydney, Department of Veterans' Affairs, January 13, 1984

9. Abraham K, Freud S, Ferenczi S, et al: Psychoanalysis and the War Neurosis. London, International Psychoanalytic Press, 1922

10. Kardiner A: The Traumatic Neuroses of War. New York, National Research Council, 1941

11. Archibald HE, Tuddenham RD: Persistent stress reaction following combat: a twenty year follow-up. Arch Gen Psychiatry 12:475–481, 1965

12. Horowitz MJ: Stress Response Syndrome. New York, Jason Aronson, 1976

13. American Psychiatric Association: Diagnostic and Statistical Manual of Mental Disorders, Third Edition. Washington, DC, American Psychiatric Association, 1980

14. Atkinson RM, Henderson RG, Sparr LF, et al: Assessment of Viet Nam veterans for post-traumatic stress disorder in veterans disability claims. Am J Psychiatry 129:1118–1121, 1982

15. Atkinson RM, Sparr LF, Sheff A, et al: Diagnosis of post-traumatic stress disorder in Viet Nam veterans: preliminary findings. Paper presented at the Annual Meeting of the American Psychiatric Association, New York, 1983

16. Erlinder P: Paying the price for Viet Nam: post-traumatic stress disorder and criminal behavior. Boston College Law Review 25:305–347, 1984

17. Goodwin J: The etiology of combat-related post-traumatic stress disorders, in Post-Traumatic Stress Disorders of the Viet Nam Veteran. Edited by Williams T. Cincinnati, Disabled American Veterans, 1980

18. Ginsberg E, Herma J, Ginsberg S: Psychiatry and Military Manpower Policy. New York, Columbia University Press, 1953

19. Frye S: Discriminant analysis of post-traumatic stress disorder among a group of Viet Nam veterans. Am J Psychiatry 139:51–56, 1982

20. Card J: Lives After Viet Nam. Lexington, Mass, Lexington Books, 1983

21. Sierles F, Chen J, McFarland R, et al: Post-traumatic stress disorder and concurrent psychiatric illness: a preliminary report. Am J Psychiatry 140:1177–1179, 1983

22. Behar D (letter): Confirmation of concurrent illness in post traumatic stress disorder. Am J Psychiatry 141:1310, 1984

23. Silver SM, Iacona CU: Factor analytic support for *DSM-III*'s post-traumatic stress disorder for Viet Nam veterans. J Clin Psychol 40:5–14, 1984

24. Escobar J, Randolph E, Puente G, et al: Post-traumatic stress disorder in Hispanic Viet Nam veterans. J Nerv Ment Dis 171:585–596, 1983

25. Haley S: When the patient reports atrocities. Arch Gen Psychiatry 30:191–196, 1974

26. Haley S: Countertransference toward the Viet Nam veteran. Paper presented at the Annual Meeting of the American Psychiatric Association, Chicago, 1979

27. Lifton RJ: Home From the War. New York, Simon & Schuster, 1973

28. Margolin Y: What I don't know can't hurt me: therapist reactions to Viet Nam veterans. Paper presented at the Annual Meeting of the America Psychological Association, Toronto, 1984

29. Fuentes R: Therapist transparency, in Post-Traumatic Stress Disorders of the Viet Nam Veteran. Edited by Williams T. Cincinnati, Disabled American Veterans, 1980

30. Smith JR: A review of 125 years of the psychological literature on reaction to combat, from the Civil War through the Viet Nam War (mimeo). Brecksville, Ohio, V.A. Medical Center, 1981

31. Hendin H, Haas A: Combat adaptation of Viet Nam veterans without post-traumatic stress disorder. Am J Psychiatry 141:956–959, 1984

6

Diagnosis of Post-Traumatic Stress Disorder in Viet Nam Veterans

Arthur L. Arnold, M.D.

6

The diagnosis of post-traumatic stress disorder in Viet Nam combat veterans should be simple, but in many instances it is both problematic and controversial. When the process of diagnosing PTSD is based upon clinical information alone, taking into consideration the developmental history, history of precipitating events, subsequent clinical course, and current status, it is straightforward. Indeed, this is a condition in which patients present with so many common factors that astute clinicians consider the presentation "stereotyped." Still, this condition is often not recognized (1–11).

To make any diagnosis, the physician must be ready, willing, and able to do so. Diagnostic ability depends mainly upon having the necessary information and recognizing patterns. Readiness requires a sufficient level of awareness to recognize patterns or clusters of information without groping. But the physician's *willingness* may be more of an issue in diagnosing PTSD than for other conditions. The problems in diagnosing schizophrenia or major affective disorders are usually substantive (12–14) rather than based upon doubts about the credibility of patients' histories of hallucinations, delusions, or depressed mood, and the rejection of a diagnosis for an individual is unlikely to be based upon rejection of the validity of the diagnostic concept itself.

While it is important to recognize that unwillingness to diagnose PTSD in Viet Nam veterans may contribute to the difficulty in doing so, the diagnostic guidelines which follow will address only the substantive issues: 1) the information that is needed, 2) methods of obtaining and organizing this information, and 3) differential diagnosis.

INFORMATION NEEDED

Specific information is needed to make the diagnosis of PTSD, and the inclusion criteria in the *Diagnostic and Statistical Manual of Mental*

Table 1.   Diagnostic Criteria for Post-Traumatic Stress Disorder

A. **STRESSORS** specifically identified and sufficiently severe to cause significant symptoms of reexperience and avoidance in almost anyone.

B. **REEXPERIENCE** of the stressor in at least one of the following modes:
   1. Recurrent and intrusive recollections of the stressor.
   2. Recurrent dreams of the stressor.
   3. Sudden acting or feeling as if the stressor were reoccurring.

C. **AVOIDANCE** phenomena by which there is reduced responsiveness or involvement with the external world in at least one of the following modes:
   1. Markedly diminished interest in significant activities.
   2. Feeling detached or estranged from others.
   3. Reduced capacity for feeling or expressing emotions.

D. **ASSOCIATED SYMPTOMS** including at least two of the following:
   1. Hyperalertness or exaggerated startle reaction.
   2. Sleep disturbance.
   3. Intensification of symptoms by exposure to reminders of the stressor.
   4. Guilt about surviving when others have not, or about behavior necessary to survive the stressor.
   5. Memory impairment or trouble concentrating.
   6. Avoidance of activities which are reminders of the stressor.

E. **SUBTYPES**
   1. Acute: Onset within six months of the stressor and of less than six months' duration.
   2. Chronic: Duration longer than six months.
   3. Delayed: Onset more than six months after the stressor.

Disorders, Third Edition (15), are a clearly stated description of that information (Table 1). Some clinicians who are fully aware of these criteria, however, report the mental status examination as within normal limits and do not diagnose PTSD even in individuals who have the disorder in severe form. Just as it is unlikely that a physical examination without a blood pressure determination and visualization of the fundi will support a diagnosis of hypertension, the signs and symptoms of PTSD must be sought for proper diagnosis, since they are often not readily apparent (1, 6, 15).

Cardinal Diagnostic Features

The three cardinal features of the diagnosis are: *history of trauma, reexperiencing of trauma,* and *avoidance phenomena.*

History of Trauma. The trauma, to support the diagnosis of PTSD, must have certain quantitative and qualitative characteristics referred to in *DSM-III*; that is, as it is of a sort which "would evoke symptoms of distress in almost anyone." The usual life stress events, such as death of a spouse, loss of a job, or accidents which have been linked to a wide range of morbidity, pale in comparison to the traumatic experiences which precede PTSD. We must take into account experiences which are grossly at variance and incongruous with one's previously established self-concepts, values, world concepts, and basic mental schema for being in the world (16). These traumatic experiences also have a shocking and unexpected quality, an unendurably prolonged quality, or both (3, 17, 18).

Reexperiencing of Trauma. Reexperiencing of trauma occurs in various states of consciousness, with varying degrees of intensity, and may have misleading diagnostic implications. This phenomenon is usually repetitive, is not voluntarily controllable, is emotionally painful, and either exactly or closely reproduces actual traumatic experiences in whole or in part. Conscious recall of trauma varies. If the trauma is one which would be overwhelming were it not for an almost immediate blocking of affect and realization, the perception of it will later return to awareness in some form. From one point of view these are "intrusive" or dreaded phenomena, forcing themselves back into attention unbidden. They may be stimulated by similar current events, on the basis of symbolic association or conditioning, or break through in unguarded moments. From another point of view these phenomena are compulsively repeated in order to complete the full experience from helplessness to mastery (16, 19). However they are conceptualized, reexperiences are pathognomonic of PTSD.

The most common form of reexperience is a sudden vivid memory which takes over full attention and is accompanied by the emotions which occurred during the original experience. When there are also visual reperceptions of the trauma, patients usually refer to them as "flashbacks."

Another very common form of reexperience is in dreams. The usual history is of wakening from a dream which reenacts the trauma, evoking strong emotions which would have been appropriate reactions to the traumatic experience itself—usually rage, terror, or grief. Others report wakening in terror without recalling the dream itself, sometimes in the act of committing violence on someone else in the bed. Both nightmares and incubus (night terrors) may be found in the same person. Observers may report shouting, screaming, and violent thrashing about which occurred during the dream. When reexperiences in dreams are intense, there is frequently a history of insomnia as well, which develops in an attempt to avoid the dreaded dreams (3, 4, 16, 19–22).

Less often reported or clearly diagnosed is reexperiencing in a dissociative state. Patients are reluctant to acknowledge such events for fear they will sound "crazy." The history given is usually of "coming to" with a memory of having been again engaged in a war experience, such as going out on patrol or driving on a road in the jungle. These dissociative episodes may last up to several hours. When they occur at night they may be difficult to differentiate from somnambulism, which is unrelated to PTSD, except for the possible recall of repetitive trauma-related mental content. These episodes are not without risk; serious injuries have occurred when veterans have prowled about backyards and alleys at night fully armed, reexperiencing a patrol in hostile territory.

At times, the reexperiencing consists of sudden "pangs" of emotion which are not accompanied by specific experiential representations either as memories or dreams. Usually the feelings are ones which bring tears and a tight throat, but they may be of fear or anger. It may be difficult to differentiate these from panic attacks or outbursts of rage which occur as overreactions or psychophysiological conditioning, but as can be confirmed when the patient reports that they are repetitive and consistent with memories and reexperiencing dreams, they are identifiable as isolated reexperiencing of affect. In some instances these are the primary reexperiences for diagnostic consideration and may be missed even by skilled clinicians since their description is extremely subtle. They may be termed "affect flashbacks" and suspected when a combat veteran refers to uncontrollable feelings.

Avoidance Phenomena. Avoidance phenomena, the third cardinal feature of PTSD, may also be subtle and easily missed. Objectively, these may appear as a remoteness of attitude, as though the patient is preoccupied, bored, or disinclined to interaction with others. Spouses and family members may consider the behavior "cold," mechanical, and lacking in affection, and they often feel rebuffed. In some veterans, the outward appearance may be of a "dropped-out" life-style or, conversely, of a dedicated workaholic. Subjectively, the patient describes an inability to feel emotion, especially toward those who are closest, or an inability to express emotions which are felt.

Other veterans express difficulty concentrating or remembering current information. These cognitive difficulties are clearly more than ennui or lassitude; they represent distressful impairments of the capacity to appreciate the essential qualities of experience. If PTSD results from trauma which overwhelms coping mechanisms and is manifested particularly by reexperiencing of the trauma, then avoidance phenomena including cognitive impairments are understandable as defenses against intolerable affective responses to the trauma.

We identify avoidance phenomena in two phases. During or immediately after a traumatic experience, a period of "numbing" occurs, in which there is diminished feeling, diminished awareness of experience, and diminished capacity for other than mechanical activity (4, 16). Later, after reexperiencing begins (hours, months, or years later), avoidance alternates with reexperiencing, apparently with a frequency and to a degree which allows the reexperiencing to be tolerated (16).

Some behaviors commonly labeled as the idiosyncracies of Viet Nam veterans probably serve an avoidance purpose and are useful in diagnosis of PTSD:

• Carrying loaded weapons or sleeping with them,
• Living in unpopulated places,
• Facing outward from a corner or wall whenever surrounded by other people,
• Drinking alcohol or using other drugs before going to sleep,
• Either throwing away uniforms and medals or wearing them regularly in civilian settings, and
• Refusing to use plastic trash bags.

Many combat veterans are always on guard and overreact when a combat-related stimulus breaks through the perimeter, so to speak. Such stimuli include the sound of an automobile backfire, fireworks, or helicopters overhead.

Affective Stress Response

But more than specific information regarding the trauma itself, reexperiencing, and avoidance behavior is needed to diagnose PTSD in Viet Nam veterans. If the diagnostic process is to initiate and facilitate successful treatment, an understanding of feelings and behavior must begin at the same time. Otherwise, a "DSM-III checklist approach" will provoke antagonism. A key to understanding lies in discovering the underlying affective stress response of the veteran. The traumatic experiences, according to their meaning for the individual veteran, set up an affective response which is usually of grief, guilt, or terror. As long as the impact of the trauma is unresolved and its significance is not integrated into the whole being of the veteran, the affective response to the stress is incompletely discharged and continues to control behavior, outside of awareness.

Significance of Associated Features

For this reason the "associated features" of PTSD should be explored beyond their superficial presentation. Depression in PTSD, for example, may be a manifestation of grief (23). Inability to mourn and work through losses of buddies, especially, may appear as continuous sadness, inability to enjoy, or vengeful rage. In addition, the grief may have an existential quality, stemming from the loss of precombat innocence and trust.

Just as frequently the depression of PTSD in Viet Nam veterans is an expression of guilt. Witnessing or participating in what would be considered atrocities according to that individual's precombat values, even despite misgivings at that time, are regularly associated with guilt and depressed mood (3, 19). Such is more severe in those veterans who, perhaps through reaction formation, came to enjoy such activities, and in those whose childhood values training had punitive themes. Similarly, while anxiety or panic attacks are not uncommon, for diagnostic purposes it is important to determine whether there was either an extreme or sustained fear of death during certain traumatic war experiences, which was unresolved and perpetuated by conditioning or reexperiences.

The irritability and explosiveness seen in many veterans having other manifestations of PTSD also should be explored for specific factors which may be trauma-related. For example, resentment of exploitive authority or intolerance for the helplessness of waiting may have occurred in combat settings and again in current life situations.

Impulsive life changes and geographic moves may also be avoidance phenomena, and thus these are important to a diagnostic understanding of PTSD. This is particularly so if they are trauma-related, such as repeated avoidance of responsibility for others by those who are reexperiencing combat deaths of subordinates and feel unresolved guilt. Part of the practical value in exploring the affective stress responses which underlie "associated features" of PTSD is in the need to include in the diagnostic process an assessment of the risk for suicide or attacks upon others.

OBTAINING NECESSARY INFORMATION

The process of obtaining the information required to diagnose PTSD is often more difficult than knowing what information is needed. A veteran who immediately launches into a detailed description of combat experiences and subsequent symptoms, with histrionic overtones, may be less likely to suffer from PTSD than one who presents with vague concern to "get my head together," with fear of losing control and "blowing someone away," or who is brought in by others in a suicidal or assaultive crisis without verbalized insight. The clinician must be aware, however, that veterans who label their syndrome and pointedly mention nightmares and flashbacks may have been unable to account for years of painful, counterproductive postwar experiences. Sudden realization of the characteristics of PTSD may have come from the media or a counseling center with a sense of relief that what had seemed to be a unique personal disaster is a named entity.

Obstacles to Communication

The manner in which the diagnostic interview is performed may facilitate or block the diagnosis of PTSD. An open and receptive, nonjudgmental attitude is essential. Preconceived negative opinions, closed-ended questions, a bored or mechanical attitude, or obvious skepticism virtually ensure that critical information will not be given by the veteran. Clinicians' expressions of shock have the same effect, since veterans then may react either by withdrawal or intimidation (24). The clinician's willingness to make the diagnosis of PTSD is the major factor in overcoming these obstacles.

Fearfulness is also an impediment. Patients who are unsure of their control over hostile and aggressive impulses and aware of their killing capabilities will have an increased likelihood of reexperiencing and a need for avoidance during the interview. Clinicians generally discover that concerned, inoffensive, and skilled professionals are usually not the target of attacks by Viet Nam veterans, even though occasionally an office wall is punched. Having someone else present or an arrangement for summoning calm assistance may provide enough comfort to allow giving the difficult task of the clinical interview full attention.

Time pressure is another impediment. If it is expected at the outset that the patient may have PTSD related to combat trauma, it is well to allow at least an hour without outside interruptions for the interview. If in the course of an examination the likelihood of PTSD unexpectedly arises and time is running short, it may be preferable to set up a second session to explore this, without giving the impression of dodging the issue.

There is another reason to allow adequate time. To develop the linkage between traumatic experience and later reexperiencing and avoidance, a sequence of associations must be allowed to occur without interruption. This is not unlike the development of a theme in literature or music. Although additional information later will augment the theme (and even change it drastically on occasion), diagnosis and the deeper understanding needed to start treatment are best accomplished in one session, within which positive rapport is also established.

Conduct of the Diagnostic Interview

Ideally, the major diagnostic interview should be conducted by the clinician who will have primary responsibility for treatment. Examinations for the sole purpose of making decisions about admission or referral or interviews to obtain social histories are not appropriate occasions for the diagnostic process described here. Most of these guidelines do apply to examinations to determine diagnosis for disability determination, however (25).

Identification of Risks

The veteran may present after recent suicidal or violent behavior. The detailed history should include evaluation of the following:

- Premeditation,
- Impulsiveness,
- Specific stimuli or provocations,
- Any injuries inflicted,
- How intervention occurred and degree of cooperation with accepting help,
- Prior history of similar episodes, and
- Whether the veteran keeps weapons, and if so what kind, whether they are carried about or stored, how often they are used and in what way.

Protection of Privacy

The guilt, suspicion, and even fear of punishment which many Viet Nam veterans feel require the assurance of privacy during the crucial initial diagnostic interview. This also frees spontaneous expression of emotion, since during the recall of traumatic experiences most veterans will become tearful, some sobbing for an extended period of time. The clinician's calm acceptance of the naturalness of this expression may be undone by the veteran's embarrassment if the interview is attended or observed by too many others, as in supervisory demonstrations or case presentations (26).

The uncovering of traumatic memories and focus upon current pain is usually accompanied by an outpouring of appropriate emotion, especially if the veteran has rarely opened up in this way, but calmly expressed support may be needed for the veteran to be able to tell of his combat experiences. "Over-talking" the veteran and interfering with expression is less likely to occur if the clinician is not too uncomfortable with the veteran's anguish or rage and with the clinician's own emotional reactions to what is heard (24).

The Primary Purpose of the Diagnostic Interview

The critical purpose of the diagnostic interview is to identify and establish the relationship between the content of original traumatic experience and subsequent reexperiencing phenomena. Everything else which is done serves supplementary purposes, such as facilitating individualized treatment, establishing credibility, and aiding differential and comprehensive diagnosis. One might begin, then, by addressing either current history or military history. Particularly in the case of veterans in crisis or concerned about current pain, the responsive therapist will begin with current life experiences. This readily identifies impairments in living which are the consequences of avoidance phenomena and disruptions in close relationships and employment.

Content of Reexperiences

One should be alert for spontaneous references to reexperiencing and, with care and consideration for feelings, pursue the content of dreams, flashbacks, or memories, especially if they are repetitive. This leads naturally to a focus upon the actual combat experiences which are repeated in the reexperiences (27). The interview can then shift back and forth among the following:

- Combat experiences which were traumatic,
- The meaning they held for the veteran,
- The immediate reaction to them,
- The reexperiences and stimuli or associations immediately preceding them,
- The affects associated with reexperiencing,
- Symptoms and behavior which manifest the affective stress responses,
- Reaction formation to affects and behavior, and
- Avoidance phenomena.

Alternating attention between "What happened then?" and "How is it affecting you now?" readily identifies the trauma and the response if the interviewer is attentive and genuinely interested. It is important to be cognizant of depression and suicidal impulses or actions, anxiety or panic, behavior which is explosive or impulsive, excessive irritability, chronic pain including headache and backache, sleep disturbances, and difficulties in concentration.

Military History

In addition to the specific traumatic experiences of combat, it is essential to obtain a comprehensive military history (28) (also see Chapter 13). This should include as a minimum:

- Family military traditions and attitudes,
- Motivations for and date and type of entrance into the service,
- Choice and significance of the branch of service,
- Training experiences,
- Military occupations specialty (MOS) acquired,
- Specialized training in guerilla or jungle warfare,
- Sequence of geographical assignments and how they were made,
- Manner of transportation to Southeast Asia or Viet Nam,
- Experiences on arrival and assignment to a unit,
- Reception by more experienced members of the unit,
- Developing relationships with buddies,
- Acquiring a nickname or reputation,
- Interactions with and attitudes toward noncommissioned and commissioned officers,
- Sequence of geographical movements and combat engagements in Viet Nam,
- Availability of sleep in the field,
- Numbers of casualties sustained by the unit and relationships with those wounded or killed,
- Killing of others (including proximity, methods, initial and later feelings, military necessity, actions in "free-fire zones" [29, 30], degree of control, whether aged, women, children, civilian, or otherwise),
- Witnessing of mutilation or torture of Americans,
- Witnessing or participation in mutilation or torture of Vietnamese,
- Being wounded,
- Providing or receiving rescues and medical evacuations,
- Experiences as combat tour was concluded,
- Whether more than one tour was served (this is very important; more than one tour in combat is highly correlated with PTSD),
- Manner of transportation back to the United States,

- Reception by public, family, and friends, and
- Date, manner, and type of discharge.

It usually must be asked specifically whether the veteran was assigned to performance of covert operations and whether or not this was in a unit so designated. Veterans often have a personal reluctance to describe these experiences, sometimes ascribed to having received official directives not to reveal them. Particularly in regard to covert operations, it is important to deal with both the official and personal rationale and the veteran's mixture of feelings prior to, during, and after active participation in such missions.

All veterans should be asked about decorations, special citations, and commendations. It is important that we in clinical settings recognize their courageous actions in combat to establish early one of the most substantial reasons for pride.

Veterans may avoid a detailed recounting of combat experiences because the clinician "wouldn't understand," perhaps being concerned about a judgmental attitude which would not be expected in a fellow combat veteran. Just as it is important not to have a moralizing attitude, it is well to realize that unfamiliarity with weapons and combat procedures may be an asset in allowing one to ask "simple" questions.

In addition to the details of the military history, it is important to learn about the veteran's life-style in Viet Nam, including the daily pattern of activities. The impact of traumatic experiences can be better appreciated by learning:

- Whether the veteran spent most of the time in a relatively secure base with only occasional patrols,
- Whether long periods of time were spent in the field in isolated positions,
- Whether there was any substance abuse and, if so, its pattern,
- Whether there was ready access to passes to cities,
- Whether there was continuous responsibility for the safety of others,
- Whether the primary role was at least nominally noncombatant (as for field medics and hospital or administrative support staff), and
- About any close association with villagers or South Vietnamese combat units (31).

Premilitary History

Not only should there be a detailed exploration of the veteran's postdischarge civilian life-style in regard to closeness of relationships, work history, values, and personal identity, but the pattern of living in childhood and adolescence must be understood in the same parameters. This may be a sensitive issue, implying for some patients that their current problems derive from early childhood developmental issues and not at all from combat experiences. If the clinician refrains from approaching this as an "either-or" issue, better cooperation and more complete information can be expected. It is important to review the following:

- The nature of significant relationships with family members and peers,
- The major influences in developing values and the way these were imparted and received,
- The role of positive and negative reinforcement in values development,
- School achievement and behavior,
- Employment and the development of work attitudes and patterns of behavior,
- Familiarity with firearms,
- Adolescent identity and ambitions, and
- Capacity for empathy and intimacy.

Any antisocial behavior should be identified in terms of persistence and seriousness, including especially fights and substance abuse (32, 33). Finally, the attitudes of various family members and peers toward the war in Viet Nam and the veteran's entry into the service and participation in the war should be learned.

Post-Combat History

A sequential review of the veteran's post–Viet Nam life will bring together many elements otherwise appearing to be isolated symptoms. This should cover both immediate experiences upon return to the United States in confronting the public and family and the subsequent life course. The degree of success at establishing close relationships and marriage, any episodes of violence toward the spouse or partner, including associated reexperiencing of Viet Nam events, outbursts of rage in response to the ordinary irritating stresses in any relationship, and unusual reactions to babies and children, should all be given particular attention.

Success or the lack of it in pursuing an education and establishing steady career development may indicate how reexperiencing and avoidance have adversely affected behavior. One should explore the reasons for terminating schooling or employment, especially. Exploring the capacity for satisfying hobbies and leisure activities may indicate grim or constricted feelings and behavior, and specific avoidances may be revealing, such as no longer going hunting, or compulsively organizing hunting trips, almost as though they were search and destroy missions.

Religious practices and beliefs, especially when compared with those during prewar years, may give insight into the patient's capacity for trust or sense of guilt. A clear picture of the patient's self-perception and identity should be developed as well as an understanding of how the world is perceived. It is important to recognize a pervasive sense of betrayal and feelings of bitterness, fearfulness of a hostile and threatening world, or disengagement from an environment with which there is no sense of connectedness (16, 33).

History of Previous Treatment

The history of previous psychiatric treatment should be reviewed; although it may be misleading for diagnostic purposes, it cannot be ignored. The veteran's own recall of the reasons for any prior treatment is often more helpful than the recall of diagnosis or treatment. If records of previous treatment are available, the narrative admission and progress notes describing patient behavior, especially those by nursing staff; quotations of the patient's statements; reports of psychological testing; and social histories are often most valuable as aids in diagnosis. One should be particularly careful to avoid being influenced by recorded diagnoses which are not fully supported by documented clinical findings and not consistent with the material noted above.

Psychological and Laboratory Tests

Psychological testing has not contributed unequivocally to the diagnosis of PTSD. A full-scale MMPI profile with significantly elevated F, 2, and 8 scales has been reported to be characteristic of combat veterans with PTSD (33–37). A 49-item subscale has also been developed, with 82 to 90 percent congruence (depending upon the cutoff level) with PTSD diagnosed by structured interviews and histories (38). Projective testing has not elicited pathognomonic features, but the content of responses often has a readily apparent resemblance to combat reexperiences of the individual. Sleep laboratories have not identified data reliable in diagnosis, although investigations of possible relationships between both REM sleep and stage 3 and 4 sleep and nightmares, incubus (night terrors), and insomnia in PTSD have produced intriguing preliminary findings. Nor have clinical laboratory findings so far been of diagnostic assistance. Dexamethasone suppression tests were normal for all patients with clinically confirmed diagnosis of PTSD admitted to a specialized unit under the supervision of this author, regardless of the severity of depressed mood present. Nevertheless, it is important to develop a multimethod diagnostic evaluation including physiological measures (39).

A number of self-administered questionnaires have been developed to aid in the diagnosis of PTSD, specifically in Viet Nam veterans (40). For the most part, the items address killing or being in danger of being killed in combat and subsequent feelings and behaviors which are manifestations of reexperiences, avoidance, or associated features of PTSD. While these instruments may be useful in screening populations at risk—for example, Viet Nam era veterans applying for any form of health care or counseling—the findings by themselves cannot be relied upon to establish a diagnosis. They would, however, justify more comprehensive diagnostic attention or statistical analysis for prevalence of PTSD.

Induced Revelations

The role of narcoanalysis or hypnosis in diagnosis merits comment. These techniques facilitate reexperiencing but are rarely necessary for diagnostic purposes alone. On occasion, when avoidance is fixed and relatively constant, and the veteran feels the need for help in overcoming resistance, these methods may be useful. Avoidance in the form of repression or suppression usually promptly returns, however, and a reinforcement of the sense of an external locus of control inherent in the original traumatic experience may occur, with countertherapeutic consequences. To some extent this is limited by videotaping the session and replaying this to the veteran while awake, until the content can be reexperienced at will. Presumably, PTSD research applications of narcoanalysis or hypnosis take place after diagnosis is established during interviews in which veterans are fully conscious (41).

DIFFERENTIAL DIAGNOSIS

The issues of multiple diagnoses and differential diagnosis should routinely be addressed (42). To be sufficiently complete to justify a diagnosis of PTSD, the examination should also justify the diagnosis of any concomitant mental disorders and rule out others. The multiple axes of *DSM-III* form a conceptual framework which, among competent clinicians, should eliminate the "either-or" debates which the diagnostic consideration of PTSD often provokes. Several Axis I and II disorders come up frequently in this regard and deserve special mention.

Antisocial Personality

Antisocial personality disorder is, not surprisingly, the principal diagnosis often made for Viet Nam veterans who have had multiple marriages or otherwise have had many unstable relationships, who have repeatedly changed jobs or had long periods of unemployment, who have abused alcohol and other drugs, who have been arrested (especially if for dangerous behavior), who have been persistently irritable or explosive, or who have had a nomadic life style. A history, not uncommonly found associated with PTSD, of inconsistent employment, unenduring attachments to sexual partners, repeated fights, and travel which is not planned and goal directed, all since the age of 18, might in fact support an Axis II diagnosis of antisocial personality disorder *if* it is part of a pattern established before the age of 15.

Personality disorders by definition begin in childhood or adolescence and are characteristic of most of adult life (43). Accordingly, it is essential to obtain a history of the degree of responsibility exercised in personal relationships, school, and work; control of aggression; and use of intoxicants in childhood, adolescence, and during active military service before making a diagnosis of antisocial personality disorder, whether in addition to or instead of PTSD. This effort is more likely to be made if the examination reveals reexperiencing of previous trauma typical of PTSD. Depression, a recognition of others' hostility, and impaired capacity for sustained intimacy are commonly associated with both PTSD and antisocial personality disorder. If the history is one of responsible behavior in childhood, adolescence, and military life, with concern for others, it is necessary to attribute the antisocial behavior in adulthood to a condition other than a personality disorder.

Borderline Personality Disorder

Borderline personality disorder is more apt to be considered for veterans already diagnosed as having PTSD, who have received treatment. When, following abreactive sessions, a patient with PTSD demonstrates a persistence of suicide attempts and self-injuring fights, substance abuse, manipulation and devaluation of professional staff, uncontrolled anger, and rapid shifts in mood between depression and anxiety, the overt behavior may be almost indistinguishable from that displayed in borderline personality disorder. This is particularly true when the veteran manifests splitting of the staff between "good guys" who care about Viet Nam veterans and "bad guys" who don't, and splitting of the self between "trained killer" and one who abhors any more killing.

The "bad" identity of the Viet Nam veteran with PTSD deserves more than superficial attention. In many instances this appears to be a reaction formation to the affective stress response of guilt for killings in Viet Nam that would be considered atrocities in a civilian setting, substituting a less painful but also less adaptive position. Here again, the question of a personality disorder necessitates the childhood, adolescent, and military histories for clarification of premorbid personality organization.

A plausible case may be made for arrest at or regression to adolescent personality development (44) to account for a current clinical picture more or less consistent with borderline personality disorder. Those who work regularly with Viet Nam veterans having PTSD see in the phenomena of recreational flirting, ambivalence toward authority, demands for independence alternating with demands for total support, romanticizing of male daring, and affectations of eccentric appearance an adolescent quality which is both frustrating and endearing. Usually they also see, however, a dysphoric staring (facial expression) which is inconsistent with an untraumatized adolescence.

In borderline personality disorder a frequent finding is an inability to tolerate being alone, with a dependence upon feedback from others to define and even verify the patient's existence. This interplay appears to have a personality development function in adolescence, but with a less compulsive, desperate quality. This is a useful differentiating feature, since in PTSD there is frequently an intolerance for interaction with others, and it is not uncommon to find that the veteran has retreated to a remote area, remains housebound, or stays confined to a room either alone or ignoring others for long periods of time. However, PTSD occurs without this degree of withdrawal, and the full clinical picture of both conditions should be considered in order to make separate diagnostic decisions regarding the presence of borderline personality disorder and PTSD, whether considered singly or in combination.

Affective Disorders

A depressed mood is so frequently seen by clinicians that it has been considered a sine qua non of PTSD by some researchers, although it is not among the *DSM-III* diagnostic criteria. It is uncommon for a major depressive episode to be diagnosed in the presence of the cardinal features of PTSD, even though many of the *DSM-III* diagnostic criteria are met (45, 46). The dysphoric mood of PTSD can usually be related to persistent affective stress responses of guilt, grief, or both, with which the content of reexperiences are consistent. It is difficult to distinguish the constricted affect of PTSD from the anhedonia in depression, but mood shifts between anger, anxiety, and depression are common in PTSD and thus a distinguishing feature. Six of the eight symptoms which make up the full affective syndrome are common findings in PTSD:

- Insomnia,
- Psychomotor agitation,
- Loss of interest in usual activities,
- Self-reproach,
- Diminished ability to concentrate, and
- Suicidal ideation or attempts.

Since these symptoms may be associated with traumatic reexperiencing or may be manifestations of avoidance phenomena, it could be difficult to determine whether both diagnoses should be made. Because of the treatment implications, it is preferable to assume provisionally that PTSD, if present, accounts for the depressive syndrome. If clinical validation studies of PTSD are reported, *DSM-III* should be revised to indicate that if PTSD is present before the onset or after the remission of the affective syndrome, the diagnosis of a major depressive episode is excluded.

Manic episodes are a different matter. There should be little difficulty differentiating these from PTSD, and usually the issue is whether to make both diagnoses independently, based on the clinical picture and diagnostic criteria. When the cardinal features of PTSD are also present, the manic patient is less apt to have an elevated mood and expansive good humor than an extremely irritable mood with suspicion and single-minded pursuit of a cause.

Alcoholism

Alcohol abuse or alcohol dependence presents few problems in differential diagnosis with PTSD, but they are of practical concern because of their treatment implications. While veterans with PTSD frequently report the use of alcohol as a "self-medication" to control anxiety or insomnia or see it as comforting during dysphoria, there is not necessarily any clear relationship between alcoholism and an affective stress response (47).

There is, of course, a reduced control of violent impulses while intoxicated, and some patients with PTSD who seek opportunities for violent acting out to avoid feelings of guilt, grief, and helplessness find barroom fights irresistible. Alcoholism rehabilitation programs which concentrate upon "primary alcoholism" may refuse to accept Viet Nam veterans with PTSD and the veterans themselves may refuse the requirement that they identify themselves as alcoholics. While when the principal diagnosis is alcohol abuse or dependence, this may reflect the main reason for evaluation or admission, if PTSD is also diagnosed during that episode of care, it may be the condition most requiring treatment to ameliorate pain and lessen disability.

Schizophrenia

A number of Viet Nam veterans acquired a diagnosis of schizophrenia, usually paranoid type, in clinical encounters prior to publication of *DSM-III*, with its clearer set of diagnostic criteria for both PTSD and schizophrenic disorders. Often it is difficult to locate documented findings in those medical records which would support the diagnosis. If diagnostic criteria for schizophrenic disorders are applied carefully, the absence of a formal thought disorder in form or content is useful in ruling out this condition. It is in the areas of perception, affect, and relatedness that the clinical picture may be unclear.

Flashbacks in which there is a vivid visual and sometimes auditory reexperiencing of prior traumatic events may indeed appear to an observer to be hallucinations of the type seen in psychoses. *The degree to which the content reproduces prior experience is the distinguishing factor;* no diagnosis of schizophrenic disorders should be made without detailed exploration of the content of hallucinations. A constricted affect, in which both perception and expression of emotion are avoided, may closely resemble the flattened affect found in schizophrenia. Patients with schizophrenia, however, seem rarely to appreciate the nature of their affective incongruity, while patients with PTSD often agonize over their inability to have the tender feelings they did in their prewar years. At other times it is obvious that those with PTSD feel and express rage quite readily. Likewise, the withdrawal from the world exhibited by patients with schizophrenia appears to be a consequence of an idiosyncratic inner-directedness, distinguishable from the disinterest in usual activities seen in PTSD. Furthermore, the psychotic-like episodes which are accompanied by turmoil and distress in some patients with PTSD are usually of short duration, and it is schizophreniform disorder which one should consider in the differential diagnosis. Certainly suspiciousness and hostility alone as seen in Viet Nam veterans are not sufficient to justify a diagnosis of schizophrenic disorder, paranoid type.

It should be clearly understood that schizophreniform and schizophrenic disorders do occur concomitantly with PTSD, and the diagnoses are made on their own merits. For example, both hallucinations and delusions of a religious nature and flashbacks of combat experiences accompanied by guilt feelings, when they occur interspersed in the same individual, prompt an evaluation for multiple diagnoses in Axis I. Ordinarily, the reexperiences of PTSD are the more persistent, and the thought disorder of schizophrenia the more episodic phenomenon over time.

Adjustment Disorders

Adjustment disorder with depressed mood is the diagnosis apt to be made when full details of stressors have not been obtained from Viet Nam veterans but clinicians recognize that there is some maladaptation following war experience. The critical issues for differentiation from PTSD are severity of stressors and temporal relationship to stressors. An adjustment disorder is an overreaction with an onset within three months of the stress experience, which impairs personal relationships or ability to work, and which improves whether or not the stress continues. Also, the nature of the stressful event is not "outside the range of usual human experience" (43, 48). When an individual clinician is told of specific combat experiences that return to awareness repeatedly and are accompanied by distress, despite efforts to avoid this, if this clinician concludes that the stressors are merely what anyone should expect in a soldier role, he or she should seek consensus with colleagues as to the stressors' severity. The clinician might ask their opinion of the stressors had they undergone such experiences themselves.

Naive assumptions about the severity of stress probably play a major role in the difficulties in recognizing PTSD in women and other noncombatants who served in Southeast Asia during the Viet Nam War. The danger and anguish of nurses in field hospitals are clearly comparable to those of combat medics (49). Similarly, prolonged duty in assignments such as bagging bodies and body fragments, even away from enemy fire, may result in unmistakable PTSD.

A more subtle issue is presented when a stressful event which is not too unusual in civilian life is followed by a grossly exaggerated reaction accompanied by reexperiences of seemingly unrelated combat stress which occurred years earlier. The grief of a veteran after a divorce or the death of a family member, for example, may be expressed with nightmares and a suicide attempt and be considered an adjustment disorder with depressed mood until it is learned that the nightmares are of the death of a buddy in combat, accompanied by survival guilt. When there have been symptoms attributable to PTSD prior to the current stressful event, diagnosis of both conditions is probably appropriate and readily made. When avoidance efforts have been successful for many years in minimizing or even preventing reexperiences of the combat stress, the principal diagnosis is probably PTSD. The recurrence of an emotion that is similar to the affective response to the original stress commonly triggers full-blown PTSD even after a long delay. Adjustment disorder and PTSD may be thought of as a continuum with interactive elements.

SUMMARY

These guidelines for diagnosis of PTSD in Viet Nam veterans have addressed issues of clinical attitudes (50), the information needed for diagnosis, the conduct of the examination, and the diagnostic process. An open mind and highly attentive approach on the part of the clinician help to overcome the obstacles to obtaining an adequate history. An exploration of three key factors—a detailed description of traumatic events, the form of reexperiences and especially their content, and indications of avoidance of reexperiences—must be made either to establish the diagnosis or to rule it out. A flexible approach which still covers all of the critical areas of intrusive and avoidance phenomena; combat experiences; life patterns during childhood, adolescence, time in military, and postmilitary years; and areas of relevant symptoms has been described, with emphasis upon relating trauma to response throughout the examination. The diagnostic process itself is one of either justifying or ruling out each disorder considered, with the result that multiple diagnoses, each independently supportable, may be made. It is hoped that these guidelines will assist in developing the critical information necessary to recognize PTSD in a manner which facilitates effective diagnosis and treatment.

REFERENCES

1. Horowitz MJ, Solomon GG: A prediction of delayed stress response syndromes in Vietnam veterans. Journal of Social Issues 31:67–80, 1975

2. Van Putten T, Emory WH: Traumatic neuroses in Vietnam returnees. Arch Gen Psychiatry 29:695–698, 1973

3. Hocking F: Extreme environmental stress and its significance for psychopathology. Am J Psychother 24:4–26, 1970

4. Rado S: Pathodynamics and treatment of traumatic war neurosis (traumatophobis). Psychosom Med 42:363–368, 1942

5. Swank RL: Combat exhaustion: a descriptive and statistical analysis of causes, symptoms and signs. J Nerv Ment Dis 109:475–508, 1949

6. Blank AS: Apocalypse terminable and interminable: Operation Outreach for Vietnam veterans. Hosp Community Psychiatry 33:913–918, 1982

7. Breen HJ: Post Vietnam syndrome: a critique. Ariz Med 34:791–793, 1982

8. LaGuardia RL, Smith G, Francois R, et al: Incidence of delayed stress disorder among Vietnam era veterans: the effect of priming on response set. Am J Orthopsychiatry 53:18–26, 1983

9. Pettera RL, Johnson BM, Zimmer R: Psychiatric management of combat reactions with emphasis of a reaction unique to Vietnam. Milit Med 47:673–678, 1969

10. Friedman MJ: Post-Vietnam syndrome: recognition and management. Psychosomatics 22:931–943, 1981

11. Grinker RR, Spiegel JP: Brief psychotherapy in war neuroses. Psychosom Med 6:123–131, 1944

12. Spitzer RL, Skodol AE, Williams JBW, et al: Supervising intake diagnosis: a psychiatric "Rashomon." Arch Gen Psychiatry 39:1299–1305, 1982

13. Williams JBW, Spitzer RL: Diagnosing psychotic disorders and affective disorders with psychotic features. Hosp Community Psychiatry 34:595–596, 1983

14. Spitzer RL, Williams JBW, Wynne LC: A revised decision tree for the DSM-III differential diagnosis of psychotic patients. Hosp Community Psychiatry 34:631–633, 1983

15. Horowitz MJ, Wilner N, Kaltreider N, et al: Signs and symptoms of posttraumatic stress disorders. Arch Gen Psychiatry 37:85–92, 1980

16. Horowitz MJ: Stress Response Syndromes. New York, Jason Aronson, 1976

17. Archibald HC, Long DM, Miller C, et al: Gross stress reaction in combat: a 15-year followup. Am J Psychiatry 119:317–322, 1962

18. Archibald HC, Tuddenham RD: Persistent stress reaction after combat: a 20-year follow-up. Arch Gen Psychiatry 12:475–481, 1965

19. Kardiner A: The Traumatic Neuroses of War. New York, Paul B. Hoeber, 1941

20. Lavie P, Hefeg A, Halperin G, et al: Long-term effects of traumatic war-related events of sleep. Am J Psychiatry 136:175–178, 1979

21. Greenberg R, Pearlman CA, Gampel D: War neuroses and the adaptive function of REM sleep. Br J Med Psychol 45:27–33, 1972

22. Kales A, Soldatos CR, Caldwell AB, et al: Nightmares: clinical characteristics and personality patterns. Am J Psychiatry 137:1197–1201, 1980

23. Shatan CF: The grief of soldiers: Vietnam combat veterans' self-help movement. Am J Orthopsychiatry 43:640–653, 1973

24. Haley SA: When the patient reports atrocities: specific treatment considerations of the Vietnam veteran. Arch Gen Psychiatry 30:191–196, 1974

25. Atkinson RM, Henderson RG, Sparr LF, et al: Assessment of Vietnam veterans for posttraumatic stress disorder in Veterans Administration disability claims. Am J Psychiatry 139:1118–1121, 1982

26. Frick R, Bogart L: Transference and countertransference in group therapy with Vietnam veterans. Bull Menninger Clin 46:429–444, 1982

27. Hendin H, Pollinger A, Singer P, et al: Meanings of combat and the development of posttraumatic stress disorder. Am J Psychiatry 138:1490–1493, 1981

28. Lipkin JO, Scurfield RM, Blank AS: Post-traumatic stress disorder in Vietnam veterans: assessment in a forensic setting. Behavioral Science and the Law 1:51–67, 1983

29. Fox RP: Narcissistic rage and the problem of combat aggression. Arch Gen Psychiatry 31:807–811, 1974

30. Horowitz MJ: Self-righteous rage and the attribution of blame. Arch Gen Psychiatry 38:1233–1238, 1981

31. Strange RE: Combat fatigue versus pseudo-combat fatigue in Vietnam. Milit Med 46:823–826, 1968

32. Yager J: Postcombat violent behavior in psychiatrically maladjusting soldiers. Arch Gen Psychiatry 33:1332–1335, 1976

33. Penk WE, Rabinowitz R, Roberts WR, et al: Adjustment of differences among male substance abuse varying in degree of combat experience in Vietnam. J Consult Clin Psychol 40:426–437, 1981

34. Merbaum M: Some personality characteristics of soldiers exposed to extreme war stress: a follow-up study of post-hospital adjustment. J Clin Psychol 33:558–562, 1977

35. Fairbank JA, Keane TM, Malloy PF: Some preliminary data on the psychological characteristics of Vietnam veterans with posttraumatic stress disorders. J Consult Clin Psychol 51:912–919, 1983

36. Foy DW, Sipprelle RC, Rueger DB, et al: Etiology of posttraumatic stress disorder in Vietnam veterans: analysis of premilitary, military, and combat exposure influences. J Consult Clin Psychol 52:79–87, 1984

37. Resnick RJ, Schulz P, Schulz SC, et al: Borderline personality disorder: symptomatology and MMPI characteristics. J Clin Psychiatry 44:289–292, 1983

38. Keane TM, Malloy PF, Fairbank JA: Empirical development of an MMPI subscale for the assessment of combat-related posttraumatic stress disorder. J Consult Clin Psychol 52:888–891, 1984

39. Malloy PF, Fairbank JA, Keane TM: Validation of multi-method assessment of posttraumatic stress disorders in Vietnam veterans. J Consult Clin Psychol 51:488–494, 1983

40. Wilson JP, Krauss GE: Predicting post-traumatic stress syndromes among Vietnam veterans, in Post-Traumatic Stress and Diseases of the Veteran Patient. Edited by Kelly WE. Springfield, Ill, Charles C Thomas (in press)

41. Brende JO, Benedict BD: The Vietnam combat delayed stress syndrome: hypnotherapy of "dissociative symptoms." Am J Clin Hypn 23:34–40, 1980

42. Sierles FS, Chen JJ, McFarland RE, et al: Posttraumatic stress disorder and concurrent psychiatric illness: a preliminary report. Am J Psychiatry 140:1177–1179, 1983

43. American Psychiatric Association: Diagnostic and Statistical Manual of Mental Disorders, Third Edition. Washington, DC, American Psychiatric Association, 1980

44. Wilson J: Conflict, stress and growth: effects of war on psychosocial development, in Strangers at Home. Edited by Figley C, Leventman S. New York, Praeger, 1980

45. Helzer JE, Robins LN, Davis DH: Depressive disorders in Vietnam returnees. J Nerv Ment Dis 163:177–185, 1976

46. Nardial JE: Diagnosis: depressive disorder. Stars and Stripes, June 23, 1983

47. Lacoursiere RB, Godfrey KE, Ruby LM: Traumatic neurosis in the etiology of alcoholism: Vietnam combat and other trauma. Am J Psychiatry 137:966–968, 1980

48. Horowitz MJ: Post-traumatic stress disorder. Behavioral Science and the Law 1:9–23, 1983

49. Vandevanter L: Home Before Morning. New York, Beaufort, 1983

50. Keane TM, Fairbank JA: Survey analysis of combat-related stress disorders in Viet Nam veterans. Am J Psychiatry 140:348–350, 1983

7

Individual Psychotherapy with Viet Nam Veterans

John Russell Smith, M.A.

7

Although the experience of Viet Nam is a thing of the past, Capps (1) has noted that the United States and its veterans are left with unfinished business. Those who know veterans realize that their experiences often remain vivid in their memories. Yet, those war experiences are 15 to 20 years old. Subsequent events during the intervening years may play as important a role in veterans' current adjustments as do their war experiences. In contrast to survivors of recent trauma, post-catastrophic coping mechanisms are well entrenched. Some veterans' histories now contain events far more tragic and traumatic than their original war experiences, complicating the clinical picture.

This chapter describes work specifically with veterans of Viet Nam. Many readers will note similarities to work with veterans of other wars and survivors of other catastrophes. Others familiar with psychodynamic, especially psychoanalytic, treatment approaches will observe parallels with what is described here. Still others may comment, "That's just good clinical practice for any client." No claim is made for a monopoly on truth or originality; this chapter represents an effort to share observations which have helped me better understand my own work with veterans—men and women, combatants and noncombatants.

PERSPECTIVE

There are several current approaches to the understanding of post-traumatic stress disorder. These include the physiological (2), behavioral (3), psychoanalytical (4), sociological (5), and cognitive (6, 7). The model described in this chapter reflects the assumptions of the cognitive/affective perspective, which was first postulated by Janet (8) and articulated most recently by Horowitz (6, 7) and Hilgard (9). However, despite differences in perspective and the apparent diversity of approaches, therapeutic interventions derived from each approach are especially effective and appropriate in particular phases of treatment.

Trauma consists of experience which an individual cannot integrate with some cherished aspect or significant notion of self, of others, of the world, or of morality. Such discrepant experiences are dissociated and placed out of awareness. They may periodically threaten to intrude or exert unconscious influence on the individual's current activities. Warding off or walling off the effects of discrepant experience also hampers or restricts current functioning. Adaptive intermediate resolution results in assimilation of some traumatic experience and the isolation of undigested experience so that current functioning remains relatively intact. Full resolution, however, involves the transformation of existing cognitive and affective structures to permit the accommodation of discrepant traumatic experience.

Janet, in his work in the late nineteenth century, recognized the existence of discontinuity between mental set and experience perceived as incompatible with it. Through hypnosis Janet identified traumatic memories forced outside of awareness. He resolved traumatic discrepancy by transforming the perception of the traumatic event. He did this by suggesting that the event really didn't happen as remembered. In the decades since then, work on hypnosis has demonstrated that memories of real events remain despite such intervention.

While recognizing discrepancy as did Janet, today we understand resolution differently. Instead of attempting to reshape discordant memory, we try to transform conscious mental set to accommodate the previously dissonant experience. Resolution then becomes a process involving cognitive structures and affective controls. It involves conscious reexamination of values and expectations and allows reconsideration and integration of previously dissociated traumatic material. While survivors most often accomplish this work independently, therapy may be helpful in many cases.

The therapist is an ally who helps clarify the steps in this process. The therapist stabilizes controls and titrates efforts at reconsideration. Fundamentally, therapy empowers the client to control symptoms, impulses, and fears. At every roadblock and juncture, the manner of structuring resolution should enhance the client's options and capacity for control.

The process of enhancing control and confronting traumatic experience does not just emphasize pathology. Equally important in the resolution of traumatic stress reactions are the recognition of integrity and honorable actions within the traumatic experience and the identification and validation of existing attempts at restraint and control.

WHO NEEDS THERAPY?

The process of resolving traumatic stress may proceed independently of therapeutic intervention. Most veterans functioned normally prior to Viet Nam and are able, determined, and motivated to function effectively afterwards.

If a person asks for help or is feeling out of control, we have no problem recognizing the need for therapy. Many veterans and other survivors will deny any problems. "I put that all behind me," "I had to get on with my life," and "It doesn't really bother me now" are common assertions about catastrophic experience. Does one take them at face value? Do we presume that such statements are manifestations of denial and resistance masking underlying pathology?

If a veteran or other survivor of trauma can remember and consider the entire experience without consuming passion or mute withdrawal, then this individual's expression of resolution can be taken at face value. The ability to face pain and grief and to recognize the honor, joy, and even excitement of the catastrophic situation indicates healthy resolution. Trauma victims who can hear and accept different perspectives on the traumatic events without rancor or turmoil demonstrate their strength, adaptability, and resolution of stress. If the client does not have these characteristics, then there is good indication that the traumatic experience is not yet integrated. Whether or not it needs to be integrated is a decision for the veteran and those close to him or her. Whether it *will be* integrated is up to the veteran.

BEFORE THE FIRST ENCOUNTER

It is a long road before the first therapeutic visit with a veteran. Spouses, friends, relatives, school personnel, or family or marital therapists are usually the first to identify the signs of stress in the veteran. Months and even years of urging precede the first contact. Veterans may pick up a pen to write or a phone to call as long as two years prior to face-to-face contact. "I've made it this far OK" or "I ain't one of those crazy vets" are common comments from new clients.

Often, it is a spouse, other family member, or friend who makes the first contact. The family and social network have long been making accommodations for the veteran's distress. Usually more information is requested so these individuals can better understand (10). Therapists must urge these concerned people to stop "understanding" and to acknowledge the burden they feel because of the veteran's distress.

The impact on the family may be evidenced in marital or family therapy, in difficulties with children, or simply by consistent complaints from family or friends. Once such difficulty is acknowledged, the veteran often agrees to come for help. In other cases, former nurses, doctors, or other professionals or more "successful" veterans read a newspaper article, hear a lecture, or attend a discussion which triggers recognition that there are unresolved war issues.

There is a popular prejudice that combat reactions reflect cowardice and abnormality. The parallel assumption is that normal veterans have no long-term adjustment problems (10, 11).

Typical coping with war trauma involves setting it aside, sealing it over, and attempting to reassume one's civilian identity. The press to make up for lost years, "to get on with life," and "to put the war behind you" defers reconsideration and resolution of trauma. The consequences of denial seem less odious than turmoil and loss of control, which veterans fear should they grapple with their undigested war experiences.

> *Shawn, a 30-year-old veteran, was in a V.A. hospital for a series of elbow operations necessitated by injury sustained in combat. Shawn's mother called a therapist concerned that he was unable to hold a job or avoid nightly brawls. As the therapist walked into his hospital room, Shawn's eyes rolled back in his head and he experienced his first grand mal seizure. Later he indicated that he had felt "some anxiety" as he anticipated this first therapeutic contact, though a neurologist agreed anxiety may have precipitated the seizure.*

THE FIRST ENCOUNTER

The first question to ask a veteran client is "What has changed?" (12). Since years have passed since combat, it is likely that some current crisis brings the veteran to therapy. Fear of loss of control during a dramatic incident often is the precipitant.

> *Lou, a 37-year-old former Marine infantryman with two tours in Viet Nam, was troubled by nightmares. His wife's fear was exacerbated when he awakened and shot at a nightstand across the room, mistaking it for an oncoming North Vietnamese soldier. A few weeks later, he woke to find that the North Vietnamese soldier he was throttling was his nine-year-old son.*

Fear that he might actually harm his wife or children in one of these episodes led Lou to seek help.

The therapist must identify current problems and determine which aspects of the veteran's life they affect. Before any checklists or standardized instruments are used, the presenting symptoms must be assessed as articulated by the veteran. Primary indicators of traumatic stress reactions may not be immediately apparent. Troubling symptoms often include rage, nightmares, emotional numbing, phobias, drinking, abuse of drugs, fighting, and conflicts with authority. The arena where problems are played out must be determined. Possibilities include the workplace, with friends, in the family, or within the veteran's mind.

Current observations (13) suggest that many veterans meet the diagnostic criteria for more than one mental disorder. They may suffer from alcohol or drug abuse, depression, paranoia, anxiety disorder, phobias, and character disorder. Just as in crisis intervention, an initial objective is to stabilize the situation, buy time, and distinguish and establish priorities for treatment of each of the separable problems.

Sources of stability in the veteran's life must be determined. These include inner strengths, modes of coping, and support resources. This information allows the therapist to determine the extent of crisis, the need for hospitalization, and the role that out-patient interventions—such as marital, individual, or group therapy—are likely to play in enabling the veteran to maintain control.

A central question is "How does the veteran see the problem; how does the veteran see himself or herself handling it?" The veteran's goals must be determined. Does the veteran want change, stabilization, or an escape? Is the veteran looking for a way out of some current legal difficulty? Is the veteran seeking compensation or a service-connected disability from the Veterans Administration? Is the veteran feeling out of control and afraid of what he or she might do? Is the veteran seeking a symptomatic relief? What, among the many areas of difficulty, are the veteran's priorities? Clarity about what the veteran seeks enables the therapist to define his or her role.

SETTLING ON A THERAPEUTIC ROLE

Since the intensity of issues of trust and the press of problems are so frequently overwhelming, as a rule of thumb the adoption of only one therapeutic role with any individual veteran client is advisable. The various roles of assessor in legal or disability cases, family or marital therapist, and therapist for an individual or a group demand different helping postures, since the client in each role is very different (14). Indeed, it is because needs arising out of different problems conflict that only one therapeutic task may be addressed by a therapist with any individual veteran client.

After settling on a role, the task is to communicate it to the veteran and reach agreement as to appropriate therapeutic goals. Identification of secondary problems and goals requires referral of the veteran to other appropriate resources.

FOUR MAJOR THEMES OF
POST-TRAUMATIC STRESS DISORDER

There are four major themes which emerge in early encounters with Viet Nam veterans and others suffering from PTSD: control, integrity, ambiguity, and personal accountability. These themes, along with the characteristic symptoms of traumatic reactions, indicate the presence of the disorder. These same issues reappear throughout treatment and the dimension of each determines the content and course of the therapy.

Control

Control is often the most significant issue in the initial session. At every stage of therapy and recovery it continues to be a crucial issue. Fear of losing control often brings the veteran in for the first consultation and precipitates nearly all flights from therapy. The depth of therapy possible is largely determined by the extent to which the veteran believes he or she has self-control or the ability to predict emerging symptoms, outbursts, or intrusive episodes.

The issue of control may manifest itself in several ways. For some, concerns about control may be related to affect. The veteran will express a fear of beginning to cry and that he or she may never stop. In others, the imposition of control, or restrictions, on behavior or activities will have only a vaguely expressed purpose: "I never go to Viet Nam movies; I don't want to get into that stuff."

Frequently, the prime factor driving a Viet Nam veteran into treatment is a recent event or an impending situation which the veteran feels has or will set him off, render him out of control, or influence him to do something he will later regret. This issue of control must be taken seriously and addressed directly, not immediately used as an opening for uncovering unconscious material. A plea for hospitalization or an expressed fear that "I am going to kill someone" *must* not be ignored.

Bill had been back from Viet Nam for 11 years. He worked in the personnel office of a large corporation and had recently been divorced. He had been meaning to call a therapist for 18 months, but it took an incident two days prior to his first session to bring him in. A woman he was dating informed him that she was seeing another man, and Bill found himself angrily stalking her on her date and barging into her apartment when after-dinner drinks lasted past 11 o'clock. Bill then invited her for a black tie dinner and, while serving coffee, pulled out an unloaded 38-caliber pistol, put it to his temple, and pulled the trigger. The terror generated in his girlfriend and his subsequent realization that he was dangerously near the edge of doing something drastic drove him to finally seek help.

The veteran's realization of the unraveling or inadequacy of previous control strategies becomes, then, the first topic of interest. Failures to adequately attend to pleas for help with control, and unheeded worries about impending loss of control, have resulted in tragic outcomes for veteran clients, therapists, hospitals, and the community.

To minimize the possibility of tragic outcome, a cardinal rule is to never uncover until the client and therapist have satisfactorily established some process for maintaining control. The greater the perceived danger of loss of control, the more cautious must be the approach to uncovering and the more initial work on control mechanisms must undergird the psychotherapeutic relationship. Strategies for enhancing control will be discussed later.

Not all veterans present with loss of control as a major initial theme. Many—especially doctors, nurses, and other professionals—maintain a facade of great self-control. They are led to therapy by complaints of spouses and family members about their behavior, somatic concerns, or difficulties remembering or concentrating. While uncovering the roots of difficulty may proceed more directly with these clients, such uncovering may unlock a core of anger, resentment, and hostility that was previously controlled only by rigidity and denial. Therefore, careful attention to developing concerns about loss of control or the expression of anger must be taken seriously, and appropriate attention should be focused on control issues before these clients either leave treatment or explode.

Integrity

During the course of initial discussion with a veteran, questions of integrity will inevitably arise. Usually the issue arises in the form of blame or criticism of an institution or individual for a lack of integrity. It may concern a medal which a veteran feels he had justly earned, but for some reason reflecting lack of governmental integrity was not awarded. It may take the form of a general complaint about the public's lack of recognition and respect for the sacrifices and hardships that Viet Nam veterans have endured. It may be an attack on the Veterans Administration for its failure to provide what the veteran sees as appropriate services. In this form, V.A. physicians inappropriately take the concern with integrity to indicate a character disorder or psychopathy in the veteran.

In more settled veterans, every apparent conflict and experience seems resolved, save one. For example:

> *"I could handle everything that happened in Nam," said Tim, a former infantryman who had married a Vietnamese woman and fathered a child by her. "But when they wouldn't let me take my child home with me, that was the last straw."*

For a career officer, the complaint may be about civilian policymakers who determined the conduct of the war "by tying one hand behind our backs," thus causing unnecessary losses among U.S. troops. Black veterans, like other minorities, were more likely to have served proudly in elite, front-line infantry units. They may express anger over a small Southern town's refusal to permit the burial of a close buddy in the local veterans' cemetery.

In still other cases, concern with integrity may appear in the form of a conflict at work over justice, fairness, or morality.

> *Bob, a graphic designer, was struggling over his reluctance to complete a design for an auto company. He was unsure whether the car had been modified to correct a potentially hazardous door lock. It emerged that the cars were of a type which had been involved in a series of accidents complicated by faulty door locks.*

Frequently, the prominence and vehemence of the challenge to the integrity of others are interpreted as signs of psychopathy. The transfer of blame to others may be viewed as the type of refusal to accept responsibility associated with character disorder. The specific theme expressed in the concern over integrity will later prove to be a direct reference to some episode for which the veteran feels overwhelming, subjectively perceived responsibility.

> *Bob, the graphic designer, had been an infantry squad leader. One day on patrol he had stopped the squad's armored personnel carrier (APC) for lunch. Bob and others ate outside, while he had the radioman stay inside at the radio. The squad came under attack, and the APC was hit with a rocket-powered grenade. Bob tried to rescue the radioman but was unable to pry open the door, which was warped shut by the heat. Bob agonized as the dying radioman screamed. His impotence to do something about this death left him feeling guilty and responsible.*

For Bob, the connection between integrity and a Viet Nam experience suddenly became apparent. The car door lock for Bob was the concrete representation of the APC door latch, which he had not been able to open. For each veteran specific forms of integrity which are of concern reflect questions about personal war experience and behavior. This is true whether veterans discuss their own integrity, lack of public recognition of their contributions, or lack of integrity in another individual.

Ambiguity

Veterans may rail against the image of Viet Nam veterans as walking time bombs. A veteran may deplore the lack of recognition of his unit's honor and integrity. "We never killed any civilians like Calley did," he may assert. But accompanying such assertions will most often be despair and anguish over what it all meant: "What did he or she die for? What good was it all? What a waste!"

Contradictory or seemingly incompatible attitudes towards the war experience are key identifiers of unresolved stress reactions. Statements like, "I'd send my son to Canada before I'd let him fight in a war like El Salvador," are accompanied by vehement assertions that Viet Nam was "the best time of my life and I wouldn't trade it for anything." An editor who has "put it all behind me" spends hours in his office researching the roots of the American decision to limit the exercise of power in the Viet Nam War effort. The internal crisis this represents is only apparent when he locks himself in his office on the eve of Veterans Day and fires a shotgun blast to his head.

One clear manifestation of this ambivalence presented itself when veterans on a stress ward demanded to be allowed to attend the Veterans Appreciation ceremonies held at a V.A. hospital on St. Valentine's Day. The group arrived to receive the recognition they had so long been denied wearing tee-shirts that read: "I'm a Viet Nam Veteran. If you don't like it, Screw You!"

The veteran's ambivalence is often powerfully illustrated in the individual's approach and avoidance of treatment.

Gary, a former Marine, was hospitalized for the fifth time. He was alienated from his wife of 18 years and his four children. His primary concern was his "mood swings," which turned out to be periodic rage attacks. He castigated his former therapists for not having helped him and for telling him that he just had to "cry and get it out." He repeatedly denied any PTSD or any connection between his problems and Viet Nam. He refused medication and examination of sources of his anger, while insisting that this was his last visit to the hospital and that he "damn well" wanted help this time.

Gary marked a dramatic change in his life from his return from Viet Nam. He continually boasted of his prowess in bar fights and reacted fiercely to any challenge to his machismo. Hypnotic relaxation attempts invariably led to recall of a traumatic episode from Viet Nam. Only much later did he finally reveal to his therapist that he had been a "coward" in Viet Nam, although he declined to discuss the episode itself for several months.

Therapy must make explicit both sides of the veteran's state of mind. The veteran must recognize the coexistence of his or her own feelings of honor and futility, joy and pain. A cognitive structure to encompass *all* experience must be developed. The sign of successful resolution of the stress process is the ability to remember and face, though not without pain, one's whole experience. This includes the good and bad, the sad and joyful. The ability to tolerantly hear of other veterans' experiences—be these veterans anti-war, pro-war, experienced in combat, or REMF (rear echelon motherfuckers)—is another prime task of therapy.

Personal Accountability

By far the most criticial issue in significant cases of stress reaction is the question of personal accountability. At the core of all cases of PTSD is some action, or failure to act, which leads to tragic or deadly consequences. For this the veteran holds himself or herself accountable. This subjectively perceived responsibility is so great that its conscious acknowledgment threatens to overwhelm cherished notions of self-respect and self-worth. Variations on this theme have been described elsewhere (15).

Common examples of perceived personal responsibility include the forward observer who accidentally called in artillery fire on a friendly unit and the squad leader who ordered grenades tossed into an enemy hut during an assault on a suspected Vietcong village, only later to discover a dead civilian family inside. The healing sanction, which traditionally shifts responsibility for such actions occurring in war from soldier to society, eroded during the Viet Nam War. This left individual soldiers alone in sorting out responsibility for such tragedies (16).

Combat provides a deadly environment in which the possibility for such choices is common. Combat itself is not the stressor but is the context in which trauma may occur. Many noncombat situations are too readily overlooked because of the emphasis on combat. The helicopter mechanic who fails to replace a critical oil seal that results in a fatal crash, or the nurse triage officer who decides against treatment of a critically wounded soldier, later discovering that he may have been saved by prompt attention, are two who may struggle with personal accountability.

In initial interviews a veteran may directly reveal guilt and agony over such an episode:

Brett, a former Army artilleryman, came to his first interview with bandaged hands, broken while beating the walls of his apartment. Almost immediately he wept. He revealed for the first time that he had called in artillery fire on a bunker full of families that he now suspects might have been civilians. He wonders whether he acted in retaliation for the deaths of his close buddies.

Revelation of a traumatic episode involving personal responsibility is more often not directly communicated. Reference to violent experience will be casually dropped as an obscure aside: "The gooks never gave me any trouble, at least not any who lived to tell about it." Frequently, the issue over which the veteran expresses fear of loss of control, the question of integrity over which he or she blames others, and the theme about which the veteran expresses a sense of ambiguity will all be vivid metaphors for an episode of personal responsibility.

There are many possible combinations of concerns which veterans present; two situations are particularly common. Paying attention to the detail of presenting concerns is important because it is inevitably linked to specific underlying concerns and to particular types of traumatic episodes.

THE TYPE I SITUATION (THE ANIMAL)

The characterization of veterans as "the animal" or "the wimp" (below) may seem extreme to some readers. As the descriptions indicate, these terms are actually mild in comparison to how the veterans actually view themselves. In the type I situation the presenting concerns reflect fear of losing control or dread of reversion to some kind of primitive or brutal animal nature. The veteran may appear overcontrolled and go to great lengths to avoid even appropriately angry responses. The veteran generally avoids fights and violence and wants to avoid being seen as dangerous or unpredictable. The veteran will generally avoid combat gear or clothing. He or she may seem somewhat paranoid and hypersensitive to criticism. A principal concern may be what the veteran will turn into if he or she responds to perceived provocation.

Another concern may be the hostile or aggressive behavior of the veteran's children, such as that typical of "the terrible twos" stage. As Haley (4) has noted, the behavior of the veteran's children may trigger concerns that he or she has passed on "evil genes."

Also typical of the type I situation are nightmares or fantasies of being under attack, captured, or punished. Veterans may express fear that attackers are coming to avenge certain acts committed during the war and as a result "hole up" at home. Noises are thought to be attackers in the yard or at doors or windows. The veteran may adopt rituals of "checking the perimeter," patrolling the house or yard before retiring or in the middle of the night. Weapons are resurrected or purchased to protect the veteran from expected invaders, but the veteran will not display them and will be quite responsive to needs to keep them safe.

Veterans in type I situations become hypersensitive to criticism. Friends and family members wonder at the intensity of response to seemingly mild correction or critique. The veteran may also appear to choke down great amounts of anger in situations which others might simply shrug off.

Underlying type I concerns is nearly always some *action* evoking feelings of personal responsibility. Generally, it is an incident viewed by the veteran as an atrocity or unjustified action that violates his or her morality and code of conduct. It is important to understand that concern about justification exists in the veteran's own mind. Indeed, the incident may well be understandable and justifiable when viewed objectively by others.

Even though the veteran may not articulate, or even be aware of, a traumatic event of the type just described, fear of losing control and feeling assaulted or criticized should alert the therapist to the possibility of such an historical event. The dynamic appears to be one in which the veteran feels himself drawn into responding to or preparing for defense against an attack, and fears the emergence of his "animal" nature.

> *Sy, a white man who was formerly a member of Marine military police, worked on a city police force in New Jersey. He came for treatment just before quitting the force because of tension. He was becoming increasingly anxious every time he was called to an incident involving a black. His anxiety peaked around the time of Martin Luther King's birthday. In therapy shortly afterward, he revealed that he and his military police unit had been called into an area where a group of black enlisted men had barricaded themselves following the assassination of Martin Luther King. Despite pleading with his commander for negotiations, Sy was ordered to assault the barricaded building. He complied, and in the resulting fire fight a number of the black rebels were killed. Fourteen years later Sy was afraid a similar incident might occur.*

The core of the type I situation is fear and trepidation over what the veteran will become when he or she slips into old patterns of behavior. It is not a concern that the veteran will not be successful, but rather that he or she will be *too* successful, too brutal, and then bitterly remorseful after the event.

In type I situations, the veteran is attempting to maintain self-respect and integrity by avoiding overreaction, anger, or loss of control because he or she knows the guilt and remorse resulting from such actions.

THE TYPE II SITUATION (THE WIMP)

In the type II situation, the presenting concern is retaliation. The target for retaliation may be the U.S. Government, the Veterans Administration, the military, or Vietnamese refugees in the United States. Highlighted in the concerns of these veterans is the notion of being wronged, especially by the failure of institutions or persons to act properly or responsively. "The V.A. failed to treat my injury properly," or "They screwed me out of my compensation," or "Those gooks fled during a fire fight where my best buddy was killed" are typical comments by members of this group.

In contrast to the type I situation, here the veteran seems eager for an opportunity to retaliate. The veteran looks for situations of injustice which he or she can correct. A type II veteran might look for opportunities to avenge the honor of an individual who is wronged or abused. In a working class veteran, retaliation may take the form of picking bar fights with those critical of the Viet Nam War. In more sophisticated veterans, it may take the form of a crusade of one kind or another.

The "wimp" will appear undercontrolled and impulsive. He or she will appear to have few controls before lashing out. He or she will resist, defeat, and undermine attempts at gaining control over outbursts. The veteran in the type II situation will more readily wear combat gear and display weapons. While the veteran may express regret at his or her "bad" image, the concern will seem superficial. The veteran appears more than a little invested in preserving the image of the tough, hair-triggered retaliator. The image is that of Clint Eastwood, the secret self-perception is that of Woody Allen.

Type II veterans may also be especially sensitive to criticism; such sensitivity is particularly acute where the criticism is generated by the veteran's alleged failure at something the veteran was supposed to do or had promised to do. Type II veterans constantly project anger, guilt, and blame onto others, deflecting any personal responsibility from themselves. They are most commonly seen as having character disorders, even when the preservice history is lacking in the essential substantiation.

Type II veterans are also withdrawn, isolated, and afraid they will not live up to their potential. Such veterans fail to complete academic tasks, and manage to avoid probable promotion, advancement, or success. They are stagnant and don't undertake resolution of current problems.

Underlying these concerns in type II veterans is some perceived failure to act or some act of cowardice or self-preservation that resulted in another's death or injury.

In contrast to the type I situation, where the driving force is remorse over an action, the type II situation is characterized by the *failure to act or to act effectively*. The dynamic of the type II situation leads veterans to recreate situations through which they can gain self-respect, by acting responsibly or properly according to their behavioral code. This dynamic is clearly illustrated in the cases of Bob, the graphic designer, and Gary, the former Marine, both described above.

In the alternative resolution of the type II situation, the veteran withdraws and avoids situations where responsibility might fall on his or her shoulders. The veteran refuses to fail and has successfully shielded from destruction any remnant of self-respect.

Jay, a former Navy Seabee, was living on V.A. disability. For years he had been unable to work and had avoided nearly all contact with neighbors and relatives. One of his complaints in seeking treatment was disgust with himself over not giving a neighbor a lift across town. In therapy, he remembered an incident in Viet Nam, in which he was detailed with an armored column to retrieve a disabled tank.

Jay was manning the 50-caliber machine gun on a tank retriever, the unit was ambushed, and two accompanying machine gunners were shot. He was unable, because of the gun mount, to fire at snipers high above in surrounding trees. Finally, under heavy fire, he leaped from his exposed position and ran behind the tank retriever. This left other members of the rescue unit without cover of 50-caliber fire.

Having sprained his ankle in his leap, Jay was medevaced with the most seriously wounded. Their moans and mutilated bodies compounded his guilt and sense of inadequacy. Unable to forgive his behavior, he increasingly avoided activities over the years. He became a virtual recluse, fearful that any demand for responsible behavior would again underscore his cowardice and capacity for failure.

The key to understanding the "wimp" or type II veteran is either his or her avoidance of action or the constant misconstrual of present situations as calling for dramatic combative action, where success never seem satisfactory. No matter how many fights or battles the veteran wins now, he or she cannot undo the past failure.

In both type I and type II situations the precipitating traumatic event generally remains out of awareness. Even if it is vaguely recalled, its relationship to present behavior is not appreciated. Nevertheless, the episode has served as a central metaphor, or organizing principle, for present behavior. The single incident is not simply repeated, does not simply dominate the life of the veteran. Rather, the traumatic episode becomes a metaphor which serves to channel the other significant, dynamic currents in the individual's life in a particular direction. It narrows the range of current opportunities and constantly focuses present reality into a recapitulation and attempted resolution of the past trauma. All of this is designed to restore, strengthen, or maintain self-respect and a sense of personal integrity.

THE TYPE III SITUATION
(THE DOUBLE-BOUND VETERAN)

Sometimes, a veteran's experience will contain both type I and type II episodes. These veterans at one time acted brutishly (in their estimation) and at another time failed miserably. In these cases, resolution of one tragedy inevitably brings the opposite to the surface and leaves the veteran torn no matter which way he or she acts.

Fred, a 36-year-old former Marine, was hospitalized for ingesting lye. On the ward he seemed challenging and provocative to other patients, was irritated by their behavior, and seemed to want to draw them into fights. Just before the inevitable eruption, he would catch himself and beg the nursing staff to place him in restraints. A review of his history revealed two significant episodes from Viet Nam.

Fred walked point for his company. He was well respected for his ability to spot ambushes and traps. One day the unit was ordered to assault what was described as a highly fortified North Vietnamese Army stronghold. In the assault, Fred saw a figure dart from one of the buildings. Firing quickly, he brought the man down. When he reached the place where the man fell and turned him over, he discovered an unarmed old man who reminded him of his grandfather. Fred described himself as "flipping out" at that point. Hearing a child cry, he located the cover over the tunnel where she lay, lifted it, and tossed in a grenade on the child and her mother.

Three weeks later Fred left for a seven-day R&R (rest and relaxation) trip to Tokyo. When he returned, still distraught from the previous killings, the first sergeant ordered him back to the field to rejoin the company. Instead, he went off on a three-day bender in the nearby town. When he returned he discovered that, during his absence, the replacement point man had led the company into an ambush in which two-thirds of the unit was wiped out. The first sergeant and the company commander blamed Fred for the disaster: "If you had been out there doing your job, this wouldn't have happened.

After his discharge, Fred found himself paralyzed to act. He was afraid of taking action and turning into the animal he had been on one occasion. Yet he constantly belittled himself for not acting. Despite his paralysis he managed to work and stayed out of the hospital for 15 years. One day Fred and his brother were working on his car. His brother, also a Viet Nam veteran, got word that someone was looking for him to settle a score. Fred knew that that the man looking for his brother was "carrying" (a weapon). When his brother asked Fred to join him while he looked for the man, Fred declined. Fred's brother went alone and was shot to death in the street. Three weeks later, Fred was hospitalized for a suicide attempt. Now Fred finds himself whipsawed by self-blame over having again failed to act, and yet fearful of the kind of animal he will turn into if he does act on his anger.

In many homicide cases involving Viet Nam veterans with apparent PTSD, it often turns out that the veterans have histories that fit this pattern. The homicide often involves a desperate attempt to resolve, in seemingly bizarre fashion, both sides of the veteran's dilemma. The following case illustrates one such example.

Peter, an Army infantryman, presented for treatment with intense rage at Vietnamese refugees in his community and frequent powerful impulses to attack and kill them. He joined a rap group and during the course of it was moved to a tearful revelation of an attack he had made on Vietnamese civilians. On guard one night, he heard movement outside the barbed wire perimeter and opened fire with a machine gun. Examination of the bodies revealed that the people Peter had killed were elderly unarmed civilians. In the rap group, Peter expressed grief over the error. Yet his symptoms did not remit following the revelation, and the intensity of his hostility toward the Vietnamese seemed to escalate. Only months later, after an incident in which he actually fired upon a group of civilians, did another episode from Viet Nam surface.

Early in his tour in country, Peter had been on perimeter watch in a foxhole with a buddy. A sapper and mortar attack was launched against the base. Rounds were landing all around them. Fearful of his life, Peter excused himself and went for more ammunition. He hid in a bunker until the attack subsided. When he returned to his post he discovered that his buddy had been killed by a mortar round which landed in the foxhole. Now, in the rap group, Peter revealed that his quickness to shoot in the incident with the civilians had resulted from his wish to undo his earlier cowardice. The group pointed out that his present actions were a continuation of this pattern. His course, they said, was unlikely to resolve either dilemma, but would end with him in jail.

Continued attention to the congruence between presenting current problems and the outlines and dynamics of reported traumatic incidents is essential to finding a route to uncovering and resolution. Failure to question and explore inconsistencies can leave the veteran to drift into disaster. Only asking Peter why he wanted to again kill Vietnamese civilians, if he had so much guilt over the previous episode, led to the uncovering of his earlier failure. Then the dynamics made sense to the group and led Peter to some understanding of himself and his situation.

ISOLATION

In severe stress reactions the degree to which the veteran has become alienated and isolated is an important consideration. While occasionally a veteran literally barricades himself in his house, surrounds himself with weapons, and awaits a Vietcong attack, this represents an extreme. Yet, isolation must always be evaluated.

Catastrophic events generate awe, curiosity, relief, and discomfort among observers. When the event involves a socially controversial issue, such as the Viet Nam War, denial of the suffering of participants may be part of the societal response. Because the public is troubled by it own ambivalence over the situation, it is unable to deal with the painful aspects of an individual victim's experience. This pushes the veteran into a more isolated position.

Veterans, and other survivors, isolate themselves and reinforce the aloneness produced by public reaction. They frequently feel misunderstood, asserting "If you weren't in my situation, you can't possibly understand." Individual veterans draw a dividing line between themselves and those who did not share their experience. Men, women, blacks, Hispanics, Green Berets, medics, nurses, noncombat veterans, and journalists will overtly or subtly convey the sense that "I am special." Though others have shared almost all aspects of an experience, some special quality—race, sex, religion, role—will enable individuals to separate their unique experiences from those of others. There is intense identification with others in the group, such as nurses, American Indians, and victims of agent orange. Within such groups individuals emphasize special characteristics which separate them from others. Consequently, they cannot share their pain or diminish their grief.

The focus on uniqueness allows members of a group to band together and blame their troubles on an external source. This, in turn, permits avoidance of the experience of personal confusion, ambiguity, and self-blame. If one is a member of a group of isolated, unique, and misunderstood victims, the individual cannot legitimately be blamed for what happened in Viet Nam, to the individual and to others.

In treatment, psychotherapists who have read, listened, and developed an understanding of the war and its participants are startled when their knowledge or understanding produces withdrawal or hostility in the veteran. The underlying message of the veteran is, "I don't want you to understand, because I am afraid to be understood or to understand myself."

Veterans who have isolated themselves and avoided contact with a support system are most likely to have difficulties with ambiguity, personal integrity, and especially control and personal accountability. The more isolated the veteran, the less adequate therapeutic work in a group and treatment aimed at uncovering will be. First, the sense of personal control may need to be reinforced, and the possibility of hospitalization must be considered. Isolation and withdrawal must not be ignored, for they indicate that there are impulses which cry out for control in the absence of effective mechanisms of defense.

THE PROCESS OF INDIVIDUAL PSYCHOTHERAPY

Psychotherapy for PTSD is a process in which the survivor integrates and masters the conscious and unconscious effects of traumatic experience. The goals go beyond relief of symptoms and include enhancing self-esteem and self-control, an appropriate sense of personal accountability, and a renewed sense of personal integrity and pride. It attempts to build on the victim's independent work in these areas.

Despite anger, rage, acting out, threats, and even violent behavior, the therapist must remain the veteran's ally, encouraging and thereby empowering the individual to take control of memories, pain, actions, and even the pace of therapy. Therapy must help the veteran recognize and structure choices involving the exercise of such control. Situations in which the therapist or institutions impose outside control should, when possible, be avoided.

Central to the perspective of this chapter is the gradual de-escalation of the use of weapons, actual or metaphorical, necessary for the exercise of control in the veteran's psychological and interpersonal domains.

There are nine major themes which the veteran and therapist will encounter in the course of therapy:

1. Trust and rapport,
2. Control,
3. Anger, rage, and blame,
4. Uncovering,
5. Transformation,
6. Relationship to other life experiences,
7. Repetition and falsification,
8. Affective articulation, and
9. Animating action and the survivor mission.

Trust and Rapport

An intriguing aspect of the veteran's way of thinking is the lack of trust. Extensive testing precedes the veteran's genuine approach to another. Burdened with pain, in a new relationship the veteran first dispenses grief or rage. Believing that no one can understand, the veteran tests the potential therapist, or friend, to confirm his or her preconception that "You, too, cannot understand."

> Ray walked into a rap group one night upset about his lack of success in establishing an intimate relationship with a woman. He appeared articulate, so the group found it hard to believe he would have such difficulty. It turned out he found it quite easy to establish initial closeness. Trouble arose when this led to the possibility of sexual intimacy.
>
> Ray would be at either his or the woman's apartment. Chatting over a glass of wine, he would casually mention experiences in Viet Nam. He was stunned when the intimate mood disappeared and the woman recoiled in horror. Pressed by the group about his particular recent experience, Ray revealed that he had recounted the story of an ambush, the death of a buddy, and his return to retrieve the corpse two days later. He revealed to the group that he had described to his date the details of the mutilated and decomposing body. The head had been severed, and the genitals were cut off and stuffed in the mouth. The group then relayed to Ray their vivid understanding of the woman's withdrawal.

The therapist must first address his or her investment and interest in the work, for the veteran may well be questioning the therapist's motives. The veteran silently or openly asks, "What's your game? What are you getting out of this? How much are you making by treating me? Where were you during the war?" The veteran's real question is, "Are you capable of listening to me or are you going to criticize me, reject me, or in some way lay your own rap on me?"

The veteran may engage in provocative behavior or threats or relate horror stories to test the therapist's perspective, commitment, and tolerance. The survivor's concerns include these:

"Can you [the therapist] get past this?"
"Can you tolerate me?"
"Can you pay attention?"
"Can you accept me? If you can, maybe I can accept myself."
"I'll tell you I'm special, but I'm not special. I'm dirt."
"Am I safe with you?"
"Can you help me with me?"

This testing process is a form of transference reaction. The therapist's personal characteristics won't necessarily prevent such behavior. The veteran is concerned with how the therapist handles himself or herself in the therapeutic relationship. The patient needs to know whether the therapist can stand being yelled at and being frightened, and how the therapist will respond to a veteran who acts out.

The therapist's reaction is important in terms of its honesty and integrity. Therapists in this situation must accept themselves, their shortcomings, their reactions, and their mistakes. This provides a model for the veteran to do the same.

Frequently a veteran will ask whether the therapist works for the Veterans Administration. Ducking the question by claiming, "I don't really work for the V.A.; I'm a consultant," or claiming shared mistrust of the Veterans Administration skirts a potential confrontation. But it also misses an important therapeutic opportunity. By responding, "Yes, I work for the V.A. and I'm here to listen," the therapist introduces ambiguity into otherwise unquestioned survivor hostility and demonstrates an ability to tolerate challenge. It also opens the door for exploration of the stereotyped assumptions which have blocked and frustrated past attempts at resolution of traumatic stress.

The therapist's reaction to physical threats and acting out are opportunities for intervention. The therapist who acknowledges fear when the object of yelling or threats forces the veteran to recognize the impact of the veteran's own behavior. The veteran also learns there is no need to escalate threatening behavior to get needed attention. Finally, this interaction causes the veteran to accept responsibility for his or her own actions. Likewise, encouraging a veteran to clean up, repair, and replace a window he's broken or a hole he's punched in a wall allows the veteran to tangibly demonstrate recognition and acceptance of the consequences of his actions.

There is an important caveat to emphasize here. Long and painfully acquired experience has taught the therapists who are most experienced with PTSD that *all* strange behavior, acting out, and challenges to the therapist must be considered symbolic action related to trauma, until proven otherwise. In addition, presenting problems and first statements and actions are a direct communication of the trauma to be addressed in the course of treatment. Of course, it is not easy for therapists to attend to such communication initially.

Control

Earlier, control was described as the single most significant issue in many cases, particularly at the outset. Many clinicians find this difficult to understand. Faced with anger, rage, and acting out, clinicians often respond with hostility and frustration and diagnose a character disorder. Sometimes, treatment will founder as the therapist's own moral code influences an effort to "correct" and control the patient's behavior. Alert to an apparent lack of guilt and sense of responsibility for current actions, these therapists attempt to set limits and induce responsibility in their clients.

Other clinicians, sensitive to concerns about trauma, will inquire about a veteran's combat history. They hear a seemingly traumatic episode related with little or no expression of injury and pain, and they correctly assume that these feelings are repressed. This provokes these therapists to attempt a metaphoric crashing of the veteran's resistance to feelings related to trauma.

Still other therapists, alert to the veteran's tension and the intensity of the veteran's efforts at control, attempt stress reduction and deep relaxation therapy.

Behind each of these strategies is an appropriate therapeutic goal. For clinicians working with character disorders, resocialization and the fostering of guilt and responsibility serve to temper and channel anger, rage, and acting out. For dynamic clinicians, uncovering and encouraging catharsis of long-isolated traumatic experience, with the emergence of intense affect and grief, are expected to bring relief. Relaxation and stress reduction are expected to lower tension and open the opportunity for deeper work.

Unfortunately, clinicians attempting each of these approaches frequently encounter paradoxical effects. Limit setting and restraint of acting out in veterans frequently seem to provoke increased acting out and, in some cases, veteran clients have actually taken over inpatient wards. Uncovering and catharsis of a traumatic episode are frequently followed by a flight from therapy. Paradoxically, relaxation techniques with veteran clients sometimes elicit a panic attack.

Treatment of PTSD requires a delicately balanced approach involving the use of control and reformulation. Appropriate attention to and reinforcement of control must precede uncovering and reformulation (17). Inadequate attention to the control issue underlies the paradoxical results described above.

Hilgard (9) has described the phenomenon of dissociation—the splitting off from awareness of traumatic memories and dissonant cognitive structures. Such dissociation, reluctance to remember, and the isolation of affect associated with PTSD are adaptive and purposeful. They indicate that present cognitive organization cannot accommodate traumatic material (7). By reinforcing control mechanisms, therapy creates psychic breathing space. Cognitive structures necessary to integrate traumatic experience may then develop.

In the following section, discussion of the control of weapons use is a paradigm for the development of self-control in the entire stress recovery process. The focus here on weapons is doubly motivated. In themselves weapons can be a most perplexing and sometimes dangerous therapeutic problem. Weapons also serve the veteran as a powerful metaphor, a tactic to ward off perceived attacks by others, and afford protection against the vulnerability the veteran feels.

Veterans are trained in and experienced with weapons. Weapons literally provide self-protection and the ability to retaliate; on the other hand, they create fear and discomfort among families and therapists. When a therapist feels comfortable with and competent in dealing with this most dangerous of control issues, there is a greater likelihood that lesser issues of control will be addressed successfully. More importantly, when the therapist feels comfortable and competent in this area, there is less chance that the therapist's anxiety and discomfort, generated by the veteran's fear of losing control, will result in avoidance of the control and weapons issues. This minimizes the possibility that violence and tragedy will unexpectedly occur.

Therapy, once it can address this most serious problem, can easily and with similar techniques deal with less dramatic issues involving self-control, empowerment, and responsibility. Thus, this discussion of the management of weapons includes principles which apply to the therapeutic management of other problems of control.

The fundamental assumption of therapy is that the veteran has the power to solve his or her problems. The therapist acts as an ally who encourages and enables the veteran to exercise power and responsibility. Should the therapist assert control and confiscate weapons, the personal responsibility which therapy intends to foster would be undercut. To aid the veteran in putting weapons aside, or temporarily creating deliberate roadblocks in the path of their potential use, fosters the veteran's responsibility for thought and action which will be the hallmark of the entire recovery process.

The therapist should not initiate a discussion of weapons. However, should weapons be mentioned or hinted at as part of a description of a troubling incident, it is obligatory to ask about them or pursue the discussion. Also, in veterans with an initial high level of concern about control, it may be necessary to gently ask if there is a concern that an explosive use of a weapon may take place.

It must be assumed that when a veteran talks about weapons he is expressing concern and the wish to discuss possible loss of control. Certainly, this wish is not unambiguous, and an authoritarian attempt to dispose of a weapon in the veteran's possession will meet with opposition. If the therapist believes the situation is labile, any attempted limit-setting must be accomplished in an empathic atmosphere. The therapist must identify with the veteran's concern over his current crisis, the rise in his distress, and his concern over control. The therapist can then stress the *temporary* need for limits and controls over weapons to prevent an unintended escalation of violent behavior. The therapist is then an ally in creating a safe space for therapeutic work to continue without tension over weapons. Finally, the worry about control must be made explicit, and the veteran's agreement secured that feeling in control and free of tension over a potential outburst is desired.

Two possible concrete alternatives have been helpful in this situation: rental of a safe deposit box in which the unloaded and dismantled weapons can be placed is one, while checking the weapon into a pawnshop is another. In either case, an arrangement is made whereby the safe deposit key or pawn ticket is entrusted to a stable and sober close friend or to a trusted family member who has a separate residence. In this regard, the weapon should *not* be held by a relative or a drinking buddy, *nor* should the key or ticket be easily accessible.

The therapist should present these options and ask for the veteran's thoughts. In discussing the veteran's choices, the primary concerns are trust in the person who will hold the ticket or key, the veteran's distance from the weapon, and the need for deliberate steps to be taken in order to retrieve the weapon. After agreement has been obtained, the therapist and veteran discuss exactly what steps will be taken. Details include approaching the people involved, securing the weapon, and requirements for retrieval of the key or pawn ticket. The purchase or acquisition of new weapons must also be discussed.

This discussion constitutes the development of a therapeutic contract. It includes safety valves, such as an agreement to make therapeutic contact should a dangerous eruption seem possible. Indeed, the therapist should be available around the clock at such times. Once this plan has been implemented, there is a noticeable drop in tension and concern and a concurrent rise in therapeutic trust.

The elements of this strategy and the benefits derived deserve reiteration. The veteran and the therapist have together identified a concern and taken effective action. The therapist, by not taking the weapon, key, or pawn ticket, avoids being placed in the middle. The veteran asserts control over the weapon by taking steps which reflect free choice. No one else takes or keeps the weapon. Indeed, the veteran has the option of repossession when the crisis is past.

In sum, the survivor has taken a major step in asserting control in crisis and in mastering his fears of loss of control. The actions are his;

the therapist has been an ally. This paradigm for therapeutic intervention permits action by the veteran, with the therapist-ally placed figuratively at the client's shoulder. It underlies the approach to therapy with the veteran who suffers from PTSD.

One final note about weapons. Some clinicians, reacting to countertransference fears and concerns, prohibit weapons in the consultation room, while failing to address the problem of control and potential violence elsewhere. While it is recognized that many, and perhaps most, therapists need to establish limits on the carrying of weapons into therapy sessions, to do this and otherwise ignore the problem clearly enhances the possibility of a serious episode of violence in the community.

Veterans use verbal threats, demonstrations of anger, swearing, and even silence or refusal to engage in the same way they use weapons. Goals include distancing people, backing them off, or fending off perceived assaults.

Psychological assault was a large part of the Viet Nam War experience. Behavior was cultivated to emphasize prowess and authority. Tagging enemy corpses with an ace of spades, or another unit symbol, was intended to terrorize enemy soldiers who retrieved those bodies.

The war sanctioned many forms of revenge. The metaphorical use of interpersonal weapons is an outgrowth of vengeful action and may persist as a learned behavior and form of defense. A task of therapy is to help the veteran recognize the range of weapons in his or her armory: guns and verbal assaults and withdrawal are all weapons. If therapy progresses, the veteran will recognize his or her vulnerability and develop responses consistent with intimacy and trust.

Several approaches have been proposed as alternative therapies for PTSD. Among these are behavioral interventions, such as implosion and systematic desensitization (3). Medications (18–20) have also been suggested for the treatment of specific symptoms such as nightmares. In addition, Brende (21) has noted the usefulness of hypnosis.

In my own view, the success of diverse treatments reflects the enhancement of self-control, accomplished in a therapeutic manner similar to the process described above. The limitations of various treatment approaches reflect their failure to address other aspects of the stress recovery process, but as elements in a program of comprehensive clinical care designed to enhance control, they are invaluable.

Paradoxically, some interventions typical of a stress reduction program can have undesired results. Collier and Miller (22) note that relaxation exercises designed to reduce stress and tension have the effect of precipitating crisis or panic attacks in some veterans. Clients with tenuous or rigid controls experience relaxation as a threat and therefore experience panic in response. Close attention to presenting issues of tenuous control must precede the use of special therapeutic techniques.

There is another strategy for enhancing control over a range of situations less volatile that those involving weapons. Veterans frequently express concern over a repetitive experience, during which they feel they may lose control. Examples include a particular argument with a spouse, a repeated confrontation with a boss or coworker, or a repetitive barroom disagreement. Indeed, a veteran may seek help because he fears losing control. The first task of therapy is to establish control, through a technique which involves discussion of the experience, identification of points at which conflict can escalate or be resolved, and development of alternative modes of action.

The central task involves discussion of the experience. The veteran will most frequently describe the origin of the incident in brief and circumscribed terms, picking up the story shortly before the blow-up, generally where there is some action by the other party which the veteran sees as precipitating the final outcome. After establishing agreement that the veteran is concerned about escalation and would like some alternative methods for handling future repetitions, the work on control can begin. Avoiding for the moment concern over who is to blame, the veteran and the therapist can focus on what choices the veteran can make to avoid the feared outcome. Frequently, a veteran's view will be to avoid work, his spouse, or the barroom altogether; he will believe that otherwise he will replay the situation to its stereotyped end. Given the choices as the veteran sees them, the first choice is generally not feasible, and so the second is inevitable. Next, the veteran elaborates the steps which lead to the patterned, undesirable final outcome. He is helped to identify the elaborate set of steps and antecedents which lead to escalation. It is of interest that the veteran will almost always be aware of a critical point prior to the final outcome when the veteran knew he or she was on the wrong track: "When my boss said that to me," a veteran might recall, "I knew where we were going to end up."

The therapist must avoid choosing sides or assigning blame and should nonjudgmentally discuss with the veteran what would have been an alternative comment or action, one which would have given the veteran control and avoided the final undesirable outcome. The client may realize that he or she is not capable of a different verbal response, but that he or she could turn around and walk away. In that case, the therapist helps to identify the red flags and signals to which the veteran must so respond.

The therapist and veteran then negotiate an agreement. The next time the situation arises and the critical point is reached, the veteran will take action: he or she will turn and walk away. The therapist and veteran discuss the possibility of failure, so that even if the unwanted outcome isn't avoided, the unsuccessful attempt is viewed as a first step.

If the attempt is successful, the therapist and veteran can then further elaborate and articulate preferred actions and alternatives that the veteran feels he or she can try. Gradually, therapy is directed toward the beginning of the conflict situation, breaking it down into its components. The therapist consistently tries to structure "small" successes as the veteran assumes responsibility for and control over his or her actions.

One useful technique in helping the veteran deal with control is to define the relevant coping strategies he or she is already using. One veteran described himself as "totally out of control nearly every night." He regularly found himself about to get into a fight. He would make a quick exit, hop into his car, dash across town, and punch another hole in the wall of his condominium. He was startled to realize in therapy that he had actually exercised enormous restraint and control via this action.

Frequently, the most effective path to control involves reflection and explicit articulation of existing but not consciously recognized controls. Recognition and elaboration may then be accompanied by hierarchical ordering of alternative strategies for coping with stressful or provocative situations. Granting permission for the veteran to defer uncovering of traumatic issues until a later session or granting permission for extra-hour phone calls or additional sessions may also provide sufficient control and relief to greatly reduce the concern.

Anger, Rage, and Blame

Anger, rage, and blame often become treacherous traps in therapy with Viet Nam veterans. Some therapists glimpse a veteran's unceasing wrath toward institutions such as the Veterans Administration and see a hopeless cycle. The veteran seems to express never-changing rage, assignment of responsibility to an external source, and self-righteousness. Correctly noting that such a posture embodies hopelessness, the clinician attempts to focus on the veteran's contribution. The veteran hears only that his rage is misunderstood, and turns it on the clinician.

Other clinicians, sensitive to the origins of the veteran's anger, encourage the veteran to ventilate and support these assertions. They hope that, once expressed, this rage will dissipate.

Each of these approaches is a trap. There are real and legitimate causes for rage in the veteran's experience of war, homecoming, and long-term public and governmental attitudes. A basic assumption concerning stress reactions is that profound guilt and self-criticism are lying beneath assignments of blame. In expressing wrath the veteran is saying, "It's all bad. . . . It's hopeless. . . . I want you to help me prove that I am stuck and there is no solution. . . . I'm so bad that you can't abide me." Or, the veteran may be so angry that the rage has turned to apathy: "I'm so angry I don't give a damn and I won't react."

Other veterans are manifestly guilt-ridden and seem to do nothing right. They constantly lose jobs and disappoint and fail their families. Yet, when someone else has clearly wronged such a veteran, he or she lashes out at the offending party with incredible, righteous vengeance.

Expressions of rage are a part of the stress recovery process. The process involves the understanding and allocation of appropriate blame and responsibility to oneself and others. Some blame is assigned to the country and the policymakers. But the real pain of PTSD lies in the oscillation between self-condemnation and furiously blaming others, and feelings of guilt and self-punishment are inevitable stages in the process. How can veterans be helped through this experience?

Veterans must understand the impact of their behavior. When they rage and threaten, the therapist must help them realize they are frightening to others. They must also realize that they do not have to escalate their angry behavior to gain therapeutic attention. The therapist must also convey the intention not to reject the patient, regardless of his or her behavior. Nonjudgmentally, the therapist must acknowledge the veteran's anger without implying either total approval or disgreement.

The therapist must ask the veteran why the wrongdoing of others is so important to the veteran today. After a therapist has established trust and rapport by listening; accepting his own mistakes; acknowledging his actions during the war, in or out of the military; and addressing honestly his motives for doing his work, he can then confront the veteran. "If these others are to blame, why do you continue to allow it to screw up your life?" "They may be to blame, but why do you have to continue to suffer for it? Are there other choices you have?"

Veterans reject one typical form of the therapeutic contract, in which problems are presented which the therapist can neutrally address. The process of stress recovery involves absolution of guilt and clarification of values. While not all experts agree, I believe that only by presenting yourself as a human struggling with your own values may you, as a therapist, make yourself available for the veteran.

Some veterans with seemingly well-developed coping skills have superficially adapted very successfully. When coming for treatment, they may have marital or other "minor" problems but present themselves as having their lives under control. Other than irritation over the incompetence of others, they may express little anger. However, careful exploration of this irritation with veterans who cannot "get it together," or with veterans who cannot help personal problems from interfering with work or life, will reveal tightly controlled anger beneath the surface.

One final caution about dealing with rage and anger. Many veterans have learned to use anger and rage as a defense against feelings of vulnerability. Danger for the veteran lies in successfully learning to handle anger. When a veteran understands his anger, knows that cowing his wife by yelling, smashing things, bolting out of the house, hopping into the car, and driving away recklessly at high speeds no longer provide either a quick release or an answer, an overwhelming depression will surface. As anger comes under control, the veteran must confront the chasm of pain it covers. The clinician, at this point, must be very alert to the emergence of despair and the possibility of self-destructive thoughts and actions. Anticipating with the veteran these feelings of depression and pain, and formulating a plan to cope with their expected emergence, can help prevent such crises.

Uncovering

So far the focus of discussion of therapy has been on trust, control, weapons, and anger, and not on the resolution of the traumatic experience. Having started by addressing presenting issues of loss of control and anger, the clinician may then begin exploring the underlying traumatic event. It is useful to wait for the veteran to allude to the importance of the trauma. This usually occurs when the veteran, in discussing current problems, talks of Viet Nam. A veteran may talk of nightmares. He may be wearing fatigues or parts of his uniform. His behavior may become strange or bizarre in relation to present circumstances. Sometimes the latter may initiate prompt appearance of a critical traumatic event:

> *Billy, a former Marine, sought treatment because his wife was complaining about the length of time he took to return home at night. It emerged that Billy drove home in a great loop to avoid a particular town. It was revealed that he had grown up there, had left to join the Marines, and had never returned. Later, Billy revealed that his best friend, who had joined the Marines with him, was buried in a cemetery along the route Billy would have driven through the town. Several months later Billy revealed*

that he had accidentally shot his friend as the friend was pulling him from a swollen stream by the muzzle of his rifle.

In the absence of such an early revelation, the therapist can begin inquiring by asking the veteran when he first noticed his problem. Frequently, the response relates onset to some time after his return from Viet Nam. Another approach is to ask if the veteran has ever noticed a particular behavior, or whether the behavior reminds him of anything. Once it has been established that something important happened in Viet Nam, a detailed military history should be obtained (see Chapter 13).

The history should include the following:

1. Events the veteran thinks of as significant;
2. Periods of time which the veteran cannot remember, especially if he or she is quite clear about other events;
3. Contradictions or glib statements about an event: "Yeah, the squad got wiped out but it didn't bother me none. . . .";
4. Areas the veteran would rather not talk about: "Yeah, I had a couple of close calls but I don't like to talk about it. . . .";
5. Important themes described in this chapter should be investigated.

Each of these topics is potentially useful in later exploration.

The therapist taking a history must hear the veteran's story and listen for the meaning it has for the individual. Often, the sensitive therapist feels that something important has happened, but recognizes that the veteran is unable to remember precisely what it was. Memory may improve in the course of discussion of peripheral events. Asking for geography, details of terrain or weather, identification of individuals by name, description of the veteran's clothing and that of the others, or description of the veteran's weapons may trigger retrieval of the critical traumatic event.

Sam, an infantryman, insisted that Viet Nam had nothing to do with his current rage reactions. Under hypnosis to find a link to this simmering rage, Sam quickly associated to a particular uniform. By tracing details, he was able to remember with great pain the lieutenant he was unable to reach and had left to die in a withering crossfire. The uniform he remembered belonged to that officer.

The veteran must determine the pace of uncovering. Careful therapeutic attention to developing agitation, anger, fear, and crying, as well as direct inquiry as to the impact of memories, help veterans stay alert to their own reactions, recognize the therapist's concern, and control the speed of uncovering and the depth of probing questions.

Transformation

The key to resolution of stress reactions is reformulation of attitudes, expectations, and cognitive set, to allow integration of what really happened. As long as memories remain dissociated and out of awareness, guilt operates covertly and influences current behavior. Recapitulation, which is at the root of the most troublesome of stress cases, occurs outside of conscious control. Not surprisingly, when memories of traumatic events are retrieved, the reaction is powerful.

As veterans remember the trauma, they relive it with the affective impact of the original experience. They cry, get angry, feel guilty, and become exhausted. Then, contradictions emerge. They will berate themselves, for having shot, for having not shot, for having hid, etc. In the course of the veterans' reactions, some distorted view of their expectations will become clear to the therapist or to other neutral observers.

Gentle questioning must then begin. Veterans may get angry, exasperated, or frustrated with the therapist's failure to concur with the veteran's guilt-ridden judgment. The therapist must plant a seed with questions, avoid absolute or judgmental statements, and indicate a willingness to be told that he or she is wrong and doesn't understand. The therapist must be willing to reexamine, to return again and again to the same topic.

Resolution of traumatic experience is not simply the result of retrieval of a traumatic memory or abreaction of emotion. Only with exploration of the discrepancy between actions taken (or omitted) during the traumatic experience and judgments and expectations subsequently made by the veteran regarding the previous behavior will tension begin to dissipate.

While the first recounting of a trauma may result in an affective catharsis, dreams, nightmares, and other intrusive recapitulations and examinations will continue. Not until these veterans can realize and live with the fact that corpsmen do not always risk their lives for the wounded; that quick reactions may save one's skin but may also result in the deaths of innocent civilians; that nurses sometimes break under the strain of tending broken, young bodies; and that a one-degree error in a mortar's elevation may be the difference between hitting friendlies and the enemy (to name but a few traumatic events)—not until then will these veterans' pain diminish.

In individual therapy, therapists will find that reassurance about the veteran's behavior, even if the therapist is also a veteran, will not be sufficient to change the patient's self-judgment. Only by thoughtful acts of reparation, or the concurrence of veteran buddies, will such shifts take place.

Relationship to Other Life Experiences

Current problems and traumatic events from Viet Nam may be linked psychologically to unresolved issues from the prewar past. But these earlier events are not necessarily the major themes of an individual's life.

Seth, a 38-year-old former Marine, had previously been treated for alcoholism, which had resulted from his attempt to control his nightmares by drinking. His first psychiatric admission came after the death of a close friend. The friend, a Viet Nam veteran, was in the habit of inviting Seth to drink with him. The friend would often pick bar fights and Seth would rescue him. One Saturday Seth had promised his wife that they would spend the evening together. When the friend asked Seth to go out, Seth declined. The friend went out drinking alone, got into a fight, and was stabbed to death.

Seth sought treatment and in short order recalled an ambush in Viet Nam that occurred right after he had medevac'd himself for immersion foot. Seth, who walked point, was replaced by a new man who walked into an ambush with the unit and was impaled on a swinging trap.

Only later did Seth connect these episodes to an earlier childhood one. As an eight-year-old, Seth and one of his friends would hop on and ride the rear bumpers of buses as they rolled down his street. One rainy day, Seth's friend asked him to come out and play, but Seth's mother refused to let him because of the weather. Seth's friend went out to play by himself and was killed when he slipped off a bus's bumper at a stop sign and the bus rolled backwards over him. Seth remembered the boy's funeral and the fact that he and the boy's corpse were dressed in the same suit. Seth remembers not being sure whether it was he or the boy lying in the casket.

It is frequently the case that such earlier episodes find their parallel in the traumatic circumstances of war. Their later recapitulation in postwar life often serves as a precipitant to decompensation.

In other cases, the individual is more clearly impaired prior to military service. Yet it is possible that such individuals can also develop post-traumatic stress reactions. At times recognition and treatment of these reactions can serve as an avenue for treatment of the earlier disorder, when previous attempts have failed.

Ed, a 38-year-old former Army radioman, was hospitalized for the eighth time. He had a chronic alcohol problem and was diagnosed as having schizophrenia and a character disorder. He was first hospitalized for a paranoid episode in Viet Nam. Ed constantly found himself in bar fights and brawls with his bosses. Whenever hospitalized he would attempt to pick fights with staff and other patients. On his last admission, a thorough history and diagnostic workup revealed borderline personality disorder and confirmed the psychotic episodes. However, in the course of treatment, Ed disclosed that after his paranoid episode in Viet Nam he was offered the opportunity to return to the United States or to be assigned to the field. He chose to return to the United States. For years he felt he had let others down and engaged in bar fights whenever anyone challenged his masculinity. Following several months of therapy, he found himself feeling less pressured to fight and decided to continue treatment for the personality disorder as well as for his marital difficulties.

Treatment of stress disorders must take the entire clinical picture into account. The decision as to which clinical entity to pursue first will depend on the individual case. However, stress disorders can occur and be treated appropriately in concert with other disorders. The relationship of PTSD to other life experiences is complex; in each case there are many possibilities, and much remains to be learned about this subject though future research.

Repetition and Falsification

In therapy, a traumatic episode will be repeated several times. Careful attention to each repetition will reveal important shifts, new details, and new characters. The action first described clearly can become ambiguous with repetition.

Dick, an army squad leader, first described leaping from a helicopter under heavy fire. Glimpsing an armed figure to his right, he quickly turned and fired a burst at the North Vietnamese soldier. Later repetitions of the story revealed that the fire was not so intense, that the soldier Dick shot may have been an unarmed civilian, and that Dick had gone off on the assault eager to avenge the recent death of a buddy. Later still, Dick revealed his concern over having failed to properly cover that buddy during an ambush.

Further repetitions, then, invariably introduce ambiguity regarding the rightness of action, the choices open to the veteran, and the moral justification for behavior.

Sometimes veterans appear to fabricate traumatic combat episodes. While frequently seen as attempts to claim compensation, experienced observers are led to a different conclusion. PTSD and accompanying moral quandries of combat elicit sympathetic understanding from both veterans and civilians. Military service, and especially combat, elicit admiration and represent an undimmed badge of character and manhood. To have suffered as a result of one's combat experience is usually thought of as noble and respectable, whereas—even in *DSM-III*—"lesser" traumas rate only as adjustment disorders, with the implication of a less hardy character.

A mystique, therefore, has grown about legitimate combat trauma and the sympathetic understanding it elicits. Consequently, some veterans who desperately need sympathetic understanding will distort, exaggerate, or even fabricate traumatic combat episodes. Of course, their response to sympathy is hollow, for they know the truth. In addition, they are usually exposed as their experience is explored. Should this occur in therapy, the therapist can be especially helpful. An important task of the therapist is to make known that there is no hierarchy of suffering, that the pain and distress of nurses and of those in the rear not directly in combat can be as devastating as that of combat survivors.

One traumatic experience can also serve as a defense against an even more painful experience. In these cases, the revealed traumatic episode is incongruent with the presenting symptoms.

During initial interviews Roger, a former career Army infantryman, mentioned fears generated by thunderstorms and his impulse to hurt Vietnamese immigrants living near him. During later interviews, Roger broke down and cried while revealing an episode in which he was a machine gunner on a convoy. After an ambush, in which two vehicles in the convoy were blown up and several people were wounded, Roger caught a glimpse of a fleeing Vietnamese out of the corner of his eye. Quickly turning and firing a machine gun burst, he was horrified to discover he had shot a teenage Vietnamese boy, carrying soda pop to sell to the soldiers on the trucks. Troubled by dreams of the shooting, he frequently compared the boy to his own teenage son. Roger described how teasing about the incident by members of his unit led him to attack one of his fellow soldiers. Despite the intense affect associated with the revelation of these stories and repeated discussions of the incident, Roger's symptoms did not diminish.

Only much later did Roger's dreams reveal an earlier incident. During a thunderstorm Roger and a buddy were on guard duty. A battle began. Afraid of the storm and the intense fire, Roger stayed huddled in a bunker while his buddy attempted to return fire. When the buddy took a round straight through the face and fell back on top of him, Roger felt relieved to be alone and guilty over his own fears and "cowardice."

In this case the original presentation—fears about thunderstorms and an eagerness to seek revenge on Vietnamese—did not match with the revealed traumatic episode of killing the boy. Only the later revelation of the earlier failure to act during an assault made understandable the impulse to act during the convoy ambush, to kill disparaging buddies, and currently to seek revenge against Vietnamese. It also made clear why there was no reduction in symptom intensity after the revelation and exploration of the first described incident, which turned out to be a cover story.

Affective Articulation

Despite the intensity of affective response as reflected in anger and rage, the range of emotions available to veterans is often quite limited. In spite of pain and extreme sensitivity to criticism, the only emotion in the veteran's repertoire is anger. Rage becomes a mechanism to cover hurt, guilt, shame, doubt, vulnerability, intimacy, and even pride. It serves to slam the door on conscious self-blame, as blame is directed at someone else. The task of articulating and learning to express a range of emotions is a crucial part of the therapy.

For many veterans, the first step is simply recognizing that they feel. Even in the midst of anger, troubled veterans may be unaware that this constitutes a feeling. Identification of an emotion frequently leads to a rejection of it: "I'm not supposed to be angry. My wife tells me anger is my problem."

The veteran's next step involves learning to tolerate these emotions. As the veteran learns to distinguish varieties of affect, anger is sorted into irritation, rage, betrayal, contempt, envy, and righteousness. By discriminating shades of emotion, the veteran learns to exercise control through the process of naming and understanding. From there, complicated relationships among feelings may be identified: "Oh, at work you feel frustrated and you get angry. At the V.A. you feel dismissed and insignificant; you get irritated at the wait and your lack of power and you find someone to blow up at."

Eventually, this exploration of feelings and behavior leads to appreciation of tenderness. Vulnerability, hurt, guilt, affection, love, and pain are recognized. Generally, after uncovering critical traumatic episodes, fears, grief, and vulnerability come into full awareness. Avoided up to that point, the feelings suddenly emerge. The danger now is that the veteran, fearful of the intensity with which these emotions have erupted, will flee from treatment.

Consequently, as affects are articulated, the veteran must be alerted to expect the emergence of long-dormant emotions and reassured that self-control is still possible. Strategies for control are discussed, and the veteran will not be overwhelmed.

Animating Action and the Survivor Mission

Almost from the moment they enter treatment, veterans express a desire to help others, to spread the word about PTSD, to assist other veterans. Lifton (23) has written eloquently about the transformation of lacerating, incapacitating guilt into such an animating force. The process of reparation and the survivor mission adopted by Viet Nam veterans represents such a force, and as such it is a direct and systematic effort at reparation in the present for what was done in the past.

Many veterans come into therapy already involved in some process of reparation. A pilot who sprayed agent orange in Viet Nam now works as a chemical safety officer, trying to prevent toxic accidents. A soldier who left the child of a brief liaison back in Viet Nam now works to secure the release of such mixed-race children.

Such behavior has two major drawbacks. First, there is no awareness of the motivation on the veteran's part. This renders the behavior ineffective in resolving traumatic conflict. Second, since the behavior usually produces no resolution, anger, rage, and accusations dominate the veteran's thoughts and affective life. An example of how this prevents successful reparation concerns the veteran who attempted to gain the release of Vietnamese orphans. He ends up raging at the U.S. and Vietnamese governments and cannot elicit their cooperation.

One of the most powerful scenes in the 1984 film *Ghandi* shows a confrontation between Ghandi and a Hindu who had killed a Moslem child during ethnic rioting. Gazing straight into his eyes, Ghandi tells the Hindu man to go out and find a Moslem orphan and raise him as his own child, but in the Moslem faith. The process of reparation and the survivor mission adopted by Viet Nam veterans takes precisely this form. The survivor mission embodies a direct and systematic reparation in the present for what was done in the past.

Veterans entering treatment are reluctant to wait for clarification in the recovery process of exactly what act they wish to repair and precisely what form such reparation might take. Rather than discourage attempts at action and repair, the therapist should explore them, explore the impulses behind them, and eventually explore traumatic episodes which undergird the veteran's system of adaptation.

When therapy has progressed to a point where critical issues of war have been identified and their influence on current behavior understood, animating action may be planned. The therapist does not plan the survivor mission. Under gentle questioning, the veteran begins to identify unfinished business related to the trauma. There may be a letter the veteran has always wanted to write, or perhaps a visit to the family or grave of a buddy who was killed in Viet Nam. Beginning the task of exploring such current loose ends makes a powerful connection between the lost past and the present. Suddenly, lacerating guilt over what can never be changed or undone can be transformed by present action. The veteran realizes that there are things that can be done now and meaningful contributions that he or she can make.

When Sy, the former member of the Marine military police described earlier, became aware of the source of his difficulty, he began his own process of reparation. He made a trip to Washington to visit the Vietnam Veterans Memorial and to pay his respects to the men who died in the fateful incident. He began to locate their home towns and visit, one by one, their grave sites. He then contacted some of the families to see if there were ways local veterans groups could be of assistance. Finally, he left his job as a police officer and began a job as a social worker, working especially with Viet Nam veterans in the prison system. He found the work frustrating, but exhilarating and rewarding. His bouts with depression and anxiety ended, and he began renewing personal friendships and dating relationships.

For most traumatized veterans, initiation of an appropriate survivor mission is the primary means of resolving PTSD. Doubt and guilt are transformed into action, integrity is enhanced, positive values are established and promoted, and an avenue is created to allow maturation and full participation by veterans in the lives of their communities.

REFERENCES

1. Capps WH: The Unfinished War: Viet Nam and the American Conscience. Boston, Beacon Press, 1982

2. Kolb LC: Gross stress reactions, in Modern Clinical Psychiatry, 8th ed. New York, Saunders Co, 1977

3. Keane TM, Kaloupek DG: Imaginal flooding in the treatment of a posttraumatic stress disorder. J Consult Clin Psychol 50:138–140, 1982

4. Haley SA: When the patient reports atrocities. Arch Gen Psychiatry 30:191–196, 1974

5. Kadushin C: Friendship and stress reactions, in Legacies of Viet Nam: Comparative Adjustment of Veterans and Their Peers. Edited by Egendorf A, Kadushin C, Laufer RS, et al. Washington, DC, U.S. Govenment Printing Office, 1981

6. Horowitz MJ: Stress Response Syndromes. New York, Jason Aronson, 1976

7. Horiwitz MJ, Zilberg N: Regressive alterations in self concept. Am J Psychiatry 140:284–289, 1983

8. Janet P: Les actes inconscients et la memoire pendant le somnambulisme. Revue Philosophique 25:238–279, 1888

9. Hilgard ER: Divided Consciousness: Multiple Controls in Human Thought and Action. New York, John Wiley & Sons, 1977

10. Smith JR, Parson ER, Haley SA: On health and disorder in Viet Nam veterans: an invited commentary. Am J Orthopsychiatry 53:27–33, 1983

11. Smith JR, Roth S: A Review of One Hundred and Twenty Years of the Psychological Literature on Reactions to Combat from the Civil War through the Viet Nam War: 1860–1980. Unpublished manuscript, Duke University, February 1981

12. Williams T: Post-Traumatic Stress Disorder Intake Evaluation. Unpublished manuscript. Indianapolis, Disabled American Veterans, 1982

13. Green BL, Grace MC, Lindy JD: Prediction of delayed stress after Viet

Nam: a pilot study. Paper presented at the First National Conference on PTSD. Cincinnati, Ohio, October 1982

14. Monahan J (ed): Who Is the Client: The Ethics of Psychological Intervention in the Criminal Justice System. Washington, DC, American Psychological Association, 1980

15. Smith JR: Personal responsibility in post-traumatic stress reactions. Psychiatric Annals 12:1021–1030, 1982

16. Smith JR: Veterans and combat: toward a model of the stress recovery process. Paper prepared for the Readjustment Counseling Service. Brecksville, Ohio, V.A. Medical Center, 1981

17. Horowitz MJ: Phase oriented treatment of stress response syndromes. Am J Psychother 27:508–516, 1973

18. Hogben GL, Cornfield RB: Treatment of traumatic war neurosis with phenelzine. Arch Gen Psychiatry 38:440–445, 1981

19. Friedman MJ: Post Viet Nam syndrome: recognition and treatment. Psychosomatics 11:931–943, 1981

20. Kolb LC, Burris BC, Griffith S: Propranolol and clonidine in the treatment of chronic post-traumatic stress disorders of war. Paper presented at the Annual Meeting of the America Psychiatric Association, New York, 1983

21. Brende JO, Benedict BD: The Viet Nam combat delayed stress response syndrome: hypnotherapy of "dissociative symptoms." Am J Clin Hypn 23:34–40, 1980

22. Collier D, Miller M: Paradoxical effects of relaxation therapy in PTSD. Paper presented at Operation Outreach Training. Portland, Ore, V.A. Medical Center, 1982

23. Lifton RJ: Home from the War. New York, Simon & Schuster, 1973

8

Rap Groups and Group Therapy for Viet Nam Veterans

John Russell Smith, M.A.

8

Just what is a rap group? The Viet Nam veterans' rap group has been defined ambiguously. The term *rap group* is applied loosely to several forms of therapy groups: leaderless groups, didactic groups, open and closed groups, topic-centered groups, client-focused ("hot seat") groups, free-floating groups, and Yalom-styled groups (1). Some groups have been very successful therapeutically, some benign but ineffective, some confused, and some downright pathological in their effects. This inconsistency has sparked criticism of the rap group concept by some observers (2, 3).

It is significant that in the midst of such diversity, expert clinicians and facilitators have agreed on the goals and characteristics of therapeutically effective rap groups (4–8). This effective rap group model accurately describes a range of self-help, peer support groups that have evolved for survivors of many different kinds of trauma (9). These groups have common characteristics in their history and process, as well as in the themes they explore.

Rap groups evolved as did groups for families of suicide victims and other survivors. Initially, therapists who had not had actual survival experience themselves attempted to run them as traditional therapy groups. These groups failed when survivors resisted being "treated." Other groups, such as Twice Born Men in San Francisco, were created by the survivors themselves without therapist involvement. Intensely

I want to thank Drs. Robert Jay Lifton, Chaim Shatan, Florence Pincus, Arthur Egendorf, and Martin Lakin for the early lessons they gave me. I also want to thank Dr. Stephen Frye, Timothy Wackerhagen, Dr. Arthur S. Blank, Jr., Shad Meshad, M.S.W., and the staffs of all the Vet Centers across the country for the privilege of working with them and the veterans. To Ann Sethness, I am indebted for many hours of rereading and comments on drafts of this chapter.

The views expressed in this chapter are solely those of the author and may not reflect the views of the Veterans Administration.

cathartic, they lacked therapeutic guidance and formal attention to group process.

In 1970, the evolution of the original Viet Nam Veterans Against the War rap groups unknowingly melded both of these group forms. Sensitive clinicians, like Robert Jay Lifton, M.D., Chaim Shatan, M.D., and Florence Pincus, M.S.S., joined with Viet Nam veterans such as Arthur Egendorf and Jan Barry to create a forum to constructively address the distress they all saw in themselves and other veterans. The clinicians brought therapeutic expertise and openness to the amalgam of often contradictory war attitudes, both in themselves and in the veterans. The veteran leaders brought to the group a developing clinical awareness and fierce adherence to the reality and personal impact of their war experience. This critical interaction combined, in a balance, the poles of clinical expertise and survivor experience. The result was more powerful than either alone. And, since then, this group model has proven useful for many types of trauma survivors.

Rap groups, like other survivor groups, encourage the bonding of survivors of similar traumatic events for therapeutic purpose. Survivors implicitly know that their reactions to the trauma are different than their reactions to previous "normal" events. The reactions and suggestions of others who have not experienced the traumatic events often confirm in the survivors a covert feeling that they are "abnormal." Therefore, survivors often look to people who have experienced the same or a similar catastrophe for validation and "normalization" of their response (9). Through such interaction they confirm that their response is, in fact, a normal response to an extraordinary event.

A recent longitudinal study of therapy with survivors of the Beverly Hills Supper Club fire found that the best results were achieved by experienced clinicians who had been exposed to catastrophe themselves (10). These results confirmed the intuitive wisdom of survivors in their help-seeking behavior. The rap group process allows for survivor behaviors and feelings to become group norms, to be marshalled for therapeutic ends.

However, there is a pitfall: the forces marshalled in this norming process can just as easily serve destructive as therapeutic ends.

The potential power of these marshalled forces has led many V.A. therapists to be concerned about rap groups. On several occasions, on hospital units where therapists brought patients with post-traumatic stress disorder together, rap groups were created. Soon the ward staffs would be stunned and terrified to see this critical mass of veterans suddenly stirring each other up, asserting control over the ward, and terrorizing the therapists and the hospital population.

Such experiences have led some therapists to disavow the rap group and to institute rigid controls on therapy groups (2, 3). Such situations underscore the importance of recognizing the liabilities, as well as the benefits, of rap groups and the need for special care when mobilizing such powerful psychic forces.

This chapter continues with a discussion of the stress recovery process as it relates to rap groups, the ways in which rap groups differ from other therapy groups, and the group process in rap groups and modified rap groups. Finally, some of the structures which define effective rap groups will be described.

RAP GROUPS AND THE RECOVERY PROCESS

A rap group is a peer group, a therapeutic means for the exposition, exploration, transformation, and resolution of undigested traumatic experience. The assumption at the heart of the rap group process is that a tension exists in a survivor between unresolved, traumatic experience and his or her "normal" expectations. Furthermore, the tension of this variance manifests itself in current cognitive and behavioral problems. The rap group model further assumes that exploration and discussion of current and past experience in a group setting with veteran peers can significantly contribute to resolving past and present difficulties (8, 11).

The trained group facilitator will see little formal distinction between the principles of group process as observed in a well-run rap group and a Yalom-style psychotherapy group. However, the intensity of the interactions, the potential for destructive subversion, and the heightened demands on the therapist do distinguish the rap group.

Like other therapy groups, rap groups operate on the premise that change must start with the individual even though others may have contributed to the individual's problem. But in other therapy groups, there is often only token recognition that something is wrong with the world while concern focuses mostly on the individual's maladaptive behavior. Rap groups recognize implicitly that forces beyond the individual—families, societal values, leaders, and even nations—may have major responsibility for the shaping of traumatic events. Rap groups differ in their fundamental view of the necessity of the group's scrutiny of the outside world. For only by appropriate recognition and acknowledgment of the role of others may the rap group create a climate in which the group can reformulate a value system against which individual veterans may accurately reappraise, evaluate, and take appropriate responsibility for their actions in the traumatic situation and since.

War is by nature an *extraordinary* human experience. It requires of its participants deeds that often violate important civilian norms. Societies temper this violation by erecting boundaries, establishing rules of war, and providing for soldiers and veterans a sense of justification and mission. Nevertheless, aspects of war experience can develop at odds with the expectations that nations and participants possess for themselves. When war experience conflicts with cherished notions of honor and integrity, symptoms then result in nations and individuals. For example, Laufer et al. (12) note that symptoms of stress response are intensified in the wake of exposure to, or participation in, war atrocities.

For many veterans, the tapestry of normal meaning and values is unravelled by the events of war. Viet Nam veterans have to find meaning for powerful personal experiences and have to acknowledge responsibility for their acts, without societal sanction and support to justify what was done. A special characteristic of rap groups is that they provide the forum in which the veterans' value system and sense of meaning can be refashioned. A new sense of self can develop and symptoms wane.

Veterans are often forced by a more idealistic sense of values shaped prior to the war to condemn themselves. Alternatively, some veterans employ denial; they assert only their integrity and patriotism and deny those aspects of their experience that might be incongruous with an heroic stance or those earlier standards. Rap groups enable participants, both members and therapists, to be true to their experiences of war; to weave a new, collective tapestry of meaning and value; to retain integrity; and to understand and take responsibility for their personal behavior in and after the war.

Some Viet Nam veterans have rigid and stereotyped attitudes toward their war experience and often seem to repeat endlessly the same stories without apparent therapeutic value or resolution. In response, inexperienced therapists and other "objective observers" frequently encourage patients to "forget it," "put it behind you," or attempt to explain it away rationally. But the veteran resists. The experienced rap group facilitator knows that the stereotyped story is frequently an attempt to resolve ambiguous questions of responsibility for the veteran's actions (13). Simple dismissals or assertions of understanding meet with objection from the veteran who directly, or by repetition, is asserting that there is more to the experience that needs to be resolved.

Consider the reflections of this helicopter pilot who damaged his tail rotor in an assault landing and barely missed losing his crew and passengers:

The original damage estimate was $10,000, later raised to $100,000. The Accident Board decided the cause was extreme, dusty conditions. They had let me off the hook. The usual verdict was pilot error. I mean if the rotor blades came off in flight the pilot was posthumously charged with failure to preflight the ship properly. . . . If you tumble down the side of a mountain while trying to land on a pinnacle under fire, it was pilot error. There was usually no other conclusion. So the Board was generous when it decided the accident was due to extreme, dusty conditions. But guess what I thought. . .the pilot was in error. (14, p. 181)

In such ambiguous questions of blame, in which the burden of responsibility seems to shift between self and others, lies the key to linking current difficulties, prewar personality, and war trauma.

All current problems in Viet Nam veterans are not the result of the Viet Nam War. But the stress recovery process shows that obsession with the past, insistence on personal responsibility or nonculpability, and bizarre and unexplained current behavior are often connected to unresolved past trauma. When current solutions fail, the veteran who comes to a rap group finds among his peers a willingness to explore possible links between present and past. At the same time, the rap group therapist must be alert and responsive to the issues of control and loss of control explored in Chapter 7.

In rap groups, the possible link between a troubling episode (or a seemingly trivial one about which the veteran seems obsessed) and the veteran's current distress is explored. By promoting discussion about the sometimes ambiguous nature of action in combat—about honor, pride, guilt, and anger—the peer group frames the veteran's dilemma. Rather than repress the painful memory, the veteran learns to recognize his or her dilemma and to live with it.

With his rap group buddies, a veteran can transform rigid and inflexible expectations that prevent recognition and acceptance of his past behavior. After this transformation, the group encourages the veteran in a survivor mission that converts guilt and a distorted sense of personal responsibility from a debilitating curse into an activating force. This process enhances the veteran's sense of personal meaning and integrity.

Rap groups provide a forum in which veterans who share personal history can examine and validate the reality of that experience and reformulate its meaning. By examining individual actions, which contrast with otherwise courageous behavior, and discrepancies in harsh self-judgments, rap group members soften calcified judgments of their own and others' guilt. From the tattered remnants of integrity and values, survivor participants forge a new world view, a redefined sense of self, and a renewed sense of personal mission.

TYPES OF GROUPS

Having described rap groups in general, the following sections will critically examine a variety of therapy groups and explore those which together constitute the rap group genus.

Open Groups

The primary work of the rap group involves building trust among members who then explore the relationship between traumatic experience and current problems. Exploration of the general Viet Nam experience occurs in the first few meetings of a rap group. As the group moves on to deal with current problems, Viet Nam emerges only in the context of specific, painful memories triggered by discussion of current issues.

When an open group is conducted on an ongoing basis, several problems emerge that threaten the integrity, continuity, and process of the group. Introduction of new members inhibits the evolution of group trust, camaraderie, and intimacy and prevents deep exploration of traumatic experience. The need to initiate new members forces the group to repeatedly discuss Viet Nam experiences in preliminary ways, and the group must forever wait for each new member to "catch up" before it can move on.

In addition, the open format relaxes the demands for attendance and participation by the group members. The potential for commitment by the members to the group, for observations of each other, and for give and take—the basis of the rap group process—all diminish in the open group. With constant changes in composition and no strong commitment, the group never gells, never grows, and the potential for the more destructive forces to emerge increases.

Having commented on the limited usefulness of open membership groups, it must be recognized that the open group format may arise spontaneously. Sometimes it plays a useful role in providing information and as a setting for beginning exploration. This function of an open group will be further discussed below.

Leaderless Groups

Leaderless groups have little usefulness for Viet Nam veterans because sidetracking of the group is foreordained. Every rap group needs a leader experienced in group process and familiar with the Viet

Nam experience. The leader must monitor powerful group forces and act to assist the group in controlling destructive or stagnating impulses.

Without someone designated and accepted as leader, the destructive forces of the group have no formal check. Everyone is free to play participant. Attention to process, tensions, or psychological damage happens only on a haphazard basis and disintegration occurs.

In rap groups with leaders, when the facilitators fail to confront the process issues, a leaderless situation evolves unplanned. By default, leadership passes to one of the group members. For example, in one group some powerful group members decided to exclude all noncombat members. Soon the group was composed exclusively of combat veterans, and members began topping each other with stories of their kills. The group leader, a veteran who harbored lingering questions about his own combat credentials, was reluctant to confront the group and risk incurring its wrath. Only when an outside observer joined a group session did the focus shift. The observer noted that the group did not discuss the happy, the sad, the painful, and the intimate aspects of combat. This observation reoriented the group, and it began to discuss a range of relevant issues.

It is not enough for a rap group leader to listen to veterans. The leader must put himself or herself on the line to challenge inappropriate group process. Frequently, facilitators become too identified with their veteran clients and fail to confront the group on significant issues.

Even otherwise excellent facilitators sometimes neglect to challenge inappropriate group process. Some facilitators who are veterans have not sorted out their own residue from combat. Rather than confront the group and risk its wrath, the facilitator lets the issue of combat bravado slide by. Failure to challenge inappropriate group process can also result when former combat veterans want to limit the group's membership to combat veterans only. Combat can become a means to avoid more intimate topics, which involve risk of vulnerability. Chaplains and former military mental health professionals, other noncombat personnel unsure of their own "combat" credentials, and professionals who avoided serving in the war can also be trapped by this issue. Rather than risk confrontation over their role in the war, their student deferment, their lack of combat experience, or their guilt over escaping the draft as a woman, they fail to confront the process, and the group becomes leaderless.

It is these demands and the personal vulnerability risked that causes some facilitators to decline rap group participation or to defeat the rap group process by narrowly circumscribing its time, its topics, or its challenges to the leaders. All group leaders fail at times; therapeutic courage lies in modeling the same vulnerability asked of the patients.

Client-Centered "Hot Seat" Groups

The client-centered "hot seat" group is often described as a rap group. In this group, each week one member is designated to occupy the "hot seat," and the group focuses on that veteran and his or her problems. In other respects, the structure and intent of these groups is not very different from what is described as a typical rap group. The advantage of this format is that it solves the potential problems of silence and inactive participation. Silent or reluctant members eventually have their day on the "hot seat." And there is no question about on whom to focus. Reluctance to talk is overcome by a battery of questions about why the veteran is silent.

Another advantage of this client-centered group is that it can help restrict irrelevant discussions. The repetitive stories and tailgating discussed below can be controlled.

These groups suffer from the artificial manner in which topics and the member's concerns are brought into focus. In regular rap groups, the focus is on pressing concerns that are stimulated by current difficulties and memories. Individual members control the timing of exploration and sharing of reactions. The leader or other group members may comment on facial reactions, body language, or even silence, but the choice of disclosure is up to the member.

The "hot seat" format can produce too rigid a set of expectations. Certain kinds of combat, certain lingering impulses, and particular types of current problems are seen as the "real stuff" and distort a more open group process. "Hot seat" group leaders have described clients who have fabricated combat histories or distorted their military background only to be subsequently found out. Indeed, the climate of these groups, while of help to some, may pressure others to distort their experiences to gain acceptance. In addition, this group climate can provide a cover for the group and its leaders, enabling them to avoid painful topics not fully practiced and rehearsed.

Topic-Centered Groups

As with "hot seat" groups, topic-centered groups are an attempt to better structure discussion. The leader or the group members select specific topics for discussion. By focusing sequentially on the significant topics, a group can systematically cover the major issues that veterans with stress-related problems need to address.

These groups can be very useful as informational or initial exploratory groups. However, as a definitive rap group experience, they are too limiting. Rap group discussions should be closely tied to current and immediate concerns of the members. The needs of the moment should determine what the group addresses. If the group process is well understood by the leaders, the members can be helped to address all significant topics and current conflicts. Questions of any member will be immediate and treated in a manner which is therapeutic for all participants.

The climate in topic-centered groups, like that in "hot seat" groups, can communicate expectations that only certain topics, reactions, or attitudes are legitimate subjects for the group. In a fully effective group, each client should feel that anything can be addressed and considered, no matter how violent, how horrible, how scary, how cowardly, or how seemingly trivial.

LEVELS OF RAP GROUPS

There are three levels of rap group experience. Each level is characterized by different goals and purposes. Many difficulties encountered by rap group leaders result from inattention to these distinctions among levels.

The Level I Group: The Informational or Introductory Group

The introductory group may take many forms, ranging from informal discussion among veterans over coffee at a weekend reserve meeting to a more structured PTSD seminar or a topic- or issue-oriented discussion group on the John Wayne image or the experience of black veterans. These groups are characterized by their openness, minimal structure, focus on identification of unresolved issues related to Viet Nam, and lack of formal therapeutic goals. This is not to say that such groups can have no therapeutic value. Rather, the level of involvement and commitment, the minimal expectation of therapeutic value, the open and mixed membership, and the lack of clear therapeutic group structure differentiate these groups from the other levels of rap group experience.

Most veterans engage the stress recovery process on their own in this fashion. They think, discuss, ponder, argue, read, write, and reflect about their experience at their own pace and use peer group discussion informally as they need it. Nevertheless, such informal group experiences do carry potential risks when they are the sole alternative to more structured therapy for stress disorders. In the treatment of impairment from stress disorders, more careful attention to rap group process is necessary to maximize the benefits and avoid the more troublesome risks.

Introductory groups help veterans by conveying information about the stress process and the links between current problems and unresolved traumatic war experience. Since the therapeutic purpose is restricted, demands concerning participation and attendance are flexible. Perhaps of greatest importance, these groups open an avenue for potential rap group participants to identify the relevant issues and come to know the means to move on to more deeply therapeutic rap groups. They also provide an opportunity for the group facilitator to evaluate the need and readiness of a potential candidate for more intensive group work.

The Level II Group: The Initial Working Rap Group

The initial working rap group brings together a group of veterans for a significant, but specified, period of time. It initiates the focused exploration of past war experience in relation to current life. This type of group is the most common form of rap group.

Criteria. In this form of rap group, the participants need to know what to expect, what is required of them, and what will be offered to them. The facilitator needs to know the capacity and the readiness of each candidate to engage in the rap group process. (For further discussion of the differential effectiveness of individual and group psychotherapy, and criteria for the use of the group approach with brief stress reactions, see Horowitz and Marmar [15].)

The following major criteria are used for admission to an initial working rap group:

1. Demonstrated willingness and ability to share aspects of one's current and past experience;
2. The identification of a current problem or unresolved issue amenable to group intervention;
3. The ability to share group time and to let others speak and respond;
4. The willingness to consider and to share in the group's reactions to the process; and
5. Sufficient social supports and backup for the veteran to be able to

tolerate the rigors of the group process and the intervals between meetings. Such supports may be provided in the community, a halfway house, or on an inpatient unit.

Frequently, therapists will encounter veterans who are in need of stress treatment but have other immediately pressing or overwhelming difficulties. In such cases, the group alone cannot adequately address these problems. Participation in a rap group must then become secondary to individual therapy, day hospital, inpatient treatment, or a substance abuse program until the veteran's controls, social supports, and ability to tolerate the group process have been sufficiently enhanced.

As implied in the criteria above, the facilitator must initially assess each veteran's social supports; current crises; recent history of anger, violence, or involvement with weapons; and use of drugs and alcohol. Even if these problems are secondary to the stress reactions, they need to be brought under some control before rap group treatment can be effective. Failure by the facilitator to focus on these criteria and attend to these issues is the most frequent cause of rap group casualties. For veterans without such preparation, the process is liable to undermine tenuous controls and precipitate an emotional or behavioral crisis.

The criteria also suggest that veterans with thought disorders, or those who otherwise lack the ability to listen adequately, are poor rap group candidates, because they cannot share in a meaningful way with the group. For example, one veteran with a thought disorder joined an open group. During a crisis, while the leader attempted to calm another group member "charged up" with the impulse to kill his wife, this psychotic veteran interrupted, free associated, and crippled the group that evening.

Membership. Among veterans who meet the above criteria for admission to a working rap group, self-determined distinctions are made in several ways. Distinctions include veterans and nonveterans, combat and noncombat veterans, officers and enlisted men. Veterans will also divide as blacks, Hispanics, whites, native Americans, or Pacific Islanders; as men or women; as Viet Nam, World War II, Korea, or Lebanon veterans; as POWs or Airborne. These distinctions are at once sources of trust and mistrust, issues of identity, and means of avoiding vulnerability and underlying war-related difficulties. While all of these differences may contribute to initial mistrust and tensions in a rap group, there is no hard rule on structuring group membership. The primary determinant is the degree of confidence and experience the group leader has in addressing and bridging members' differences in the beginning weeks of a group. After years of experience, some rap group leaders can take any mixture of clients and successfully synthesize an effective group. Less experienced leaders find the chances of success increased in a more homogeneous group.

It is the leader's responsibility to select members with whom he or she can work. Significant differences among members in an introductory group may be less important than in a working rap group. However, with an especially troubled set of veterans, it may be helpful to minimize differences in the group's membership. In all cases, though, the leaders must be willing to risk confronting members' differences and the powerful feelings these engender as they arise in the rap group process. Otherwise, the group perpetuates the problems it intends to cure.

Restricting membership of the initial working rap group is more appropriate than in a long-term group. In the initial group, members should face some of their differences directly, but diversity should not foreclose the development of group cohesion. As will be described below, while members of a long-term group may have many diverse characteristics, they have all honed their empathic skills in an initial working group. This constitutes a powerful unifying trait.

Preliminary Work. Once the facilitator has established that a candidate would be an appropriate group member, that individual needs to be prepared for what will be expected of him and what he may expect from others. The facilitator meets with the candidate to explain expectations of attendance, participation, confidentiality, and responsibility to the group. General expectations, which eventually become the informal ground rules of the group, are reviewed with the candidate and agreed upon. It is important to establish understanding and agreement about control of weapons, drugs, alcohol, and physical violence toward group members.

At this time, the leader should stress the importance to the group process of bringing private reactions to the group—as well as out of group contacts with other members—into group discussion.

These preliminary meetings should convey the expectation that the primary work of the group occurs between members. It is the feedback they give to and receive from each other that makes the group effective. The expectation must be reinforced that answers lie within themselves, not with the leaders.

Before the start of the group, the establishment of clear expectations, and the delineation of acceptable and unacceptable behavior in the group, facilitate the creation of group norms later. It also helps reduce the necessity for rigid leadership and the later imposition of rules by the leader.

Group norms enable subsequent behavioral violations to be used as part of the group process. When a veteran comes in drunk or high or misses a meeting, he is confronted, not by the leader, but by the other group members. Their disappointment over his inability to contribute or reflect adequately on their problems becomes the focus. He is then answerable to the group, not to the leader or to some abstract rule.

Preliminary meetings are also important opportunities to anticipate reactions to the rap group process. For example, the candidate is advised in advance that emotionally charged topics are likely to be brought up, discussed, and resolved. More importantly, the prospective member must know that in the wake of such powerful discussions, veterans sometimes feel like fleeing and not attending group for several sessions. By anticipating such reactions, later crises are modulated. By helping a veteran understand his reactions in advance, the leader and the group begin to normalize the process and offer alternative means of using group members and leaders, as well as the group process, to weather these expected storms.

The Opening Meeting. The initial working rap group has closed membership, is time-limited, and is designed to open exploration for its members. The principles which govern this type of group apply equally well to the initial weeks of an open-ended group.

The first session of an initial rap group is an anxious and exciting time. Clients and leaders are eager and apprehensive: eager for the comradeship and sharing, and apprehensive about the exploration of long-guarded experiences. Introductions center on one's branch of service, unit, and time of service in Viet Nam; one's current status; and the issues that bring each veteran to the group. Good-natured bantering and comments accompany these introductions. Initial bonding begins with identification as veterans single out those other group members with similar war experiences or common current problems.

The role of the facilitator is especially important in setting the tone in the opening moments. The group forces bent to therapeutic purposes have an equal capacity to derail the process and for destructiveness. For example, one group began with a combat veteran pulling a ski mask over his face and feigning a holdup. Another group began with members citing the number of their kills, establishing a macho hierarchy, and driving out the noncombat veterans. The creation of a "bad" atmosphere can serve to test therapists and what they can handle. It also shields veterans from their fears of vulnerability by causing others to feel afraid. The therapists' willingness to point this process out early on—and to serve as models of vulnerability and gentle strength—will set the tone for the weeks to come.

Disclosure of personal war experience and motivation for group membership is encouraged. The facilitators' own disclosures are critical to setting the tone. Brief, straightforward disclosures of the leaders' own veteran or nonveteran experiences, and of their own motivation for being in the group, acknowledges that the issues at hand are broader than individual psychopathology. It also demonstrates that the issues involve the therapists as well as the members, while reinforcing the therapeutic purpose of the group. Ideally, the therapists serve as guides and are not distant, aloof, or overly invested. The extreme posture of the aloof Tavistock leader will not facilitate the rap group process, but equally disturbing to the process is the overly invested therapist who is working out his or her own concerns about Viet Nam and identifications with the veterans. The fate of the therapist who uses the group to explore his or her own conflicts and pain is illustrated by the story of Bill.

> Bill was coleading his first rap group. He came from an Army family and had served in the Army during the Viet Nam War, but he had never gone to Viet Nam. Now, armed with a counseling degree, he wanted to work with veterans. Opening up the first meeting, he launched into a lengthy discussion of his guilt and sense of loss over not having gone to Viet Nam. The first session of the group became a therapy session for him, with the group finally forgiving him for not having gone to Viet Nam. Despite his growth and demonstrable effectiveness in the 12-week group, Bill's interest waned afterwards, and he ceased his work with veterans.

The leaders should acknowledge their reactions, "own" their own motivations, yet convey the sense that they will attend to the process, pass along observations, and permit the group to choose its course knowingly.

Along with the initial credentialing and identification process begins exploration. Group members are asked about current problems and to discuss aspects of their military experience that they still find unsettled and unsettling. Although guarded, many members will talk. One or two may immediately plunge into painful material and bring the group to its first opportunity for insight.

The initial response to such early revelation is often *tailgating*. As one veteran describes a troubling experience, it will trigger recollections in another member who feels compelled to immediately press his story on the group. Others follow sequentially. Rapid-fire movement from story to story precludes exploration of the pain of any one member. The leader's responsibility is to gently remind the group of the unfinished business of issues raised by the first member who spoke. If the members are reluctant to respond, it is important that the leader point out concrete examples of the shifts away from pain and feelings of vulnerability.

If possible, this last intervention best includes questions or comments on the reactions of group members as they listen. Wetness in the eyes of one, a nod from another, a quick look of disgust, or a roll of the eyes provide the leader the opening to focus on reaction to an earlier revelation. By using the members' behavior, the leader reminds the group that the members' reactions are central to the process and reinforces the realization that the themes are theirs, not some that are concocted by the therapist. By helping the group identify important emerging themes, by tagging significant reactions that were rushed past, and by following up with a silent member, the group leader establishes the tone and the models for a successful rap group.

Some rap group facilitators use these opening moments to comment on and teach the group about PTSD, its symptoms, and the stress process. It is more effective to let the group develop this knowledge from the revelations of its members. However, the leader does assist the group in defining the themes as they emerge. The observations made should be tentative or formulated as a question for the group to ponder, rather than as a statement of fact.

During this initial period and in the following weeks, themes of guilt, grief, betrayal, pride, respect, anger, integrity, isolation, control, rage, frustration, and confusion will emerge. (For an additional discussion of the themes and topics of the rap group, see Chapter 7 and Scurfield et al. [8].) If a group member introduces powerful and heavy material right away in an initial session, respectful silence among other members should be encouraged. Anticipation and discussion of the members' possible responses to the powerful material—manifested in desires to flee, avoid talking, or stay away from meetings—will help preclude early casualties or dissolution of the group. As always, anticipating and discussing possible responses helps temper later reactions. In addition, many members must relearn respect, empathy, and concern when faced with another's pain.

In an initial group, or during the early weeks of an open-ended group, intervention focuses on encouraging members to understand not only content but group process. During this early period, the leader is much more active as a model, inquiring about a veteran's story and noting other members' reactions, resistance, silence, and body language. Whatever the leader's own observation during the opening phase, the cue to appropriate intervention is the appearance of a similar reaction in others. By body language, an aside, a subtle phrase, or some other comment, members communicate their response. The leader's goal is to encourage group members to say what needs to be said. Therefore, the leader encourages others to make their reactions explicit; for example, "Hey, George! How do you feel about what Phil is saying? I see you've turned your back on him."

The entire life of a time-limited, initial rap group—and especially the early weeks—is characterized by unevenness of process. Intense and deep disclosure will alternate with silence and reluctance as the group develops a pace and style. Important material is often dropped like a bomb in the closing minutes of a meeting. The leader must interpret such behavior and label it for the group to discuss.

Subsequent Weeks: The Uncovering of Trauma. After the initial meeting period, resistance will stiffen. Challenges to the leaders, attacks on the Veterans Administration or military, posturing war stories, hostility to nonveterans, and questioning of the group process all signal attempts by members to limit the range of exploration. Avoidance of powerful affect may be reflected in efforts by group members and even the facilitator to interrupt, to talk the others out of their anger, or to otherwise deflect it. Some members will attempt to split cotherapists, often by flattering a therapist-veteran and attacking or denigrating a nonveteran therapist.

Veterans with significant PTSD-related problems often use anger and threats to back others off when they feel threatened or upset. Not surprisingly, they try this on facilitators and other group members. The anxiety they generate is what keeps many therapists from wanting to work with them. Other therapists respond by wanting to impose massive controls to keep the veterans in line. Failure to confront such anger leads to further escalation; the imposition of external controls may attenuate the frightening behavior in the group, but an increase in acting out outside the group is almost ensured.

Group members are accountable for the consequences of their actions, including the fears they generate. Those fears in family members are often what led veterans to seek treatment. An essential part of the treatment is to help group members recognize the impact of their behavior on others. It is essential to explore the impact and meaning of angry outbursts on each group member. The feelings of members concerning anger in themselves must also be explored and understood. An examination of alternative ways of expressing and manifesting the anger can be promoted. These methods are useful in diminishing resistance in the group and enhancing in each veteran a sense of self-control.

Because anger can seem so raw and so intense, even experienced therapists sometimes tend to blunt, deflect, or defer it. Some therapists do so by ruling anger out of bounds, others by limiting the length or number of group sessions. Both of these approaches fail to deal with a group member's anger adequately. Physical violence or destruction cannot be tolerated. A collective effort must be made to create a safe atmosphere in which to examine long-hidden pain. Violent or destructive actions threaten group safety for all members. However, rather than rule anger and its consequences out of bounds, it is preferable to use members' reactions and the impact on the group process as important reasons for addressing and containing the anger. Most anger and frustration in veterans with PTSD result from feeling "stuck" with rage. If the rage is expressed, the veteran fears losing control; if it is repressed or tolerated, it breeds corrosive resentment or escalation. What is most productive is some *verbal* expression accompanied by exploration of its meaning to the veteran. Directly addressing the anger, verbally exploring what might happen if the anger really were expressed, looking at its effect on the individual, listening to group members' observations, and examining earlier episodes and the detailed personal meaning of anger are all useful avenues for deepening the group's process while tackling such resistance.

For example, the veteran who began the first group meeting by feigning the holdup of the group was confronted with the impact of his behavior. He immediately became compliant, sheepishly remarking that it was the first time in years that anyone had stood up to him. Later he remarked on how out of control he felt: "I'm not like you. When someone hits my switch, I'm on. I can't turn it off." By standing up to him, the group helped give him some control he hadn't had in years.

The keys to handling anger, resistance, and repetitious war stories are usually not deferral or deflection but detailed explorations. Asking for clarification when the listener is confused, questioning ambiguous terms or sliding meanings (16), and requesting even peripheral detail and specifics in order to round out the picture all help to break the seemingly smooth and gapless cycle of anger and obscurity.

The critical task for the facilitator is to involve the group in the intervention. By helping members tackle issues, share a reaction, and identify a roadblock, the leader enlists the members as cotherapists for one another. This process also shifts the dynamic of the group to one of mutual responsibility.

In groups where a clinician has been attacked by a group member, the same pattern recurs. The clinician has set himself or herself up as the omniscient therapist. Interactions in this type of group are between the therapist and individual veterans, sequentially with each member. When one veteran gets angry or acts out, the group galvanizes behind the angry member, escalating his anger and promoting acting out. If the group is enlisted as allies for each other in healthy ways from the start, when an angry interchange starts the group can be enlisted to defuse and normalize the situation rather than to escalate it.

On Uncovering "The Trauma." The relationship between anger, current "problem" behaviors, the trauma of combat experience, and preexisting personality is often dramatically illustrated in early discussions in the group. Inevitably, it becomes clear that much of the anger directed at others also represents a displacement of rage against the self over behavior in Viet Nam.

> *Tom, a former Army infantryman, first presented as a tall, bearded, fierce-eyed veteran wearing a bush hat and fatigues. Overtly antiwar and angry at the government, he found himself unable to remain in college or at a job. He railed at the irrelevance of college and described frequent blowups at his bosses at work. Tom told of how he repeatedly quit jobs because of a violation by the employer of some principle that was important to him. As a critic of government policy toward veterans, he had become an effective although outspoken veterans' advocate. His initial outbursts in the group centered on the government, Army policy in Viet Nam, and the Veterans Administration.*

Like many veterans, Tom demonstrated some projection, paranoia, and antisocial behavior. Psychological testing revealed an MMPI profile suggesting a character disorder. Rather than challenge, confront, rationalize, or talk Tom out of his anger, the group encouraged Tom to channel his criticism into effective action.

Over several weeks, Tom considered his anger with the aid of the group. He began to recognize that his self-righteousness and his insistence on "mea culpas" from government officials often left potential allies unable to join him in achieving his goals. The group also invited Tom to reflect on the source of the intensity of his reactions.

Tom soon revealed to the group an episode he had suddenly "remembered" during the past week after having not thought about it for several years.

> *After several months of differences with his commanders over treatment of Vietnamese civilians, Tom stood by as other members of his unit toyed with a group of Vietnamese refugees at a garbage dump. The soldiers fired tear gas cannisters to corral the villagers. Then they shot at their feet, making them dance as in the old western movies. The actions were a retaliation for the soldiers' frustration over the villagers' apparent complicity in helping conceal a North Vietnamese tunnel complex. Tom felt dishonored by his failure to stand up to the commander and to honor his personal commitment to understand and protect civilians caught between two warring sides.*

What is striking about Tom's case is the adherence to the repeated pattern of a wartime action or failure that lies at the core of a veteran's current guilt and rage. Tom's subsequent history revealed actions, projections, anger, and reactions with the same apparent goal of undoing his presumed failure. Simultaneously, he shifted some of the burden of his guilt to others. Refutation of the projection of blame served only to highlight his perceived personal liability. Banished from awareness, it foreclosed examination of his conflict, forcing the sequelae to operate indirectly on him constantly.

The primary goal of the rap group process is the creation of an environment in which the revelation, exploration, conscious reexamination, and transformation of such trauma can take place. In the presence of supportive peers, a tightly bound and rigidly evaluated episode, locked firmly away, can surface and be gently reevaluated until finally the lacerating judgments are softened.

Criteria for Evaluating Initial Group Graduates. The initial rap group of 10 to 14 weeks is an introductory period. Lingering difficulties from Viet Nam will not be resolved in that period. Some veterans may learn important lessons from this group and continue the process of resolution on their own; others may want more assistance.

The therapist must decide whether the veteran wanting more help will best obtain it from a long-term rap group or another form of therapy. There are certain criteria which signal the readiness of a group member to continue. These criteria are supplementary to behavioral changes reported in the veteran's life outside the group.

Each successful group graduate will identify and clarify the outlines of one or more unresolved issues linking the present to the past. Some formerly confusing or ambiguous themes about the veteran's war experience will be clarified. Simplistic and dogmatic views should have softened, and more nuance will characterize the veteran's attitudes.

However, there is a way in which to judge the readiness of an initial rap group graduate to continue group therapy. If an initial rap group member has demonstrated the ability to hear out another member, to delay tailgating or starting in on his or her own story, and to question and explore the details and meaning of another veteran's difficulties, he or she is ready for a long-term (over six months) group.

Veterans who cannot listen, delay, or explore their peers' issues usually manifest some other significant problem. Most often, these veterans have a drug or alcohol problem which they have yet to get under some control. Chipping between meetings, coming high to a group session, or repeating a stereotyped, circumscribed revelation all characterize limited group involvement. Veterans with fabricated or embellished stories also fit in this category, as do veterans whose group interactions have been briefly intense and are then followed by silence or absence. These veterans are often out of control and in intense difficulty during the intervening periods between groups. All of these members probably would have been screened out of the group if this information had been known prior to the start of the group. These veterans' problems exceed the capacity of the group alone to address them. Reexamination of treatment strategy and consideration of individual therapy, substance abuse counseling, and family or vocational work lead to alternative, immediate actions. Later, participation in another initial rap group may be useful.

The Level III Group: The Long-Term Rap Group

Once a group of veterans has had a successful introductory experience, the veterans are then prepared for participation in a long-term rap group. In this level of group, since some of the initial issues of trust and reluctance have been addressed, a more diverse group membership can be tolerated. Having demonstrated the ability to share their own experience and to listen helpfully to others, combat veterans can now be more successfully mixed with noncombat veterans, minorities with whites, women with men, officers with enlisted personnel, and veterans of other generations with Viet Nam veterans.

It is not an accident that families of suicide victims, cancer patients, abuse survivors, rape victims, assault victims, and concentration camp survivors and their children have all developed this same self-help, peer group model, in which a powerful, similar experience links group members initially. Another striking feature about the model is that the most successful groups use some combination of a therapist and a survivor of the same events as leaders of the initial groups. Those groups led by only therapists without survivor experience, or by only survivors without therapy experience, seem to fare less well.

In long-term rap groups, the veterans become primary therapists for each other. The leader's role is even more clearly that of the facilitator who observes the group process and helps the group members note, verbalize, and explore their reactions to each other and to the process.

In long-term groups, the emphasis shifts more dramatically to present concerns. The war and earlier experiences come into sharp focus in highly detailed and sharply defined episodes with immediate bearing on present issues. Rather than merely indulging in a round of war stories, members engage in deeply felt and often emotionally draining revelations that draw the group together, enlisting all in an intense exploration.

Jay, an Army combat veteran, was collecting disability. His inability to leave the house or let anyone depend on him was his primary problem. This behavior was in sharp contrast to his beatings of his brother-in-law when he had abused Jay's sister. On those occasions Jay became vehement about retaliation. Discussion in the group focused one night on Jay's shame over not being able to be a Boy Scout leader for his son. Exploration of the episode soon led to an episode from Viet Nam in which Jay had been the machine gunner on a rescue tank and had leapt off the tank and abandoned the gun during an intense attack. The injury suffered in the leap had led to his current disability. It became clear to the group that Jay's reluctance to take responsibility now, as well as his impulsive retaliation against his brother-in-law, were both extreme reactions to his perceived abandonment of responsibility on the tank.

Resolution of present problems and war experience is not simply abreaction or catharsis. Considerable affect accompanies the surfacing of these issues. But conflict between rigid expectations and judgments and painfully incongruent, actual experience becomes resolved as the group helps transform and reevaluate judgments and self-valuation. Acceptance by the group of frailty, and concurrent emphasis on retained honor and integrity, fuel the reconsideration and integration of new perspectives. Different behavior and alternative strategies are explored, attempted, and reinforced. Reliance of members on their peers is strengthened.

As in the case of Tom (already described above), the function of current behavior and solutions are examined in the light of painful early experience and personal style.

Tom, the Army infantryman, was referred to a long-term rap group. After several months he revealed two childhood episodes. Both incidents involved street fights between neighborhood gangs and hooting denunciations of Tom's fear and unwillingness to join in the fighting or the gangs.

Soon thereafter, Tom explored the effect of these episodes on his later decision to join the Army and request assignment to Viet Nam. Tom realized that the war for him was an attempt at redemption from the earlier fears which he saw as failing.

It became clear to the group and to Tom that much of the current intensity in his stand as a veteran advocate reflected the same effort.

The path to resolution is never linear. Veterans in the groups seem to make clustered changes, then plateau. Intense work may be followed by a period of absence. Follow-up must be accompanied by tolerance for varying phases of involvement.

Survivor Mission. Long-term rap group members take on a survivor mission. One pays a visit to "the wall"—the Viet Nam Veterans Memorial in Washington, D.C.; another visits the grave site of a dead comrade; a third volunteers to work with other troubled veterans; a fourth becomes dedicated to a career change. All of these actions promote reinvestment in values abandoned because of painful war experience. This mission breaks the final hold of the past on the present as it opens the road back into the community. The war experience is never forgotten, but it becomes one that the veteran can live with, as reflected in the following passage by Robert Jay Lifton:

> The veterans also make clear that young people, even when considerably confused, can take powerful steps toward new integrity. I think of the My Lai survivor able to call forth at a crucial moment his idiosyncratically derived ethical forms (from military chivalry, catholic principles, and the habit of autonomy) to refuse participation in that atrocity. I think of the former grunt whose company was virtually wiped out, appearing at early rap groups in a dissociated state, close to breakdown, emerging as a man still highly conflicted, but able to mobilize extraordinary sensitivity in furthering his and others' renewal. I think of the former Naval NCO undergoing a series of debilitating personal crises, and through them all, evolving a personal commitment to a vision of integrity so palpable as to provide a nurturing standard for the entire group—and later, through various kinds of writing and consulting, becoming a leading, national interpreter of Vietnam veterans' aspirations and needs. (17, p. 406)

Termination. There is concern among some therapists that dependency needs lead veterans to interminable therapy. The corollary is the belief that once veterans develop a trusting group relationship, they will remain with the group forever. These views fail to recognize that veterans, like other survivors, have no desire to wallow in their traumatic experiences.

The underlying problem is not a termination issue but rather is a problem with veterans or rap groups that are stuck. The issue is not that the group cannot stop, but rather that it did not or cannot start properly. The focus of concern in a rap group with a termination problem often centers on a veteran who seems "hung up" on, or wallowing in, an experience. Such a veteran retells seemingly pointless war stories, dresses in fatigues, and appears unwilling to move on.

One response of therapists to such a situation is to press for termination, to try to focus on the here and now, and to encourage the veteran putting the war behind him. "We're stuck; let's move on" is the message. But termination is not the issue; getting on with the therapy is the issue. The fatigues and the war stories are messages from veterans that they are stuck, hung up on Viet Nam. The task is to resolve the hang up, not to try to shove it away. They have tried to put it away for 15 years and it hasn't worked.

The solution is to dive in, not run off. These "stuck" times act as messages that the group is uncertain about where and how to go. Rather than discourage the war stories, the leader can deepen them, ask for more detail, and attend to new figures or characters and subtle changes in the plot. These aspects will be the keys to the underlying or hidden meaning. Fleshing out the details, inquiring why a story is important, and exploring the group's reactions to the story and to the veteran yield the material that holds the answers.

When a long-term group is effective, the behavior of its members in the outside world will change. There is a desire to consolidate gains, a wish to make up for lost time, and an ability to deal with present concerns effectively. Such changes in state of mind and accompanying behavior will be integrated into stable patterns after 12 to 18 months of group participation. At that point termination of the long-term group is in order.

CONCLUSION

Many veterans are helped by rap groups. However, change and recovery can happen without therapeutic intervention. Not all veterans need rap groups. And in many cases, what begins in a rap group is concluded by veterans on their own. The process is a life-long one.

Rap groups are controversial. In part, this situation stems from the variety of inappropriate group therapies mislabeled rap groups. An even more significant source of professional concern reflects recognition of the powerful forces at work in rap groups. These forces can generate destructiveness as well as therapeutic results. Recognition of this potential leads some therapists to dismiss the modality or to be overly restricting of the groups.

Rap groups are a special form of group therapy. While they follow the same rules of group process as any effective therapy group, the strong forces reflecting traumatic experience at work in rap groups distinguish them from other groups. Rap groups for veterans, like peer groups for other survivors, depend on the special bonding that occurs between victims of a particular trauma. The groups fail when that bonding is diminished, but reliance on this bonding and the norming of reactions that occurs among survivors demand more from the therapists who lead them. Since the group's process depends on the members acting as therapists for each other, skill at eliciting, guiding, and tempering the interaction of these unskilled participant-therapists is at a premium.

Rap group therapists are also called upon to confront their own vulnerability to traumatic reactions. They must consider how they would have acted under circumstances similar to those experienced by their veteran-clients. They also expose themselves to the wrath of group members.

Not all therapists should lead rap groups. To do so may require facing questions that would be unnecessary elsewhere. The difficulty of confronting one's own avoidance of Viet Nam service and the emotional drain of responding to tales of agony and violence force many to decline.

This chapter has reviewed three levels of rap groups. For some veterans with PTSD the rap group may form the core experience of the stress recovery process.

Rap groups offer a powerful therapeutic alternative for the treatment of stress reactions, but the forces at work demand critical attention in order to buffer their more destructive potential. We have only barely begun to study and document the advantages and liabilities of rap groups. It is not clear yet how, why, and for whom the groups work. What is clear is that the power and emotional impact of this form of therapy makes the groups attractive to many therapists. The rewards of watching and aiding the transformation from victim to survivor are great. But the demands in energy and vulnerability exceed those of many other groups, both for clients and leaders. That veterans and therapists are willing to take the risk is a tribute to the capacity of healers and survivors to assist each other to emotional growth and, where necessary, to health.

REFERENCES

1. Yalom ID: The Theory and Practice of Group Psychotherapy, 2nd ed. New York, Basic Books, 1975

2. Walker JI, Nash JL: Group therapy in the treatment of Vietnam combat veterans. Int J Group Psychother 31:379–389, 1981

3. Walker JI: Comparison of "rap" groups with traditional group therapy in the treatment of Viet Nam combat veterans. Unpublished paper, 1981

4. Egendorf A: Vietnam veteran rap groups and themes of postwar life. Journal of Social Issues 31:111–124, 1975

5. Williams T: Psychological readjustment of Vietnam veterans. Washington, DC, Disabled American Veterans, 1979

6. Williams T: Post-Traumatic Stress Disorders of the Vietnam Veteran. Cincinnati, Disabled American Veterans, 1980

7. Harrington DS, Jay JA: Beyond the family: value issues in the treatment of Vietnam veterans. Family Therapy Networker 6:13–45, 1982

8. Scurfield R, Corker T, Gongla P, et al: Three post-Vietnam "rap/therapy" groups: an analysis. Int J Group Psychother, in press

9. Coates D, Winston T: Counteracting the deviance of depression: peer support groups for victims. Journal of Social Issues 39:169–194, 1983

10. Lindy JD, Green BL, Grace M, et al: Psychotherapy with survivors of the Beverly Hills Supper Club fire. Am J Psychother 37:593, 1983

11. Smith JR: The roles, stages, and structure of rap groups in the treatment of post-traumatic stress disorders. Paper presented at Dartmouth Medical School, November 1980

12. Laufer RS, Gallops MS, Frey-Wouters E: War stress and trauma: the Vietnam veteran experience. J Health Soc Behav 25:65–85, 1984

13. Smith JR: Personal responsibility in traumatic stress reactions. Psychiatric Annals 12:1021–1030, 1982

14. Mason RC: Chickenhawk. New York, Viking Press, 1982

15. Horowitz MJ, Marmar C (eds): Personality Styles in Brief Psychotherapy. New York, Basic Books, 1984

16. Horowitz MJ: Sliding meanings: a defense against threat in narcissistic personalities. Int J Psychoanal Psychother 4:167–180, 1974

17. Lifton RJ: Home from the War. New York, Simon & Schuster, 1973

9

Family Therapy for Viet Nam Veterans

Candis M. Williams, Psy.D.
Tom Williams, Psy.D.

9

In the 1980s, extensive clinical attention and research have been focused on male Viet Nam veterans, but very little attention is given to their family members and close friends. The best information available (1) indicates that more than 60 percent of male veterans have primary relationships with women. Now the inclusion of women partners and families is increasingly considered as crucial to successful psychological treatment, as discussed by Figley (2), Williams (3), Scarano (4), and Gruter (5).

Unfortunately, the veteran's primary family system is still ignored by many clinicians. Even so, family systems can sometimes, without assistance, reorganize to accept the veteran's behaviors. However, there is resulting strain on all members.

When the primary family system has not been addressed, veterans revert to old behaviors and show an increase in stress disorder symptoms. Our clinical experience shows that veterans often get symptom relief from individual or group therapy, but that unless planned interventions are done with family systems, the possibility of permanent change of behavior is reduced.

The purpose of this chapter is to acquaint mental health professionals with the usefulness of family systems theory in the assessment and treatment of Viet Nam veteran families, where the veteran shows a stress disorder due to combat experiences.

We will first outline key characteristics of veteran families. Clinically, such families show differences from families which do not have a member who has experienced extreme trauma. We will indicate the effects of systems and socialization on families, and particularly on women partners. We will also present guidelines for treatment in women partners' groups. Specific strategies of working with Viet Nam veteran families will be offered, and finally we will describe a multimodal approach which integrates family therapy with other treatment modalities. Unfortunately, although somewhere between 7,000 and 35,000 women veterans served in Viet Nam, we have not worked with their families, and, therefore, will not be referring to them.

Figley (2) has written on families of veterans, and work by Silver (1) is based on survey data of some 400 Viet Nam veteran families that received service through the Disabled American Veterans Outreach Centers. Silver's findings (1) are not unexpected. He has found that the most powerful predictor of post-traumatic stress disorder is combat exposure, and second to that is impaired family functioning. These results fit with those found by Frye and Stockton (6) in a survey of Viet Nam veteran officers. In the latter study, the degree of ease in discussing Viet Nam experiences with one's spouse best distinguished the stress disorder–symptomatic group from the symptom-free combat exposure group. Family functioning is apparently more highly significant than either developmental or personality factors. This research affirms what our own experience has indicated—that there is a strong correlation between PTSD and family dysfunction. The importance of family is further reinforced by findings from the Center for Policy Research (7), which show that combat veterans who are doing well are in supportive relationships with women. Seemingly, then, marital support is a crucial factor in the successful adjustment of many veterans. How does PTSD affect the family? Let us look at some of the characteristics of Viet Nam veteran families.

CHARACTERISTICS OF IMPAIRED VETERAN FAMILIES

In clinical work (3, 4), impaired veteran families show significant differences from other families. The following issues regularly appear and contribute to dysfunctional family patterns.

Veterans Viewed as "Identified Patients"

If one family member is identified as a "patient," as is often the case with veterans, then other family members expect the veteran alone to do all the changing. Family members usually do not understand how their own behavior can perpetuate dysfunctional patterns in family relationships. The veteran may need special attention, but frequently the family system or family substitute should also be targeted for intervention. The psychological unit is not just the individual; it is the individual in the larger social context. So long as veterans are identified as "patients," they can be maintained as scapegoats in the family or seen as the exclusive source of difficulty.

Post-Traumatic Stress Disorder

The pattern of PTSD symptoms is idiosyncratic, since not all PTSD veterans suffer from the same symptoms. But certain primary symptoms such as alienation, depression, and emotional numbing will understandably isolate veterans from their families. Present stresses often precipitate or exaggerate PTSD symptoms. The veteran as well as family members may avoid intimacy, because all seem to get hurt when they allow closeness or vulnerability.

Substance Abuse

Substance abuse, most frequently alcohol, has a negative effect on financial stability and family relationships. Therapists should explore the possibility that partners may actually share in the substance abuse or may be acting as "enablers." Enabling partners may cover for veterans' abuses by making excuses for their behavior or by simply denying that there is any problem at all.

Violence and Rage

Cyclical outbursts of rage are characteristic of some war veterans. These may reinforce a fear of going crazy and of losing control of behavior. The rage may also induce fear and helplessness in family members who neither know when to expect it nor how to control it. Violence and battering occur too frequently. Although we have no national studies on battering, in a review of cases at the Vet Center in Fort Wayne, Indiana, about one-third of 600 men admitted to striking women partners or children. Not surprisingly, violent reactions are often associated with the use of alcohol.

Inappropriate Responses to Loss and Illness

One of the most painful and problematic features in Viet Nam veteran families is that the veteran often does not sympathize with illness or pain of family members, but rather becomes hostile and distant. Such a reaction may occur even though the veteran has strong underlying loving and empathic feelings and reactions. This may be part of the emotional numbing which is common to PTSD; it also impedes the veteran's ability to grieve for actual losses. Psychic survival in combat required cutting off feelings. The effect of this withdrawal on significant others is that they may feel hurt, rejected, unsupported, and sometimes angry and resentful about the veteran's inability to reciprocate for the care and support which they have provided.

Unspoken Rules

Frequently, there is an unspoken rule that veterans will not talk about their war experiences. They say that others, including wives or partners, could not understand. This has a kernel of truth in that others can by horrified by the behaviors and experiences of soldiers in combat.

Horowitz (8) believes that veterans need to share their feelings around what happened to them in Viet Nam, but not necessarily the actual experiences. We find that giving veterans this reassurance when explaining family therapy makes it more likely that they will come into treatment. Part of the veteran's reluctance to talk about the war with their families is this: the war happened a long time ago and therefore should not disturb the family now. Such unspoken rules encourage veterans to repress their memories. But when ordinary life stresses come up, the memories return because the veterans have been unable to integrate their behavior during the war with their identity in peacetime. The "no talking" rule keeps veterans emotionally isolated from significant others and perpetuates a tendency to see themselves as different or special.

Effects on Children

Clinicians are just beginning to assess the effects of veterans with PTSD on their children. Children may act out family pathology with depression or with behavioral or school problems. They may seem immature for their ages. In many veteran families, mothers do most of the parenting. Veterans can be over-protective and over-demanding of their children. They may complain about being unable to be emotionally close to their children. This ambivalence may be a result of the veteran having witnessed, and having been involved in, the killing of children in Viet Nam. Whatever the etiology, there is frequently estrangement and emotional distance between fathers and children. Occasionally, veterans are able to express affectionate feelings toward their children while unable to do so with adult partners.

Mate Selection

Most veterans are in relationships that have developed since the war. Satir (9) believes that, in marriage, one hurting person generally looks for and finds a similarly hurting person. Each partner has a low opinion of himself or herself. Consequently, both are very needy and demand more from the other than is possible for any one individual to provide. Often partners have superficial expectations of each other. When these expectations are not met, couples can become disappointed, resentful, and angry. There is little satisfaction, support, or fulfillment in such relationships.

Isolation, Mobility, and Alienation

For the past 15 years, clinicians and researchers have noted that some Viet Nam veterans are alienated and isolated from others. Our observations reveal that this sometimes occurs for the whole family unit as well. We have noted that women partners frequently complain that veterans are jealous and do not tolerate their having social activities external to the family unit. In deference to the husband's pleas, these women cut their own ties also. Additionally, some veterans are uneasy staying in the same town or the same job and move frequently from one job to another and from one city or state to another. This keeps the family disrupted and maintains isolation.

Women as Mainstay

In troubled families of troubled veterans, women partners are often the primary financial and emotional support. They may be the major and most reliable breadwinners, and they may be almost totally responsible for child care and household chores. This leaves a rather uncertain role for the veteran and undercuts responsible functioning. Such patterns, especially when entrenched, may be seen by the clinician as due to passivity or infantile behavior in the veteran. However, chronic PTSD may lead to the same picture; differentiation of the personality disorder from the stress disorder etiology is crucial.

VETERANS AND THEIR FAMILIES

The veteran may be the identified patient, but the problems which he or she experiences do not occur in isolation from other persons. The problems occur and are perpetuated partly as a result of interactions with other people and with social, familial, vocational, political, and other systems in the environment. Often negative patterns develop over a number of years. Viet Nam veterans who are dysfunctional due to stress disorder belong to primary support systems—families— which frequently are also dysfunctional. Usually, one cannot change one member of a family system and expect that other family members will simply fall into line. Assessment of long-term and systems effects is essential in the treatment of PTSD.

The success of any treatment of PTSD in combat veterans is problematic in the absence of educational or treatment efforts directed toward the various systems within which they live and which influence their behavior. Family systems operate with ritualized patterns of interaction and established roles. If one member attempts a change, the result is additional stress on other members. The latter are likely to respond according to previous patterns of behavior in an attempt to restore stability to the family system.

Many veterans feel that if the partner understands what the veteran is experiencing, that is all that is needed. The partner's understanding *is* necessary, but to the extent that it does not promote positive change in a maladaptive system, it is insufficient. Family members may be locked into negative and habitual ways of responding to each other. According to reinforcement theory, the more one person gives in to the other's unhealthy patterns of functioning, the less chance there is that either can learn to relate in a healthy manner or effect positive change in the other's behavior. Total sacrifice of the woman is characteristic in dysfunctional combat veteran family systems, which do not afford personal autonomy to family members. Further, there is not the give-and-take or the flexibility which a family system requires to adapt to external stresses.

WOMEN PARTNERS

Unfortunately, a woman partner often thinks that a veteran partner's problematic behavior is her fault. As with men influenced by the male-oriented military system, women often seem to conform to culturally conditioned and stereotypical sex roles. To the extent that they have been affected by the stereotypes, women partners will have special problems which are different from, and more subtle than, the trauma of war for veterans. The concept of "walking the tightrope" (3) identifies a dilemma for the woman partner who must try to maintain a precarious balance between supporting another person without sacrificing her own needs versus not supporting the veteran enough, thereby risking being labeled as selfish. These women, paired with a veteran who relates in a negative manner, are more likely to conform to cultural expectations which include a stance of total responsibility for the veteran. Such women feel compelled to always give a little more and to tolerate greater deviant behavior from the veteran. Thus, a negative cycle of the woman being "responsible" and the veteran being "irresponsible" is perpetuated.

Women partners have some special problems of their own. Many have distanced themselves from others because of the veteran's problems and suffer from social isolation, so they also lack adequate social support systems. This adds pressure to primary relationships to supply all needs and increases the unhealthy dependence on the veteran partner, thus reducing the possibility of a healthy relationship.

Many women complain of helplessness and anxiety. This can be a result of the impossibility of satisfying the veteran's needs as well as his erratic and unpredictable behavior. Such women are often unable to control or effect any change in their husband. The response to feelings of helplessness may be withdrawal or counterhostility.

Most women complain of anger; sometimes it is evidenced initially, but more often it surfaces later in treatment. The woman partner's anger may derive from many factors, including the veteran's hostility, lack of emotional responsiveness and caring, and inability to change. The woman's inability to produce change in the family, and her allowing life to revolve around the veteran's demands and behaviors, also makes her angry. Such problems for women partners result in a mixture of feelings of worthlessness, helplessness, withdrawal, and depression.

GUIDELINES FOR GROUPS WITH WOMEN PARTNERS

Women's groups are never viewed as a women's auxiliary. They should not be created for, nor should they be tasked with, the supportive function of maintaining or rescuing the veteran. Group treatment for women needs to validate the fact that women partners have their own problems and concerns which are worthy of attention and treatment.

Although most clinicians realize the importance of prescreening veterans who are invited to groups, women partners are often invited to groups simply because they happen to be in relationships with Viet Nam veterans. Prescreening is indicated for all individuals for group therapy. Aside from personal dynamics, we have noted three special reasons for not referring a woman to a partners group.

1. Women who are severely dysfunctional in certain areas—for example, those who are suicidal—may need to have a different form of treatment.

2. Sometimes women who are in relationships with veterans who are extremely explosive and physically endangering should be offered family violence counseling.
3. We have found that some women who are currently not in a relationship with a veteran (because of a separation) may not fit in well with other women partners unless special care is taken to ensure that they are not perceived as models or misfits. The focus remains primarily on them, secondarily on their relationships.

Participants should agree to attend a specified number of meetings so that group cohesiveness is ensured and an atmosphere of trust and sharing is possible. Ten to 20 weekly meetings lasting from one-and-a-half to two hours are usually the minimum required for accomplishing basic objectives. At the end of each sequence, women may choose to continue, but continued attendance should also be time-limited and goal-oriented. At least one of the group leaders should be a qualified mental health professional.

We believe that it is important for all group participants, including the leaders, to be women. As noted by Brodsky (10), many women have limited opportunities to see other women in leadership positions and may tend to be inhibited and unassertive in the presence of men. This is not true of men's groups, where there are advantages to having women leaders. A male veteran leading a women's group usually subliminally reinforces a focus on the problems of the veteran. This serves to reinforce stereotyped cultural expectations that women are responsible for the welfare of veterans. In group treatment, women partners first need to be considered as individuals in their own right with their own needs, problems, and issues; this frequently should take precedence over work on the relationship with the veteran.

Leaders should have a solid clinical understanding of PTSD and know the psychological impact of the Viet Nam War and its differences from other wars. Information should be provided to group members either in the form of a limited didactic presentation or handouts, with time allowed for discussion. This frequently prompts a positive discussion and interaction between veterans and women partners.

When both partners are concurrently in group treatment, there should be a continuing dialogue between the leaders of the men's and the women's groups, so that groups do not work at cross purposes and the problems of the various couples are kept in view. Both clients and therapists need to be aware of the necessity for this communication and informed to the same degree of its content.

Group Process Objectives

Phase I. Phase I is a time for sharing, support, and trust building. Women derive immense relief and strength from knowing they are not alone and their problems are not unique. This phase includes discussion of issues of commitment, confidentiality, individual and group objectives, and the effects which change may have on their relationships. Information must be provided on PTSD and the effects on significant others. The women should be allowed to talk about the symptoms of their partners but should progress to discussing the functioning of their relationships and the effect that this may have on their own behavior.

Phase II. When group cohesiveness, support, and trust have been established, it is time for individual and group problem-solving and a positive behavioral change orientation. During phase II, it is best to avoid repetitive venting or scapegoating of male partners so that constructive work can take place. The women begin focusing on how they see themselves and what needs they have, such as social support systems. They need to establish and reinforce assertive behaviors directed toward meeting those needs.

Women, like men, often need to learn how to "act" rather than to just "react"; in other words, they need to take some initiative and control of their lives. As women in the group become fairly supportive of one another, they can begin to understand and be less defensive about how their own behaviors contribute to dysfunctional patterns of relating to their partners. It no longer becomes the men's problem alone, but their joint difficulty.

Successful work in an all-woman group produces increased self-esteem, feelings of personal autonomy, and development of outside support systems. When these occur, the woman partner gains greater capacity for action. When a woman partner begins to recognize that she cannot be responsible for the veteran, but that her own behavior does affect relationship interactions, it is time to consider whether marital or family therapy is desirable (if not already in process) or whether treatment may be discontinued.

SPECIFIC FAMILY TREATMENT STRATEGIES

The following strategies are directed at increasing cooperation between family members and enhancing certain life skills.

Removal of the Veteran from the Identified Patient Role

The therapist should convey to family members that they must share responsibility for bringing about change. Problems should be described as systems problems by pointing out how members interact with one another and how interactions are constructive or destructive. Feelings that the veteran is abnormal because of reactions to Viet Nam experiences should be explored and disallowed. The veteran is encouraged to talk with the family about Viet Nam experiences, to the degree that this is tolerable to all parties.

Rage Episodes

The family's methods of handling anger must be assessed. Rage episodes are sometimes brought on by substance abuse, primarily alcohol. Therefore, agreement to monitor substance abuse may be necessary. Next, the therapy should provide alternative strategies for coping with anger both for veterans and for other family members. The counselor or therapist should ask the veteran about episodes when he or she became violently angry. Usually, particular episodes can be recalled. Frequently, veterans are very afraid of a recurrence of violent episodes. Thus, they cope by withdrawing from any situation in which rage threatens. It is crucial that the veteran learn that he or she can control angry behavior through the experience of some success at control. Successive approximations to healthy, coping behavior may be necessary in learning to deal with anger. For example, veterans may progress from family violence, to putting holes in the wall, and eventually to jogging or other exercise as a coping response to stress.

War Experience as "Ghosts"

The therapist and family should attempt to determine whether unresolved issues from the past are interfering with the present. Most veterans have attempted to repress memories of Viet Nam, to "put it behind them." But pain not worked through and suffering from PTSD do not diminish simply because they are ignored. To some extent, painful experiences need to be verbalized, cognitively restructured, and integrated into veterans' self-identities. This requires an understanding of the context of war and the atypical behaviors which war elicits.

Education

Education is frequently a part of psychological treatment, but with this population it is particularly important. Veterans and family members often need help in relinquishing the view that the veteran is peculiar, different, or crazy. Education, including reading, will reinforce constructive change and action toward getting better control of symptoms, toward attaining greater intimacy, and toward the veteran talking more about experiences and feelings with nonveterans.

Mutual Support

The treatment should focus on partners supporting each other and building a commitment. Since there may have been hurt and distrust in the relationship, it may be advisable to start by working on motivations for staying together, before exploring the more explosive issues in the relationship. A suggested technique is Richard Stuart's "Caring Days" concept (11).

Skills Training

Skills training is important for overcoming specific deficiencies. Communication exercises such as effective listening, giving feedback, self-expression, request-making, and assertiveness training may be important. Assignments and homework tasks may be required.

Negative interactions as well as positive interactions tend to have a high degree of reciprocity. Therefore, it may be necessary to separate veterans and women partners when domestic violence is probable. The intervention may involve letting family members or the marital dyad know that it is important not to ignore conflicts. The therapy then teaches the family how to actually contain and resolve conflicts. Stuart (11) suggests some ways of teaching these skills.

It also may be important to teach couples new ways of telling each other when one is simply stressed and needs a nonjudgmental listener, as opposed to when one has a real disagreement with the other person.

Parent skill training is often required. An advantage of using this approach is that parents become united in the mutual effort of parenting. Consistency in parenting is crucial and may mean redefining roles and forming new alliances in support of one another.

Other skills concerning relationships and stress management techniques are often taught in a couple or family setting. These skills assist the family in developing alternative, positive coping strategies.

Roles and Values Clarification

In Viet Nam veteran families, there is often over-attachment to culturally stereotyped roles. In our society, tremendous role changes have occurred in the family during the past decade. Additionally, some veterans' experiences with war and the military system tended to burden stereotyped male-female roles. Obviously, a healthy relationship requires that neither spouse be unduly dependent on the other. The therapist must point out that family members need not necessarily agree with one another on issues, but each person does need to know how the others feel and be able to respect the opinions and positions of others.

Essentially, effective treatment in the veteran family system means helping veterans, women partners, and families break through learned helplessness, self-defeating patterns, and dysfunctional interactions which are likely to have developed through the years.

MULTIMODAL THERAPY: INTEGRATING FAMILY THERAPY WITH OTHER MODALITIES

Therapeutic intervention involves looking at the interactions within the family system. The treatment model usually advises veterans and partners to begin treatment in separate groups. Prior to this, individual therapy may be necessary. At such time as veterans and their partners join groups, couple or family interactions are not addressed per se, nor are radical changes in interactional patterns sought. Rather, the objective in groups is to take the pressure off the primary relationship by providing members with support systems external to the family.

This relieves pressure on the primary relationship, in that veterans and partners no longer feel as though they must have all of their needs met within the primary relationship. Groups allow members to experience the relief of finding out they are not alone and that other people share similar problems. This enhances self-respect, restores self-confidence, provides a feeling of strength, and prepares the individuals to recognize and verbalize feelings, acknowledge problems, and begin constructive problem solving.

Only when each partner gets to the point of accepting responsibility for both positive and negative aspects of their lives does the therapist open up the therapeutic system, by encouraging a focus on the primary relationship, and move into marital or family therapy. There is sometimes an advantage to remaining in a support group even after family or couples therapy has begun. Separate groups should, however, remain time-limited, with the goal of developing other support systems.

When deciding on the appropriate treatment modality, one possibility is to use Minuchin's concepts of enmeshment and disengagement (12). If a couple is "enmeshed," greater individual autonomy is needed, and it probably makes sense to separate them into women partners' and veterans' groups. If the couple is very disengaged, then it may be best to bring them in for family or marital work so they can start learning to relate to each other better. Lazarus (13) discusses pragmatic multimodal therapy.

Individual Counseling

The intake interview is usually the beginning of treatment. The intake often is the first opportunity for the veteran to talk about Viet Nam and learn about PTSD. Crisis counseling is often required, and hospitalization or medication are occasionally indicated. The goal is to resolve any crisis, build trust in the therapist, and arrange for continuing treatment. Short-term individual counseling can be a precursor to group or family treatment. The spouse, if not the entire family, should always be encouraged to attend the intake interview.

Group Therapy

Veterans. Group work includes PTSD education, grief work, desensitization, cognitive restructuring, teaching interpersonal skills, developing support networks, problem solving, learning adaptive coping skills, stress management, conflict containment and resolution, reinterpretation and integration of experience, and discrimination of current life-style behaviors from war context behavior and personality. (See Williams [14] for a further discussion of group treatment of veterans.)

Women Partners. As discussed earlier, these groups focus on PTSD information, women's issues, building social support systems, assertiveness training, problem solving, and coping and life-planning skills. Such groups are most beneficial if the veteran is in treatment at the same time. (See Williams [3] for further discussion of partners' groups.)

Multiple Couples Groups. These groups of reasonably healthy couples concentrate on development of social support systems, interpersonal and communication skills, conflict containment and resolution skills, parent training skills, and assistance in being mutually supportive.

Family or Marital Counseling. This treatment may include the children if they are part of negative interactional patterns, or other relatives or significant people in the psychological unit. Obviously, the goal of such groups is not necessarily to ensure that the marital couple will remain together, but rather to reduce the possibility of undue suffering and the unpredictability of working with only one member of a family system.

Community Education and Outreach. Therapists can help create receptive community systems which facilitate rehabilitation for veterans and their families because they are no longer treated as outcasts. This may include providing literature on stress disorder and on available services. This is accomplished by offering community workshops, open houses, and professional presentations. All of these will help sensitize the community and enhance the possibility that veterans can feel at home again.

REFERENCES

1. Silver SM: The impact of post-traumatic stress disorder on families of Viet Nam veterans, in Trauma and Its Wake. Edited by Figley CR. New York, Brunner/Mazel, in press

2. Figley CR, Sprenkle D: Delayed stress response syndrome: family therapy implications. J Marriage Fam Couns 6:53–59, 1978

3. Williams T: The veteran system with a focus on women partners, in Post-Traumatic Stress Disorders of the Viet Nam Veteran. Edited by Williams T. Cincinnati, Disabled American Veterans, 1980

4. Scarano TP: Family therapy: a viable approach for treating troubled Viet Nam veterans. The Family Therapist, December 1982

5. Gruter L: Families of a post–Viet Nam stress syndrome. The Family Therapist 2:16–17, 1981

6. Frye JS, Stockton RA: Discriminant analysis of post-traumatic stress disorder among a group of Viet Nam veterans. Am J Psychiatry 139:52–56, 1982

7. Egendorf A, Rothbart G, Sloan L, et al: Legacies of Vietnam: Comparative Adjustment of Veterans and Their Peers. Washington, DC, U.S. Government Printing Office, 1981

8. Forgotten Warriors: America's Viet Nam era veterans. Disabled American Veteran Magazine 22:8–17, 1980

9. Satir V: Conjoint Family Therapy. Palo Alto, Calif, Science and Behavioral Books, 1967

10. Brodsky A: The consciousness raising group as a model for therapy for women, in Female Psychology: The Emerging Self. Edited by Cox S. Chicago, Science Research Associates, 1976

11. Stuart R: Helping Couples Change. New York, Guilford Press, 1980

12. Minuchin S: Families and Family Therapy. Cambridge, Mass, Harvard University Press, 1974

13. Lazarus AA: The Practice of a Multi-Modal Therapy. New York, McGraw Hill, 1981

14. Williams T: Group treatment, in Post-Traumatic Stress Disorder of the Viet Nam Veteran. Edited by Williams T. Cincinnati, Disabled American Veterans, 1980

10

The Place of Narcosynthesis in the Treatment of Chronic and Delayed Stress Reactions of War

Lawrence C. Kolb, M.D.

10

To enhance both the diagnostic and therapeutic potentials for treatment of the seriously impairing repetitive dissociative reactions in Viet Nam combat veterans with the chronic or delayed forms of post-traumatic stress disorder, I have used in some cases a modified narcosynthetic technique. The results that I have had with this technique indicate that most men who have such symptomatology and who have been so treated suffer a persisting conditioned emotional response to sounds approximating those of their battle experience in addition to the well-recognized clinical symptomatology of chronic or delayed PTSD (1). Through the use of a videotape technique, the abreactive response during narcosynthesis has been recorded and then used later to confront the patient in a fully conscious state as an initiating move in continuing psychotherapy.

This technique has been applied in treatment of those with severely impairing recurrent dissociative states in whom the usually effective avoidance defenses have failed. Such symptom complexes, often precipitated through startle phenomena, were found in Viet Nam veterans with high exposure to combat stress who sought hospital assistance. While uncommon in frequency of occurrence, their recognition and attenuation are important to control recurrently destructive social behaviors, probably the most damaging symptom complex seen in the chronic states of PTSD in terms of social adaptation.

HISTORY

Abreactive therapy induced in an altered state of consciousness while under the influence of a parenterally injected pharmacologic agent achieved its greatest clinical usage in the treatment of the acute post-traumatic states during World War II. Freud et al. (2) initially described the alleviation of the acute symptoms of this condition through abreaction induced under hypnosis during World War I. As the result of the work of Blackwenn (3), who first published the use of barbiturates to effect prolonged narcosis as a method of treatment and management of excited, agitated, and insomniac patients, as well as Lindemann's (4) report of the serenity and well-being induced by subnarcotic dosages of these agents in both healthy and mentally ill persons, the technique of drug-induced abreaction was tried during World War II in treatment of the acute combat neuroses by the medical corps of the allied armed forces. Sargent and Slater (5) and Mallinson (6) described the rapid resolution of acute symptoms of stupor, mutism, confusion, and a variety of conversion-type paralysis in treatment of acute war neurosis. Applying psychoanalytic insights to the treatment, Horsley (7) designated the procedure as narcoanalysis, and now it is used to describe drug-induced recall of repressed material. The therapist provided both psychodynamic interpretations and posthypnotic suggestions. Grinker and Spiegel (8) introduced the term narcosynthesis. In so doing they implied that the derepressed material through the abreactive experience becomes consciously available for later integration and synthesis by the personality. The necessity for "working through" material exposed during narcosynthetic abreaction in later psychotherapy became recognized. Soon therapists, notably Horsley and his followers, engaged their patients in a lengthy (several hours) narcoanalytic treatment or repeated the experience a number of times.

Following World War II the technique has been applied by some in the treatment of the acute post-traumatic states of civilian life when patients exhibited evidence of seriously impairing symptoms such as those rapidly resolved during wartime (stupor, mutism, confusion, agitation, amnesia, and conversion phenomena). The hopes that narcosynthesis might offer a widespread and effective uncovering treatment of major psychiatric disorders proved groundless. Attempts to apply the techniques to treat the chronic post-traumatic states induced in victims of the Holocaust also proved unsuccessful.

The administration of intravenous barbiturates to facilitate resolution of amnestic states and to aid in recollection of memories from the accused as well as victims and witnesses of crimes had a short-lived vogue in criminal and legal circles. Redlich et al. (9) brought forward data to show that the veracity of the material disclosed was open to question. Redlich's experiments demonstrated the likelihood that those with neurotic makeup are less able to maintain a falsehood under the influence of a drug than those whose personality organization is more stable.

THEORY

Emotional catharsis is thought to provide the process by which the initial therapeutic effects of narcosynthesis are achieved. Catharsis as a means of relieving suffering probably had its beginnings in the centuries of human experience during which medicine men and shamans carried out their rituals to aid those who came to them for help. In Europe, emotional catharsis induced by hypnosis evolved as a well-recognized therapeutic tool for the treatment of certain disorders of behavior during the 19th century.

Catharsis was thought to bring about symptom relief by allowing the discharge of dammed-up emotion, thus inducing a reduction of inner tension. Bibring (10) has discussed extensively the use of abreaction as one of the major psychotherapeutic techniques. The single abreactive experience was regarded as useful in the early 1900s in the treatment of "traumatic hysteria." It was hypothesized that this condition was caused by massive repression of affect which found outward expression in the abnormal behavior. Catharsis through hypnosis was considered insufficient to bring about permanent relief in other hysterias where splitting of consciousness took place. In other than "traumatic hysteria," abreaction with discharge of affect was thought to provide incomplete relief as partial dissociation persisted and additional therapeutic "working through" was needed to effect a therapeutic change.

Massive repression of affect is assumed to have taken place at the time of the emotionally overwhelming catastrophe. This repression is postulated to provide escape from reexperiencing of the primitive affects of fear, rage, desperation, and helplessness and the anxieties consequent to conflict between id and superego drives experienced as shame and guilt. Dramatic acting out of the life-threatening scene during cathartic derepression allows both the expression of the affects mentioned beforehand and usually embellishes the historical recall of the action. Observing the abreaction makes possible for the therapist a more certain interpretation of the psychodynamics of the patient's problem.

Little attention has been given to the interpersonal relationship of the subject, who submits to catharsis either through narcosynthesis or hypnosis, and the observers. I perceive a "set" on the part of the subject to act out emotionally before another whom he or she trusts to accept and understand, one whose intent is to relieve distress and whose knowledge will provide a realistic interpretation of what has taken place within the subject. Thus, the therapist acts as an alter ego. In writing on abreaction, Bibring commented on the sufferer's sense of "being understood and accepted" and also the narcissistic gratification the sufferer receives through the personal exposure of his or her experience before the therapist (10).

In the acute traumatic states, abreaction relieves the sufferer of the tension inherent in the effort to repress and suppress the intensely held emotions as well as anxiety, guilt, and shame. Yet the very forces which have led to the massive repression continue to act in those with the chronic and delayed forms of PTSD. Psychodynamic forces, as well as the impairing effects of the use of the pharmacologic agent used in narcosynthesis, lead to a sizable failure to recall the drug-induced reenactment. It is for this reason that I confront my patients in a fully conscious state following the initial treatment with the video-taped reproduction of his action. This confrontation, carried out in the presence of the therapist, offers a conscious reproduction of the acceptance by the therapist of the expressed behavior as well as the opportunity for the therapist to provide empathic interpretations of that exposed behavior.

INDICATIONS

During the past four years, I have personally examined 100 Viet Nam combat veterans who had the symptoms of the chronic or delayed form of PTSD (as defined in *DSM-III* [1]). In addition, another sizable population of men has been seen in consultative interviews in other V.A. hospitals. Of this number 19 were treated in a single narcosynthetic session as an initiating phase to continuing individual therapy, group therapy, or both over a prolonged period of time.

Narcosynthesis was recommended for and carried out in hospitalized patients and outpatients with recurrent behavior symptoms, which suggested the breakthrough of dissociated and strongly repressed affective states. Such affective states were judged to exist when a history was given that included any of the following indicators:

1. Recurrent episodes of abnormal behavior in which the individual became aggressively threatening or violent, sometimes identifying himself as being in Viet Nam or identifying others as enemies in Viet Nam, followed by amnesia for the event. Such states have been denoted as unconscious flashbacks by Blank (11) (see Chapter 14). Often such episodes seemed precipitated by exposure of the individual to environmental situations simulating combat through some sensory experience. Frequently the individual had been drinking beforehand.
2. Persistent amnesias related to the combat experience.

3. Absence of affective response in recounting devastating combat trauma.
4. Repetitive panic attacks unrelieved by prior therapeutic efforts.
5. Chronically persistent and recurrent pain complaining behavior.

On the basis of my follow-up studies, I would still regard the first three categories of behavior as primary indicators for use of this initiating therapeutic technique. Panic attacks and pain complaining behavior might also be considered sufficient indicators if the currently standard group of nonintrusive individual psychotherapies and the use of pharmacotherapies yielded insufficient symptomatic response.

As an additional precaution, I do not prescribe either narcosynthesis or hypnotic abreaction to dispel amnesias which one might suspect concealed acts of atrocity leading to massive shame and guilt. Here the more conservative approach is through individual treatment (in my experience group or rap sessions seldom uncover such acts). Even then the likelihood of verbal exposure is obtained only after the patient has developed a firm trusting relationship with the therapist, which requires the development within the therapist of the capacity to respond helpfully to the recounting of atrocities. Preliminary therapy in an appropriate combat-related group setting seems helpful in those with severe difficulties in verbal expression.

CONTRAINDICATIONS

Psychological risks center around the potential breakdown of the patient's psychological defenses with occurrence, after abreaction, of a psychotic regression. This potential is presumed to exist in those with a prepsychotic personality configuration or those who have exhibited a previous psychotic illness. A careful diagnostic study, including psychological testing, is necessary to screen patients with such potential.

I have never encountered such a response in a combat veteran with PTSD, although many have shown widespread impairment of ego defenses, as indicated by MMPI results.

A closely allied phenomenon is the prolonged abreactive response, in which the patient acts out over many hours. In our 19 narcosynthetic trials this has occurred twice. The duration of the first was found after termination to coincide in time with the duration of a terror-ridden ambush experienced by the patient in Viet Nam. The content of this abreaction was fantasy (not fact) of capture, torture, and mutilation with acting out of pleading to be released. In the second instance of prolonged abreaction, the acting out consisted of cries of sorrowful disbelief that his close buddy had been killed on a mission; the two had decided on the toss of a coin who should take the assignment. This bout of crying out was terminated after 90 minutes by administration of a hypnotic dose of Valium given intramuscularly.

The major physiological risk in undertaking narcosynthesis with use of barbiturates is the possible occurrence of respiratory delay or paralysis. Preliminary physical examination is therefore necessary. It is advisable to exclude all persons with disease involving the cardiorespiratory systems, liver, or kidneys. Narcosynthesis is absolutely contraindicated when the patient has porphyria.

TECHNIQUE

As my intent has been both to identify the abreactive response as specifically induced by a meaningful sound stimulus associated with the experience and also to be certain that it would be possible to circumvent later denial of the response through lack of memory by presentation of that response through an audiovisual confrontation, certain modifications have been made in the standard narcosynthetic technique. Furthermore, to ensure the safety of the patient, I have regularly called upon my colleagues in the Department of Anesthesiology to administer the intravenous medication and to be on hand with necessary equipment to support any respiratory or cardiac incident.

For ethical and legal reasons, each patient is advised beforehand of the clinical reasons for undertaking the treatment, the risks involved are explained, and the patient is requested to sign two releases: one granting permission for administration of the intravenous medication and a second allowing audiovisual recording. At a later time, after the patient has reviewed his abreactive response so that he might determine whether the videotape recording be destroyed or limited in some way as to whom it might be displayed, the latter permission is reviewed again.

The critical changes from the standard technique used here are the following:

1. The abreactive response is induced by exposure to an auditory tape recording of a sequence of 30 seconds of quiet musical sounds, followed successively by 30 seconds of silence and then 30 seconds of combat sounds. The sound level of the noise approximates in the 70 decibel range in the neighborhood of the patient's head. The combat sound sequence consists of a succession of noises of helicopters, mortars, automatic rifle fire, and the scream of a wounded

man. This avoids the verbal suggestion to regress in time and place as was done during World War II to induce abreaction in treatment of the combat-induced acute post-traumatic states.

2. A videotape recording is made of the abreactive response.
3. After full recovery of consciousness the patient is brought to review the videotaped recording of his behavioral response in the presence of the attending psychiatrist, who offers therapeutic interpretation. The patient is asked whether he wishes to expose his responses to others. Many willingly agree to do this; once again, the psychiatrist attends the viewing and offers supportive and clarifying interpretative statements in the presence of the patient.

SUBJECTS TREATED

All of my patients were patients at the Albany V.A. Medical Center. Of those brought to abreaction, four were in consultation on the psychiatric inpatient service, seven were attending the Mental Hygiene Clinic, three were being treated by the alcohol and drug abuse service, and five were being treated by the medical and surgical services combined.

The predominant clinical problem in nine cases was repetitive dissociative episodes in which explosive, violent, or threatening behavior occurred; seven patients had repetitive panic attacks and explosive aggressive behavior; and three cases exhibited overdetermined pain complaining behavior.

The age range at the time of treatment fell between 29 and 34 years. These individuals were between 17 and 21 while in combat duty in Viet Nam. Currently, nine are married, nine divorced (three living with girlfriends), and one single. Educationally, all but one had completed high school or were in the last year of high school when they enlisted. One was in college. Seven were regularly employed, three were occasionally employed, and nine were unemployed.

A history of mental illness in families existed in two instances. Another had two epileptic brothers. One was an adoptee and another lost his parents at age seven, while a third was reared by grandparents. Prior to induction none had known psychiatric disorders.

During their military service 10 were wounded. Only one suffered a permanent mutilating and deforming wound of a leg; another suffered a head wound complicated with a post-traumatic convulsive disorder. On the Center for Policy Research Combat Scale, 15 out of 19 scored on the high range and the remainder scored on the middle range.

THERAPEUTIC RESULTS

One may assess the effects of the narcosynthesis in terms of immediate response—that is, the success in induction of abreaction, the early postabreactive response, and the later prevention or change in various target symptoms.

As concerns induction of abreaction with use of the described technique, 14 of 19 patients responded with emotional abreaction and time regression to a psychologically traumatic Viet Nam combat experience. These responses were dramatically vivid but varied. Some men were immediately alerted; others were deflected to crying or attempting to fight or to flee. All then verbally relived their experience, exposing a variety of affective states: fear, indignation, rage, sadness, and guilt and shame.

Of the nonresponders to the stimulus, two stated that the combat sound stimulus was meaningless to them. A man who valued his role as a nonemotional hero and who was receiving haloperidol at the time was exposed to the soundtrack used in the first few trials and correctly identified the World War II combat noises, which he stated were not significant to him. The second who stated that the Viet Nam combat sounds did not startle him had been severely wounded shortly after his arrival in Viet Nam. Two other nonresponders had both been chronically alcoholic. A satisfactory level of light narcosis was not achieved because both patients, after large doses of sodium pentothal, fell into a deep, nonarousable sleep.

To monitor physiological reactivity electroencephalographic and electrocardiographic records, as well as respiration, were recorded simultaneously during the last 15 abreactions. Fast wave activity occurred in the EEG typical of barbiturate intoxication. There were no significant changes in the rate or character of the EKG or in respiratory rhythm.

In the immediate postnarcosynthetic period the patients reported a reduction in tension. Some degree of sadness and depression but also an increase in self-acceptance and self-esteem took place after the confrontational review of the videotaped recording. Many of those who had their family members review the recordings expressed a sense that they were then better understood by the viewers.

An assessment of change in symptomatic expression and social adaptation was made two years after the narcosynthetic treatment. Since most of these patients were engaged in group and/or individual therapy of varying durations and intensities, as well as receiving anti-

depressant medication, these outcomes may not be assessed as consequent to the initiating narcosynthetic treatment alone. There has been
no recurrence of major dissociative states or panic attacks in 14 of the
15 men who abreacted. The one man who has acted out violently since
has stated recently in individual treatment that there still exists a
persisting amnestic period for events of several weeks immediately
preceding the acute catatenoid response which led to his removal from
combat. The man with associated post-traumatic convulsive disorders
has continued to have complex seizures with progressive amnesia but
no combat-related dissociative violence. Further efforts to continuously explore these amnestic periods are underway. All abreactors
who were secondarily alcoholic have ceased drinking.

Depressive affect was diminished. The constant symptoms of PTSD,
startle response with irritability, the potential for explosive rages, and
the sleep disturbance with repetitive combat dreams have persisted
although attenuated.

Two patients were lost to follow-up at two years. One, a nonrespon-
dent to abreactive stimulation, has been chronically alcoholic since his
combat experience and dropped out of treatment. The second, a
responder, continued intermittently in individual and group therapy
for six months, had no further panic attacks, expanded his interpersonal contacts, and entered college. Previously divorced twice, he
decided to move to another community when a growing closeness to a
young woman threatened him.

ADDITIONAL FINDINGS

The intense and dramatic abreactions observed in men some 10 or
more years after their psychologically traumatic experience suggested
that there might coexist abnormal physiological reactivity in various
organ systems, as well as the perceptual sensitivity to a short but
meaningful sound stimulus. Our attempts to discover such changes by
EEG, EKG, and respiratory monitoring during barbiturate subnar-
cosis were obscured by the drug effects. To explore this potential
further, 11 men with the clinical symptoms of PTSD (five of the 11
were also in the group treated earlier by narcosynthesis) were assessed
physiologically in a fully conscious state in the Stress Laboratory of the
State University of New York at Albany by Blanchard et al. (12).
Testing occurred during and after exposure to the same sequence of
sounds, played at different intensities, that was used to induce abreaction. Their responses were compared to those of 12 noncombatant,

same-aged, postgraduate university students, who were similarly exposed. The physiological responses monitored on a Grass Model 7D polygraph were heart rate, systolic and diastolic blood pressure, frontal muscle activity, peripheral skin temperature, and skin resistance. Both groups were stressed also with a mental arithmetic problem. When presented with the latter, both groups of men responded similarly. However, when presented with the 30-second exposure to combat sounds, the combat veterans—in contrast to the college students—displayed statistically significant increases in heart rate, systolic blood pressure, and forehead muscle activity.

While there is a need to extend this study and examine other control groups, including noncombatant Viet Nam veterans and those without clinical symptoms of PTSD, the findings suggest the existence of a persistent conditioned emotional response to sounds associated with combat, verifying an earlier study of Dobbs and Wilson on World War II veterans (13). In their clinical study of World War I veterans with the chronic form of war neurosis, Kardiner and Spiegel (14) offered conditioning as an explanation of those symptoms they identified as constantly present. These symptoms are 1) irritability and the startle pattern, 2) fixation on the trauma, 3) atypical dream life, 4) proclivity to explosive aggressive reaction, and 5) contraction of the general level of functioning, including intellectual functioning. Others also hypothesized the existence of a conditioning factor in the etiology of startle phenomena and some other symptoms expressive of the condition (5, 11).

DISCUSSION

This therapeutic experience has clarified the indications for narcosynthesis in the treatment of chronic and delayed PTSD resulting from war experiences. The follow-up studies suggest narcosynthesis as valuable in attenuating the risk for recurrent dissociative states, which are associated with socially destructive, acting out behavior. Confrontation of the denied and unrevealed emotionally charged experience from which the dissociative behavior has been derived, through viewing of the audiovisually recorded abreaction, has been useful in initiation of later continuing group therapy, individual psychotherapy, or both. The emotional associations of such experiences, as well as many details of the experience which provided understanding for actions taken or avoided, had not been revealed in earlier diagnostic or therapeutic efforts.

Thus, the single narcosynthetic treatment has relieved tension and reduced associated depression and has attenuated but not terminated the so-called constant symptoms of PTSD (psychotherapeutic and psychopharmaceutic treatment have likewise not abolished the latter). Modifications of individual character structure and defensive styles were in focus only in later psychotherapeutic efforts.

From these studies I have postulated the existence of an altered state of consciousness (15). This state particularly involves perceptions; excessive arousal derives from impairment of the capacity to discriminate conditioned stimuli signaling life-threatening crises. The related emotional response then occurs. To attenuate the conditioned emotional response which seems to drive the so-called constant symptoms in this group of seriously impaired men, in recent months I have prescribed use of the adrenergic blocking agents—propranolol or clonidine. Insufficient time has elapsed to evaluate the usefulness of these drugs, but in the short term many of the 40 men so treated have reported relief in the form of reduction in irritability and explosiveness, physiological arousal subsequent to startle or associated with combat dreams, as well as greater capacity for self-control. These effects seem less clear in the previously alcoholic patients, who were also more difficult to bring to abreaction.

This diagnostic and therapeutic approach has been modified over four years of work. In the few who present with the symptom complex which suggests prescription of narcosynthesis, I first examine them for hypnotic trance potential. If hypnotic potential is high, I attempt abreaction first with this technique. In the two men with high potential for hypnosis, abreaction attempted in this state was much less intense than that obtained when abreaction was induced by drug later.

In some patients, in whom major trance-like states have not occurred, resolution of amnestic dissociation has been attempted first through individual psychotherapy. These patients were advised that uncovering might be approached through individual psychotherapy, but if it became apparent that resistance remained fixed a move toward hypnotic or psychopharmaceutic catharsis might be made. As an example, after one man with long-standing recurrent psychophysiological symptoms developed an emerging awareness of an amnestic period which followed a traumatic combat experience, he requested psychopharmaceutic catharsis and has been so treated. In abreaction he reenacted experiences of massive grief at the loss of a close buddy; this loss had led to intense and prolonged denying behavior, induced by shaming responses by others in his platoon.

From the observations made upon the patients treated by narcosynthesis, the assumption may be made that the majority with continuing flashbacks are at high risk for cognitive dissociation in drug-altered states of consciousness, when exposed to stimuli associated with the traumatic experience. Clinical histories suggest that appropriate visual and olfactory stimuli might initiate cognitive dissociation with time regression and defensive behavior inappropriate to the current reality. In addition, social situations which arouse the affective states of fear, rage, and helplessness (the conditioned emotional response) may induce dissociation.

From the preventive standpoint I now regularly caution these veterans against drinking alcoholic beverages or the taking of any other mind-altering drugs. Also, these men are advised to inform any surgeon or dentist of this dissociative propensity if procedures involving anesthesia are recommended. A number of PTSD sufferers have reported that they "went crazy" during anesthetic induction or termination, according to reports made to them by their surgeons or dentists.

From the earlier studies of Kardiner and Spiegel (14) and Dobbs and Wilson (13) of severe chronic and delayed post-traumatic stress reactions to war, as well as from the experiences reported here, it is apparent that the phenomenology of the severe war-induced stress conditions derives from multiple sources. The chronic and delayed forms of war-induced PTSD are not, as Freud stated in 1921 (2), a simple traumatic neurosis.

As Kardiner postulated, there appears to exist in this population a basic physioneurosis determined on the principles of classical conditioning and generating constant irritability, explosive rages, and intermittently repetitive startle phenomena.

These recurrent physical expressions of alarm lead to the sufferers' attempts to control the sense of helplessness and fright induced by these symptoms. From the perspective of ego psychology, the problem becomes one of relating to one's body when a stable body ego no longer exists. These individuals experience interpersonal conflicts which derive from their irritability and irrational aggressiveness, which in turn follows from their misperceptions of attacks by others. Their attempts to control anxiety related to such interpersonal difficulties lead to the development of avoidance behaviors, including social withdrawal, alcohol and drug abuse, or—in the most severely traumatized—a terrified catatenoid existence. As the traumatized sufferer reflects further upon the catastrophic event, there evolve overdetermined affects of guilt or shame over presumed actions or failures of actions. These actions or failures are judged as contributing to disaster. There is also denial of relief at survival. In those who experienced overwhelming grief, rage, or utter helplessness inducing confusion at the time of breakdown, amnestic or catatenoid (16) responses may occur. Horowitz (17) has described the variations in symptomatology of the stress disorders in terms of defensive styles of the particular traumatized person.

Freud's statement, "The war neurosis may proclaim too loudly the effects of mortal changes and may be silent or speak only in muffled tones of the effects of frustration in love," (2) seems vindicated when we examine the later social consequences of those with combat-induced PTSD.

Many yearn for love and support from others, yet their fear at once again being exposed to the agony of loss prevents intimacy in marital, parental, or other love relationships. Beyond the initial mistrust in exposure of actions or inactions now perceived with shame or guilt, anxiety arises also when the attempt is made to engage in individual psychotherapy, because the patients fear close attachment to their therapists. Close therapeutic relationships may only take place over time. Such difficulties in engagement in individual psychotherapy have been noted earlier by Niederland (18) and others in the victims of the Holocaust.

Therapy must be undertaken with realistic goals. Relief of severe depression, guilt, and shame-ridden anxiety may be gained through psychotherapy. Attenuation of the fixed and recurrent symptoms of the altered psychophysiological state may occur through prescription of psychopharmaceutics. In those uncommon cases where states of repetitive dissociation or amnesia persist, derepressive techniques such as those reported here seem indicated.

REFERENCES

1. American Psychiatric Association: Diagnostic and Statisical Manual of Mental Disorders, Third Edition. Washington, DC, American Psychiatric Association, 1980

2. Freud S, Ferenczi S, Abraham K, et al: Psychoanalysis and War Neurosis. New York, International Psychoanalytic Press, 1921

3. Blackwenn WJ: Narcosis as therapy in neuropsychiatric conditions. JAMA 95:1168–1171, 1923

4. Lindemann E: Psychological changes in normal and abnormal individuals under the influence of sodium amytal. Am J Psychiatry 11:1083–1091, 1932

5. Sargent W, Slater E: Acute war neurosis. Lancet 2:1, 1940

6. Mallinson WP: Narcoanalysis in neuropsychiatry. Journal of the Royal Navy Medical Service 26:281, 1940

7. Horsley JS: Narcoanalysis. Lancet 1:55, 1936

8. Grinker RR, Spiegel JJ: Men Under Stress. Philadelphia, Blakiston, 1945

9. Redlich FC, Ravitz LJ, Dession GH: Narcoanalysis and truth. Am J Psychiatry 107:586–593, 1951

10. Bibring E: Psychoanalysis and the dynamic psychotherapies. J Am Psychoanal Assoc 2:745–770, 1954

11. Blank A: The unconscious flashback to the war in Viet Nam veterans: clinical mystery, legal defense and community problem. Paper presented at the Annual Meeting of the American Psychological Association, Montreal, 1980

12. Blanchard EB, Kolb LC, Pallmeyer TP, et al: A psychophysiological study of post traumatic stress disorder in Viet Nam veterans. Psychiatr Q 54:220–229, 1982

13. Dobbs D, Wilson WP: Observations on persistence of war neurosis. Dis Nerv Syst 21:40–46, 1960

14. Kardiner A, Spiegel H: War Stress and Neurotic Illness, 2nd ed. New York, Paul B. Hoeber, 1947

15. Kolb LC, Mutalipassi LR: The conditioned emotional response: a sub-class of chronic and delayed post traumatic stress disorders. Psychiatric Annals 12:979–987, 1982

16. Krystal H: Trauma and affects. Psychoanal Study Child 33:81–115, 1978

17. Horowitz MJ: Stress Response Syndromes. New York, Jason Aronson, 1976

18. Niederland WG: Clinical observations on the survivor syndrome. Int J Psychoanal 49:313–315, 1968

11

The Veterans Administration's Viet Nam Veterans Outreach and Counseling Centers

Arthur S. Blank, Jr., M.D.

11

Vet Centers—Viet Nam Veterans Outreach and Counseling Centers—were established by the Veterans Administration in late 1979 to treat the emotional wounds of war and impeded postwar social readjustment in veterans. This system of 189 Vet Centers, situated in all parts of the United States—from Bangor to Honolulu, and from Anchorage to St. Croix—has turned out to be the leading edge of the nation's response to postwar psychosocial difficulties in veterans. Vet Centers, fundamentally created by Viet Nam veterans themselves, are a highly successful focus for veterans (and family members) gathering together for vital debriefing and emotional processing of war events, in a context which also provides expert counseling (both peer and professional) and psychotherapy for post-traumatic stress disorder and other readjustment problems.

As of late 1984, Vet Centers had seen over 330,000 persons (veterans and significant others) for counseling, psychotherapy, referral, and related assistance.

The following sections will outline the origins of this enterprise and indicate what resources it provides to veterans and those who assist them. Particularly for mental health professionals, Vet Centers provide a point of organization of treatment services and coordination.

HISTORICAL PERSPECTIVE

For approximately 15 years prior to 1980, veterans returning from Southeast Asia who were experiencing PTSD and various life dislocations were in general unable to obtain effective therapeutic assistance,

---

The views expressed in this chapter are solely those of the author and do not necessarily reflect those of the Veterans Administration.

either from the Veterans Administration or within the private sector. This extraordinary breakdown in health care delivery was one feature of a complex repudiation (both active and passive) directed at many of the approximately 3.8 million men and women who served in the war zone. As a social and psychological phenomenon, these difficulties of veterans in obtaining treatment were caused by many factors, of which at least eight have been identified in the clinical and epidemiologic literature (1–7).

Diagnosis. Prior to 1980, the American Psychiatric Association provided inaccurate guidance on the matter of traumatic neurosis or PTSD. The Association's first *Diagnostic and Statistical Manual of Mental Disorders* in 1952 indicated that extreme stress could produce a distinct mental reaction but that such a reaction by definition was transient (8). The second edition of the nomenclature, *DSM-II* (9), dropped a clear reference to extreme stress and repeated the notion that any significant reaction to stress was inherently transient. Not until 1980, in *DSM-III* (10), did the mental health professions receive official guidance that traumatic stress produces a discrete and unique mental reaction which may occur independently and is clearly distinguishable from other mental disorders.

The Predisposition Theory. Concomitant with the lack of a clear diagnosis prior to 1980, many health professionals had a disinclination to believe that war veterans who had been generally normal before the war would develop a traumatic stress condition whose etiology was not *primarily* preexisting personality weakness or defect. The predisposition theory—the notion that war neurosis is primarily caused by prewar personality characteristics—has been steadily undermined by accumulating military psychiatry experience since the middle of World War II, and by the published clinical writings of therapists who had actually treated World War II, Korean War, and Viet Nam War veterans. Nonetheless, clinical evaluations of Viet Nam veterans with stress disorders during the late 1960s and 1970s typically ignored the history of war trauma, in favor of a focus on etiology in the arenas of childhood and adolescent experience. (In my own review of 75 cases, evaluated at one V.A. Medical Center during 1972 to 1980, the military history was ignored and the diagnosis of PTSD was missed during some period of psychiatric contact.)

The Generation Gap. During the 15 years prior to 1980, many Viet Nam veterans, who had been on the average 19.5 years old during their duty in Viet Nam, were situated across a generation and cultural gap from middle- and senior-level clinicians. This estrangement was forced in particular by the rapid changes in style and substance in American society, which accompanied the Viet Nam War.

Negative Stereotypes. During the early and mid-1970s, numerous television crime programs and movies portrayed Viet Nam veterans as violence prone, drug-ridden, or both. Although such stereotypes have developed around veterans of other wars (World War II, for example [11]), the peculiarities of the Viet Nam War may have created such images to an unusual degree. This was manifested, for example, by showing the films *Taxi Driver* and *First Blood* on nationwide television over the weekend of Veterans Day in November 1984. Both emphasize the murderousness of Viet Nam veteran protagonists.

Conflicts Within Clinicians. Intellectual, emotional, and moral tensions and conflicts about the Viet Nam War have persisted in the minds of many mental health professionals. Clinicians may have worked hard to avoid the draft or to avoid assignment to Viet Nam if in the military, or they may still experience unresolved conflicts about the nature of the war and its meaning to our country. Such tensions can interfere with the ability to hear about the war in graphic detail from its veterans.

The Inherently Painful Quality of Traumatic Experience. Treatment of war veterans requires the therapist to hear about events outside the realm of ordinary human experience. These include intense fear, horror, and sometimes gruesome human butchery, to name just three. Because of this unique content, most often some unique background or training is required for psychotherapists to be interested, and effective, with war veterans. During 1965 to 1980, mental health training in the United States emphasized no such special preparation or identification of especially talented clinicians.

Political and Historical Dimension. The highly problematic character of the Viet Nam War produced alterations in the citizen identity of many veterans, who were left with deep questions about the meaning and conduct of the war (12). This brings a political and historical dimension to most diagnosis and treatment, an element of value conflicts, and the need for such matters to be smoothly fitted in with more traditional approaches. Such a variation from one's usual peacetime practice of treating persons who have never directly participated in a national tragedy has proved to be beyond the measure of many clinicians.

Survivor Missions. The psychological recovery of most Viet Nam veterans with PTSD, as for most survivors of traumatic stress, usually requires the discovery and fulfillment, during and after therapy, of a survivor mission. This mission consists of productive activities in the real world, wherein the survivor creatively applies lessons learned from traumatic events. This may manifest itself, for example, as intense activity in a veterans' organization, working on a Viet Nam veterans memorial, assisting other veterans, or political activity on an issue related to the Viet Nam War. Clinicians unfamiliar with the central role of survivor missions in recovery from PTSD may react negatively to a perceived conflict between the mission and the requirements of formal treatment. For example, they will object to a need to reschedule or miss hours because of survivor mission-related activities.

The foregoing factors account for much of the nationwide nondelivery of postwar readjustment services to Viet Nam veterans prior to 1980. In addition, expert clinicians and researchers during that period discovered that some veterans with PTSD—and some with only equivocal constellations of stress symptoms—had vocational, social, educational, and family problems that were closely interwoven with core psychic symptoms (2, 4, 6–8). This resulted from social pressure toward suppression of direct PTSD symptoms and their subsequent emergence in an indirect manner, which affected general life functioning. Another factor was that some returning combat veterans have difficulties in reentering peacetime life processes, regardless of psychopathology.

DEVELOPMENT OF VET CENTERS

Throughout the period of nonprovision of services just described, the foundations of an ultimate response to these problems of Viet Nam veterans and American society was being laid down.

In 1969–1970, at the initiative of Senator Alan Cranston (D-California), the Senate Subcommittee on Veterans' Affairs held hearings on the status of servicemen returning from Viet Nam. There followed a 10-year legislative struggle to provide definitive federally sponsored psychological treatment and readjustment assistance. Between 1969 and 1978, the U.S. Senate four times passed legislation which would have led to Vet Centers, but the House of Representatives would not take up the matter, and the initiatives were not supported by the Veterans Administration.

However, concomitant with this legislative struggle, clinical and research documentation of the need for a special program and the activities of Viet Nam veteran self-help projects increasingly focused national attention on the status and needs of veterans.

Critical psychiatric reports during the 1970s demonstrated homology of stress disorder in Viet Nam veterans with the war neurosis of earlier wars (1, 3, 4, 13–15) and the various unique, but surmountable, obstacles that stood in the way of effective treatment. At the end of the decade, the preliminary reports of the first nationwide psycho-social epidemiologic survey of Viet Nam veterans, carried out by the Center for Policy Research, provided evidence of significant stress disorder and other readjustment problems (7).

Throughout the 1970s a number of projects started by Viet Nam veterans to help other veterans also emerged and flourished, particularly insofar as they provided a locus for the intensive discussion of wartime experiences and current emotional reactions. These projects included group therapy sponsored by *Vietnam Veterans Against the War* (2) and self-help organizations such as the *Veterans Service Project* in St. Louis, *From Swords Into Plowshares* and *Twice Born Men* in San Francisco, *Project Return* in Portland, the *Seattle Veterans Assistance Center (SEAVAC)*, and *Flower of the Dragon* in Santa Rosa, California. There were also numerous other organizations.

In 1979, these various threads were woven together in Public Law 96-22. Again at the Senate's initiative—and finally with the support of the House, the major veterans organizations, and the chief of the Veterans Administration, Max Cleland—the new law established that veterans of the Viet Nam era were entitled to "readjustment counseling." Specialized counseling centers located in communities around the nation were established. This legislation (subsequently reaffirmed by the Congress in 1981, 1983, and 1984) has cast into law the recognition of 1) persisting life-readjustment and stress disorder impact of war zone military experiences and 2) a national responsibility to provide veterans with therapeutic services for such problems.

Wisely, the service delivery structure is community-based and detached from Veterans Administration medical facilities (though working in close collaboration with them). Also, there is no requirement that veterans obtain a formal determination of service-connected disability to obtain counseling or psychotherapy. (The latter feature avoids institutionalizing secondary gain.)

ORGANIZATION

Vet Centers are operated by a national directorate in the Veterans Administration's Central Office in Washington, D.C., through regional management staffs located in the six Veterans Administration medical regions. They receive administrative support from local V.A. medical centers, with which Vet Centers also collaborate on treatment services.

The prototype Vet Center has a staff of four persons, including one mental health professional (psychologist, social worker, psychiatrist, or nurse), two professional or paraprofessional counselors, and one office manager. Nationwide, the staff mix includes approximately 60 percent Viet Nam theatre veterans, 20 percent Viet Nam era veterans, and 20 percent veterans of other eras or nonveterans. Centers typically attract significant numbers of professional and nonprofessional volunteers and trainees. A unique administrative feature, developed at the inception of Vet Centers, is the provision of absolute confidentiality of any personal or clinical data obtained on clients.

THE THERAPEUTIC MODEL

Multi-Service Centers

Within the limits of the skill range which can be assembled in a small staff, Vet Centers provide a broad span of services. This includes counseling and psychotherapy (group, family, and individual), vocational and educational counseling, community and family education about the nature of the Viet Nam War and its impact on veterans, community networking, referrals, general advocacy, and conjoint treatment with V.A. medical facility staff.

Holding Environment

Housed in storefronts, large houses, or shopping centers—and not connected to other government buildings—Vet Centers were designed and furnished according to the needs of Viet Nam veterans and their friends and families. Vet Centers ordinarily provide a safe, peaceful, comforting, nonbureaucratic, and dignified context in which veterans can contemplate and talk about their Viet Nam experience and its meaning in their lives. Combining these features with formal counseling and psychotherapy, and with an integrated program of referral and assistance on a wide range of veterans issues, creates a holding environment connected to the deepest levels of psychological development.

The emotional power of this setting is extremely important for many veterans. Vet Centers provide 1) effective help for long-buried difficulties, 2) a sense of shared pride and simple reality about the Viet Nam experience, 3) a safe place for the retrieval of prematurely shut-away memories and unfortunately neglected memorabilia from Viet Nam, and 4) constructive personal alliances with comrades who must also confront the hostility or discomfort of others about one's identity as a Viet Nam veteran. All combine to encourage completion of a long inner journey back from Southeast Asia.

The Vet Center Counseling Staff

A Vet Center staff functions as a team and includes at least one mental health professional; usually at least two staff members are themselves Viet Nam veterans. Staff immersion in the Viet Nam experience, when combined with professional skills and experience, is directly or indirectly crucial to the effectiveness of services offered. The staff mix and personal veteran background provide for a flexible response to a veteran's oscillation among engagement in formal treatment, development of a personal survivor mission, and community and family readjustment.

PRINCIPLES OF INTERVENTION

The Viet Nam Experience. In counseling or psychotherapy veterans are provided, as a first condition, with a listener who has the unflinching ability to listen to, confront, and contain memories of experiences in Viet Nam. Many (but not all) veterans with PTSD or other readjustment problems eventually find it useful to review certain war experiences in detail.

Affect. It is anticipated in the structure of the program that emotions connected to war events may be intensely reexperienced (or experienced for the first time).

Impact of the Character of the Viet Nam War. It is assumed that veterans and family members may require assistance in resolving value, ego identity, and citizen identity conflicts deriving from the Viet Nam War experience and the peculiarities of the homecoming. Counselors and psychotherapists are particularly aware of the unusual features of postwar family and social situations and how these may have contributed to the persistence of PTSD.

Training. Staff training, both initial and ongoing, addresses not only skills and development of techniques, but also full and effective working through of the staff member's personal history concerning the Viet Nam War.

Rap Groups and Group Therapy. Most Vet Centers provide group therapy for veterans, and some include groups for significant others as well. Group treatment relies, for effectiveness, on 1) a leader who served in Viet Nam, or who is deeply attuned to the Viet Nam experience because of personal qualities or experience; 2) membership composed of peers—other Viet Nam veterans; and 3) a theoretical understanding of the principles of group treatment for survivors of traumatic stress (see Chapter 8). The group program is a critical element in Vet Center services, and for some veterans participation in the program is a critical step in recovery from PTSD and resolution of other war-related problems.

Medication. All Vet Center services are organized around the professional consensus that PTSD is a freezing of the normal traumatic stress reaction and recovery process, and that the condition is therefore ordinarily most effectively addressed by psychological and psychosocial interventions. Psychotropic medication is not viewed as a central modality of treatment. However, in certain cases clients may be referred for medication as a useful adjunct to counseling services.

Avoidance of Nonspecific Drug and Psychotherapeutic Treatment. It is recognized in the Vet Center program that nonspecific treatment methods used with Viet Nam veterans with PTSD—as commonly practiced in V.A. hospitals, community mental health centers, and elsewhere in the private sector prior to 1980—are ineffective and sometimes counterproductive or even dangerous (1, 3–6). This includes the range of standard approaches (psychotherapy, counseling, drugs, etc.) if they do not include a specific understanding of the etiology of PTSD, sufficient attention to the military history, and recognition of the meaning of symptoms of traumatic reactions.

Integration of Psychological Services with Other Assistance. Vet Centers provide psychological counseling and therapy along with educational and employment counseling; the counselors are knowledgeable about many veterans' needs and issues. The decompartmentalization of services is based on the view that the psychological symptoms derived from PTSD and various postwar life-functioning defects (such as failure to resume higher education or chronic underemployment) interact closely and synergistically and require integrated services.

Stress Reduction. General stress reduction techniques, including guided relaxation, meditation, biofeedback, and hypnosis, are of value in some instances and are provided either directly or by referral, depending on staff qualifications.

Outreach. All services are conducted within an outreach context. Reaching out in various ways is a responsibility of the Vet Center staff, so that difficulties in the way of utilization of services by veterans are removed.

SUMMARY OF SERVICES PROVIDED

1. Counseling and psychotherapy—individual, group, and family;
2. Educational and employment counseling;
3. Vocational and educational testing at certain locations;

4. Psychological testing at certain locations;
5. Counseling concerning Veterans Administration and other government benefits and procedures, which may include technical information concerning discharge upgrade, benefits, etc.;
6. Community education about the Viet Nam experience and the problems and strengths of Viet Nam veterans; and
7. Consultation with professionals about PTSD and other war veteran readjustment problems.

FEE/CONTRACT PROGRAM

The legislation that authorizes the Vet Center system also authorizes a mechanism whereby counselors and mental health professionals in the private sector can apply for private contractor provider status. If so designated, these professionals can be reimbursed for consultation and therapy with veterans. The types of problems authorized to be treated, and the types of treatment, are the same as those encountered in the Vet Centers. Clients may be seen in the fee/contract program if referred by a Vet Center staff member or V.A. medical center mental health professional.

REFERENCES

1. Van Putten T, Emory WH: Traumatic neurosis in Viet Nam returnees. Arch Gen Psychiatry 29:695–698, 1973

2. Lifton RJ: Home from the War. New York, Simon & Schuster, 1973

3. Haley S: When the patient reports atrocities. Arch Gen Psychiatry 30:191–196, 1974

4. Figley CR (ed): Stress Disorders Among Viet Nam Veterans. New York, Brunner/Mazel, 1978

5. Blank AS Jr: First training conference papers (mimeo). Readjustment Counseling Service, Veterans Administration, Washington, DC, 1979

6. Figley CR, Leventman S: Strangers at Home. New York, Praeger, 1980

7. Egendorf A, Kadushin C, Laufer RS, et al: Legacies of Viet Nam. Washington, DC, U.S. Government Printing Office, 1981

8. American Psychiatric Association: Diagnostic and Statistical Manual of Mental Disorders. Washington, DC, American Psychiatric Association, 1952

9. American Psychiatric Association: Diagnostic and Statistical Manual of Mental Disorders, Second Edition. Washington, DC, American Psychiatric Association, 1968

10. American Psychiatric Association: Diagnostic and Statistical Manual of Mental Disorders, Third Edition. Washington, DC, American Psychiatric Association, 1980

11. Leed EJ: No Man's Land: Combat and Identity in World War II. New York, Cambridge University Press, 1979

12. Louis Harris & Associates: Myths and Realities: A Study of Attitudes Toward Viet Nam Era Veterans. Washington, DC, Louis Harris & Associates, 1980

13. Horowitz MJ, Solomon GF: A prediction of delayed stress response syndromes in Viet Nam veterans. Journal of Social Issues 31:67–80, 1975

14. Shatan C: Post–Viet Nam syndrome. The New York Times, May 6, 1972

15. Solomon GF, Zarcone VP, Yoerg R, et al: Three psychiatric casualties from Viet Nam. Arch Gen Psychiatry 25:522–524, 1971

12

Inpatient Treatment of Viet Nam Veterans with Post-Traumatic Stress Disorder

Arthur L. Arnold, M.D.

12

Not all Viet Nam veterans with post-traumatic stress disorder require inpatient treatment as a medical necessity. However, those who present sufficiently serious problems of risk management should be considered for inpatient admission just as would others with a range of mental disorders. The clinical decision between inpatient and outpatient treatment is more complex when both provide adequately for risks of suicide or assault.

INDICATIONS FOR ADMISSION

Viet Nam veterans usually come to clinical attention because of a crisis. They may fear imminent loss of control of hostile impulses. A reported urge to "blow everyone away" or to commit a specific attack on particular people should be taken seriously enough to consider immediate inpatient admission. Some are brought to a hospital after already acting on such impulses. Others are suicidal. They are more likely to be intercepted during actual suicidal behavior by others who bring them to the hospital than they are to present themselves with a complaint of suicidal ideation. Since they are likely to have lethal weapons and are experienced in their use, it is unwise to assume that the risks are low simply because previous episodes have not been fatal.

Most lethality assessment protocols for suicide and assault developed for psychiatric patients include factors which would place many veterans with PTSD at high risk. These include the following:

- Potentially lethal methods,
- Having sustained significant losses,
- Having inadequate social supports,
- Previous similar episodes,

- An attitude of helplessness and hopelessness, and
- Being male (1–4).

The withdrawal of a spouse or partner, especially one who has sustained mental or physical abuse, combined with unresolved grief at the loss of fellow soldiers in combat is a common precipitant of crises in Viet Nam veterans. Some veterans engage in dangerous behavior during reexperiences of combat, particularly dissociative or fugue states. For these patients the necessity for inpatient psychiatric admission is usually obvious; the problem may be to convince the veteran.

On the other hand, Viet Nam veterans who present general complaints of not fitting their concept of themselves or their role in the external world, and who have the cardinal features of PTSD but are not an imminent risk, may be candidates for either inpatient or outpatient treatment. The decision often depends upon availability of facilities.

CHOICE OF INPATIENT OR OUTPATIENT TREATMENT

If, after the diagnostic interview (see Chapter 6), the patient and staff agree that treatment specific for PTSD will be undertaken, the options should be reviewed. The patient needs to work with a clinician to confront, reexperience, analyze, and come to terms with the trauma underlying continuing distress. If there is ample opportunity for shared recollection and mutual support with other Viet Nam veterans —in such a way as to be coordinated with psychotherapy—and if inpatient admission can be assured in the event of a crisis, the preferable approach is outpatient treatment. If, however, the patient's day-to-day functioning is tenuous, with disturbing explosive outbursts and repeated indications of risk (such as suicidal ruminations or repeated fights), and there is unreliable interpersonal support, inpatient treatment is preferred. Only a treatment program which meets the specific needs of patients with PTSD should be initiated, whether on an inpatient or outpatient basis.

SPECIFICITY OF TREATMENT

A patient with PTSD following any trauma is ill-served by any treatment which does not specifically meet the needs of that condition. Psychotherapy, whether individual or group, that focuses only upon symptoms such as depression (5), maladaptive responses to here-and-now issues, self-defeating interpersonal patterns of behavior, or early life phenomena having current significance *instead of* the meaning of traumatic experiences and their consequences is ineffective (6), may be harmful, and is an invalidation of the patient's psychic wounds or a rejection of the patient.

CRISIS RESOLUTION

For patients in crisis, admission to a general acute psychiatric ward is appropriate, with the goal of resolving the immediate crisis and restoring stability. Even for achieving these short-term goals and the application of nonspecific techniques, it is important that staff of all disciplines have an understanding of stress disorders. The clinical leaders of the treatment team, at least, should be familiar with PTSD in Viet Nam veterans, and countertherapeutic attitudes should be confronted by staff who are empathic role models.

Some cannot work effectively with Viet Nam veterans or with patients having combat-related PTSD. In any hospital setting, if exceptions are to be made to the usual staffing pattern, the question of selective assignments or participation should be settled either in advance or as each admission arrives on the ward. This requires sensitivity and mutual respect. For example, the potential for oriental staff members to stimulate combat flashbacks or nightmares, for authoritarian staff to evoke "fragging" impulses (7), or for staff who are themselves Viet Nam veterans to overidentify with patients and perhaps even themselves decompensate should be discussed and understood in terms of the patient's best interests.

CONSIDERATE ADMISSION PROCESS

If admission procedures are expedited and straightforward explanations of expectations are provided, the inpatient stay is more apt to achieve its purpose. The participation of a Viet Nam veteran who is trusted and who is familiar with the hospital is valuable. Staff of Viet Nam veteran counseling centers are often involved with the rescue and transport of the patient to the hospital. If possible, they should walk through the admission process with the patient.

INITIAL RISK ASSESSMENT

A careful risk assessment should be performed promptly, and appropriate precautions should be initiated to minimize the likelihood of suicide, assault, or premature departure. Weapons must be removed, including those carried habitually for a sense of security (8). Recent or repeated hazardous behavior should be evaluated. These past actions are more reliable in predicting risk management problems than are the patient's assurances that once in the hospital no disturbed behavior will occur, no precautions are necessary, and all rights and privileges should be retained. After further observation, increases in freedom from protective controls are easier to arrange than are greater restrictions.

STAFF AUTHORITY

If the unit operates with clear hierarchies of authority based upon professional discipline, the mode of exercise of staff power to control patients should be apparent (9, 10). If possible the input of mental health professionals who are themselves Viet Nam veterans should be considered nondefensively. Some veterans may not be able to tolerate the perception of being given orders concerning picayune rules or the risk of being physically or chemically overwhelmed if they disobey, because this too closely resembles wartime experiences. The most effective staff members are those who are most open, straightforward, secure, and able to humanize and individualize the care they provide. These attributes are most essential in nursing staff, with whom the patients will interact most often. It should also be recognized that veterans with PTSD may not accept a psychiatric patient role. This is not surprising since they usually are not psychotic, are doubtful of their worth, and are fearful of submission.

Patient Government

If the ward is operated as a therapeutic community, the degree to which patients assume responsibility and the manner in which peer influences are exercised greatly affect Viet Nam veteran patients. If there is an organized patient government, nonpsychotic Viet Nam veterans often assume elected roles as officers (11), but at the other extreme others may avoid participating altogether.

Challenges to Authority

In either case, many veterans with continuing distrust of authority will challenge staff who have the power to control patient behavior. The purpose is to determine the degree of staff caring and strength, both of which are needed, rather than to undermine authority itself. Suicide threats are also made as part of this testing process. It is important that staff persevere in demonstrating concern for the veteran, while requiring the veteran to act in the best interests of the peer group.

The maintenance of ward discipline reflects staff credibility. The parental approach which may be effective with patients with schizophrenia or cognitive impairment is anathema to patients with PTSD. Viet Nam veterans need to avoid feelings of fear or helplessness. They distrust unfamiliar authorities and have wounded self-esteem (both derived from combat realities), so they are apt to respond to the hospital staff with hostility. It is difficult for staff to avoid overreacting with force as they feel intimidated. Uniformed hospital police should be prudently utilized to restore order, and then only in a restrained manner.

DIAGNOSIS

Even for a relatively brief crisis resolution admission, an accurate diagnostic workup is essential (6, 12) (see Chapter 6) in order to provide the basis for further treatment. The rapport which will be required for more definitive treatment as well as the evolution of a data base, will be possible when careful attention is given to specific combat experiences when obtaining a military history; the content of nightmares, flashbacks, and other reexperiences is explored in the psychiatric history; and there is expression of a genuine desire to understand how these are related.

MEDICATIONS

If the purpose of a crisis-related admission is to reduce distress, medications may be utilized (13). Chronic PTSD is characterized by traumatic reexperiences with painful levels of affect alternating with avoidance phenomena (14). If upon admission the intolerable affective stress response is one of depression with guilt or grief, antidepressants with rapid onset of action may be helpful. If agitation and anxiety are most prominent, neuroleptics may be preferred on a low-dose, as-needed regimen. Benzodiazepines are problematic because of habituation and occasional enhancement of rage. Haloperidol tends to produce akathisia and dystonia especially of the neck and throat muscles in these patients. Both panic attacks and nightmares often respond to tricyclic antidepressants (15, 16). It may be useful to discuss the judicious short-term use of medication with the patient soon after admission, without making this an unnecessary confrontation. Viet Nam veterans who complain that they are overmedicated as well as those who threateningly demand medication appear to see in both situations a rejection and forced helplessness (17).

INTERACTIONS WITH OTHER PATIENTS

Even during short inpatient stays, veterans with PTSD may be critical of psychotic patients on the ward and even react with hostility to any annoying symptomatic behavior. When Viet Nam veterans are assigned to share rooms with each other, there is mutual empathy, and informal support networks are promoted which are invaluable after discharge.

Staff are sometimes fearful that Viet Nam veterans will gang up on them if the veterans are encouraged to associate with each other. As with anything which benefits patients, the opportunity for veterans to relate to each other usually promotes more, not less, cooperation. As veterans settle down, with a sense of legitimacy and belonging, it is often possible for those with PTSD to become helpful to psychotic patients by acting as guides in a ward "buddy system"; the experience is mutually beneficial.

ACTIVITIES

Physical exercise, organized team sports, and outdoor activities are important physical outlets for any young adult with emotional tension, and these should be provided for veterans with PTSD as soon after admission as practical. Occupational therapy of the busywork arts and crafts type are often rejected, but masculine hobbies popular in adolescence, such as constructing models of cars and aircraft, are popular among male veterans. One of the purposes of the crisis admission is to reduce traumatic reexperiences, and organized activities play a part in this process.

PATIENT EDUCATION

Viet Nam veterans can benefit from learning factual information about PTSD. This often reduces anxiety that something inexplicable or untreatable is happening to them. This requires not only an informed staff capable of effective patient education, but staff attitudes in which patients are expected to learn about themselves as part of a healing process, rather than in an effort to obtain compensation.

SUBSTANCE ABUSE

Issues of alcohol and other drug abuse often must be addressed, both in patient education and referrals for appropriate treatment (18–23). When substance abuse occurs as a result of self-medication to reduce the intensity of combat nightmares and other traumatic reexperiences, veterans may reject standard substance abuse rehabilitation programs, which do not address PTSD. Nevertheless, while crisis management of PTSD may not require the initiation of substance abuse rehabilitation, any subsequent, more definitive treatment of PTSD must preclude nonprescribed use of mind-altering drugs. Referral should be made to alcohol or drug rehabilitation programs when indicated. The success of such substance abuse treatment, however, may require simultaneous treatment of the PTSD.

PSYCHOTHERAPY

The psychotherapy specifically required for treatment of PTSD is too lengthy a process to attempt during an inpatient admission of a few days or weeks, but the groundwork for it can be laid. If appropriate treatment for PTSD is available, diagnostic interviews may be used to introduce the veteran to introspection and trust, so that a referral for treatment is likely to result in a good start.

COORDINATION WITH OUTPATIENT TREATMENT

When veterans who are already involved in outpatient psychotherapy specifically for PTSD have intercurrent crises requiring brief inpatient admissions, it is good practice for the therapist to maintain regular contact and, if possible, to advance the therapy during this time. The outpatient therapist and the inpatient staff should communicate to minimize the splitting which so often occurs in this situation, with the veteran playing off the "good guys" who understand and the "bad guys" who impose restrictions. Splitting may well make the inpatient staff feel undermined and ineffectual, and this impairs effective risk management when a Viet Nam veteran is in a life-threatening crisis (24). The outpatient therapist can be helpful in potentially dangerous situations and also when a veteran wants to leave the hospital against medical advice.

FOLLOW-UP

Every effort should be made to refer patients with PTSD to appropriate follow-up when they are discharged from the hospital. One cannot assume that a general purpose program will focus upon the veteran's PTSD pathology. Vet Centers operated by the Veterans Administration and other outreach counseling centers which have been established to serve Viet Nam veterans are an invaluable resource in planning for follow-up after discharge. This is particularly true if the hospital has no established link with a clinic providing a specialized outpatient program for PTSD. Informed clinicians in the community, who understand the problems of veterans with PTSD and know how to treat them, can also be a valuable resource.

SPECIALIZED INPATIENT UNITS

Inpatient treatment of veterans with PTSD is indicated in many instances even when an immediate crisis is not present. Specific treatment which has as its goal accelerated progress in working through and resolving the personal impact of traumatic experiences in Viet Nam (23, 24) can be accomplished on an inpatient unit. For those veterans whose lives are chronically unstable, who have no reliable personal support system or whose behavior has jeopardized their supportive relationships, or who are unable to function adequately on a day-to-day basis (in other words, for veterans who cannot be treated safely and effectively on an outpatient basis), a specialized inpatient treatment program is indicated. These are not widely available; there are only 12 such units in V.A. hospitals at this writing, although work underway at several other facilities may increase this number (25).

The existing units are highly effective according to informally reported clinical impressions. Most are continuously at capacity and have waiting lists for admission. However, the desirability of specialized inpatient treatment units for Viet Nam veterans with PTSD is not universally accepted. There are those who object to anything which would make these veterans think they are "special," as though this would be a capitulation to demands for such care or somehow legitimize antiauthoritarian attitudes. Others express concern that nothing must impede the veterans from leaving the Viet Nam War behind them and reentering the mainstream of society, and they assume that when Viet Nam veterans are treated with the mainstream of primarily psychotic inpatients reentry into society is somehow facilitated. It is, of course, widely accepted that some patients are best treated in specialized units. These include geriatric, adolescent, alcoholism, forensic, and medical-psychiatric wards. The assumption that in many situations specialized expertise makes it possible to provide the best care is common in medicine. The rationale for specialized units for combat-related PTSD reflects the same assumption.

THE BASIC PRINCIPLES OF TREATMENT

The specificity of treatment for PTSD derives from the nature of the disorder and the natural course of its resolution. Exposure to sufficient trauma produces an affective response which overwhelms usual coping mechanisms (26, 27). The trauma is reexperienced repeatedly, avoidance mechanisms being utilized when the recurring affect becomes intolerable. As these cycles are repeated, there is the potential for mastery of the traumatic experience and integration of its significance into a changed self (14, 28). Treatment which facilitates this phasic process in a protected setting is appropriate and essential.

As inpatients spontaneously reexperience trauma in such forms as nightmares, flashbacks, and recollections, they are supported in confronting and coming to terms with their meaning. When they are unable to tolerate the painful feelings this produces, they are supported in resting and putting it all out of awareness. If they persistently avoid reexperiencing their trauma, they are confronted with reminders to deal with it. Within the treatment process there is implosion, abreaction, and catharsis, and all require the utmost in empathic, creative, and courageous listening.

At times the treatment process is like working with a patient to repeatedly incise and drain an old infected wound that is poisoning the entire system. Although the process is often painful, eventually the wound heals, until only a scar remains. The physician's goal is to heal the infected wound with as little pain, impairment of function, and disfigurement as possible. Likewise, careful treatment of PTSD supports mastery of the unimaginable to allow the veteran to become a stronger and wiser survivor.

Individual Psychotherapy

Individual psychotherapy of veterans with PTSD is similar whether conducted on an inpatient or outpatient basis (29). Anger and tears come naturally as the trauma of war comes back to mind, each time with another nuance, meaning, or perspective. Interpretations are not always needed to assist recognition of the meaning of fantasies and symbols. The recall of reality is often in focus. Missing memories are often remembered. In this most serious effort to incorporate the unacceptable into oneself, responsive listening is crucial.

Inpatient Group Psychotherapy

It is in the use of most intensive group psychotherapy that specialized inpatient programs are distinctive. Several times a week, or even daily, the group members support and confront one another, sharing in the catharsis and integration of their similar past and recent experiences (25, 30). The mutual support of survivors makes possible the painful disclosure and self-examination which can lead to healing and growth. A number of technical issues are important to consider:

- It is well for there to be two therapists to allow each some mental time out when needed.
- The number of members should be kept manageable; most therapists find 10 or 12 the upper limit for individualizing the impact and assuring the active participation of everyone.
- Role playing may get across a point when a dead buddy becomes "part" of the group.
- Some limits are necessary: no physical attacks can be allowed, and neither can unexplained verbal attacks.
- The contract for participation should make it clear that those who must be asked to leave, to preserve the therapeutic opportunities of others, have effectively removed themselves.
- A buddy system to provide support after sessions, during the night, and on weekends is beneficial.
- Any focus upon current problems assumes that they are based on combat issues, which are then explored (30).
- Sessions shouldn't become "can you top this?" paroxysms of war stories, which parody the intensely personal experiences which give the group its purpose.
- Frequently, inpatient groups must be "open," with patients joining and leaving the group as they arrive on, and leave, the unit.
- In the group, "new guy" and "short-timer" roles in combat are

reinvoked, with an opportunity to experience greater unity and more thoughtful transitions than in the war.

- Such groups provide for visible cooperation between ward clinicians and Vet Center counselors serving as coleaders, thus reducing patient splitting of medical center and Vet Center staff.
- If sensitively handled, rotation of coleaders is a valuable learning experience for new staff and trainees.

Journal Therapy

Veterans often benefit from keeping a journal in which they make daily entries of their combat memories, the meaning these have for them at the time of writing, and the working through process (31). This facilitates a cognitive approach to traumatic experience. As journal entries are voluntarily shared in a separate weekly group session, further bonding among survivors takes place. As veterans review their journals from time to time, they can see where they have been and where they are going.

Therapeutic Community

Organization of the unit as a therapeutic community is necessary, not just a token concession to democracy. Basic to the injurious effect of psychic trauma is helplessness and the inability to control events. Through the therapeutic community veterans share real responsibility for their situation. This internalizing of the locus of control is difficult for many, who find it more comfortable to place demands on the facility staff and repeatedly express dissatisfaction. Particularly for those who feel responsible for the deaths of others in their unit, or for participation in killing which (at least in retrospect) had little military necessity, there may have been a decade-long avoidance of responsibility affecting employment, marriage, and parenting.

For others the therapeutic community may offer an opportunity to understand the wish to wrest control from the authorities and to fulfill fantasies or repeat actions which occurred in combat.

Participation in the therapeutic community encourages a shared self-help ethic, practice with negotiation and compromise, and the realization that decisions for the good of the group must be balanced with the needs of the individual. When the staff sufficiently trusts the process, the community itself may share in making decisions about discipline and even share in developing protective measures for risk management (22).

The experience of organizing benevolent projects and acknowledging spontaneous acts of caring has a gentle healing effect on those who are preoccupied with their own pain, consumed with a desire for revenge, or isolated from feelings and intimacy. While someone on the staff must assume ultimate responsibility and have the authority to overrule actions of the community, it is essential that careful thought and open communication go into that process. Betrayal of noble expectations is part of the trauma many Viet Nam veterans still feel and must not inadvertently be repeated.

Medications

There are a number of other program elements which contribute to the effectiveness of specialized units for PTSD. Medications may be less necessary in the control of symptoms than in general psychiatry crisis management (16). Other methods, combined with the support of staff and peers, are often effective in reducing distress enough to allow the veteran to endure it while confronting the combat experiences which are its cause. Nevertheless, specific use of medication should sometimes take place, and mention has already been made of this. In addition, when anxiety levels are persistently so high that participation in therapeutic reexperiencing is seriously impaired, the use of β-adrenergic blockers such as propranolol, or calcium channel blockers such as verapamil, may be considered. It has been hypothesized that neurophysiological conditioning accounts for the persistence of exaggerated autonomic reactions to stimuli in some instances of PTSD, and these agents may have specific effects in deconditioning. Monoamine oxidase inhibitors can control agitation and depression, but before using these care should be exercised in assessing the veteran's life-style regarding food and alcohol control (32).

Illicit Drugs. Illicit drugs are readily available and may have been utilized to blunt affective stress responses. Such drug use interferes with the confrontational aspects of the treatment process and should be prohibited. Veterans who are unable to become drug free may not be ready for a PTSD treatment program (21, 33, 34) and should be referred to a specialized drug treatment program. In that case, however, some simultaneous PTSD-specific treatment may have to be provided in order for the patient to tolerate becoming drug free.

Dream Groups

Dream groups facilitate confrontation and understanding of stressors which are reexperienced in dreams and, in addition, help veterans to see nightmares, however painful, as natural opportunities to return to and cope with traumatic events they have been unable to leave behind (35).

Stress Management Techniques

Stress management and relaxation training, including biofeedback techniques, provide additional means of controlling distress. These methods can be practiced unobtrusively in situations when veterans unexpectedly face reminders of particularly stressful aspects of combat (36–42).

Family Counseling

Family and marital counseling may be vital in preserving relationships strained by violence, mystery, and estrangement. Family groups provided with information about the Viet Nam War and PTSD, and a chance to supportively share experiences, are effective (43).

Religious Counseling

Religious or spiritual counseling has been very helpful to some veterans, but great sensitivity is required to arrange it. The clergy have an acknowledged legitimacy in the area of morality, but if the tenets of faith of a particular clergyman stress sin and punishment or portray expected human nature as being incredibly pure, veterans having serious problems with self-acceptance may reject the counseling which is offered. On the other hand, nonjudgmental guidance in dealing with combat experiences in moral terms may lead to the formulation of a new personal moral position which enhances productive living.

Vocational Counseling

Vocational counseling should be readily available. Work is often problematic because of repeated job loss, the lack of career course, and intolerance for the work environment. The veteran may be 10 or 15 years past the usual starting point for training or entry level employment in fields which are most suitable, and educators' or employers' prejudices may be difficult to overcome. Notwithstanding these and other challenges, an organized effort should be made to help the veteran succeed in having an occupational identity, a proud position in the family and society, and a reasonable income. Bitterness about competition with Asian refugees and draft-deferred Americans is better dealt with in psychotherapy; vocational rehabilitation should be geared toward results.

Substance Abuse Rehabilitation

Alcoholism and drug abuse, when coexistent with PTSD, are not usually amenable to treatment and rehabilitation on specialized PTSD treatment units. Referral to alcohol or drug rehabilitation programs before commencing definitive treatment of PTSD is preferable. In order to maintain abstinence, the group counseling and sobriety principles of a group such as Alcoholics Anonymous should be incorporated into the PTSD program. As noted above, PTSD-specific treatment may be a necessary component during a stay on a substance abuse unit.

Medical and Surgical Treatment

Similarly, care for physical problems should be provided as part of the overall PTSD program, except for procedures which may require short stays on medical or surgical wards. Many Viet Nam veterans with PTSD, perhaps a majority, are hospitalized for medical or surgical treatment (44), and even when sleep disturbances, agitation, hostility toward staff, and persistence in behavior which exacerbates the physical condition are marked, no psychiatric consultation is requested. Active case finding by empathic staff may enable veterans to consider entering a PTSD treatment program if the stigma of mental disorder can be avoided.

It is interesting, in this regard, that Viet Nam veterans with amputations and hospitalization for other significant orthopedic problems directly after combat appear to have fewer PTSD difficulties. It has been speculated that their informal and spontaneous rap sessions in hospitals allowed a working through of acute combat-related stress responses for many of them.

STAFF ORGANIZATION

The unit staff organization should be explicit in order to coordinate these components. Reliable clinical decision making requires a treatment team leader recognized by team members as having credible clinical authority. The skills of psychiatrists, psychologists, social workers, nurses, activity therapists, chaplains, vocational counselors, substance abuse counselors, and Viet Nam veteran outreach counselors are all needed, and representatives of at least the first four disciplines should work on the unit full time. The number of staff should allow for sufficient individual psychotherapy and dual leadership of all therapy groups. Ideally, all professional staff should be voluntarily assigned after screening and acceptance by at least the core professional group.

Staff members who are themselves Viet Nam combat veterans make a critical contribution to the effectiveness of the unit through their commitment and their unique ability to establish rapport. Care should be taken to support these valuable staff members, since the usual high stress of this work may be specifically traumatic for them and undo even seemingly solid resolutions of their own PTSD. Former combat medics may be particularly vulnerable to reexperiencing their Viet Nam frustrations. The integration of team members whose qualifications primarily stress their Viet Nam military experience should be openly addressed.

As the staff team gains experience, it becomes increasingly apparent that sharing of staff Viet Nam experience with the veterans treated on the unit contributes toward substantial understanding and trust. The clinical team should encourage and perhaps formalize a buddy system to ensure mutual support among themselves and to provide for appreciation of each other's work.

Staff Attitudes

Staff attitudes are the single most critical element in a specialized program for PTSD. Psychologically secure people who are honest and open, natural, and self-disclosing are certainly the most effective, but they also appear to be most subject to burnout because of their sensitivity. Mutual staff support is essential. Independent operators antagonize patients and staff alike. Similarly, risk-taking nonconformists may set up situations which easily get out of control: staff who glamorize or romanticize the recalcitrant warrior behavior of some veterans do nothing to encourage self-reflection and promote acting out.

Those staff members who are themselves honestly self-reflective are perhaps most vulnerable to painful experiences when veterans cause them to face their own fears, vulnerabilities, loss of control, and moral dilemmas (43–48). This is, of course, part of the opportunity for personal growth of clinicians who do this work.

ADMINISTRATIVE CONSIDERATIONS

The administration of specialized PTSD treatment programs becomes more effective with experience. There are as yet few published guidelines to follow. A number of administrative issues deserve specific mention, such as space, time, patient flow, and staff support.

The most effective treatment program is carried out in its own well-defined space. If a PTSD program must share space on a general psychiatry ward, however, border clashes may be minimized by arranging for a separate block of sleeping rooms, separate staff assignments for the core team disciplines, separate therapeutic community organizations with an effective liaison group, and separate access times for group rooms and game rooms. Even if there are sound clinical reasons for different sets of rules of patient privileges, disagreements will occur and almost constant conciliation is needed.

WORKLOAD IMPACT

The length of stay, which on a PTSD unit is usually two or three months, may impact significantly upon the patient turnover of all other wards of the inpatient psychiatric department. Bed occupancy is usually high, and this may create a high workload for other units.

RISK MANAGEMENT

Even if the admission and discharge criteria are explicit, individual circumstances require judgment that is best shared by several staff members. A screening group—preferably kept small with rotating membership, including both inpatient and outpatient staff as well as Viet Nam veterans outreach counselors—should regularly review all applicants for outpatient and inpatient admission and discharge. A waiting list is inevitable in most locations, and priorities regarding urgency, previous cooperation, court charges, and geographical factors require group discussion. Efforts to maintain contact with veterans who leave against medical advice should be made. Instances of factitious PTSD should be explored carefully to determine the best approach to discovery (49).

UNIQUE MANAGEMENT CHALLENGES

Viet Nam veterans who habitually carry or sleep with loaded firearms or jungle knives may feel the need to have them on the unit, or even to display them for intimidation. Clear statements that no weapons are allowed must be repeatedly expressed, and responsibility for enforcement should be shared with the patient government. Some veterans want to wear combat fatigue uniforms and insignia everywhere, and this issue requires periodic attention to ensure that legitimate needs for pride are recognized while other patients are protected from disturbing reminders of traumatic experience.

Current attitudes toward the "system" often take political form, and where this becomes a harangue which interrupts the treatment of others, it should be redirected outside to more appropriate and constructive forums including veterans service organizations.

DISABILITY COMPENSATION

Compensation is an ever-present concern for many veterans with PTSD. Resolution of the issues of personal recognition, validation, and indemnification are important to the therapeutic process, but the procedures for submitting claims and performing disability examinations should be kept separate from treatment activities.

This may be difficult. Information necessary and sufficient to document a claim ordinarily will be available from a treating facility. If there are few professionals available locally with sufficient expertise to carry out examinations for disability claims adjudication panels, the claimant's treatment staff may be asked to participate. A question of conflict of interest may be raised.

The most reliable approach would utilize the best available specialized staff, even if they participated in treatment. The development of sufficiently detailed documentation to allow independent verification is necessary (50). This arrangement, which may be difficult for claims adjusters to accept, also places the treatment staff in a bind with patients. It may increase the tendency of patients to introduce specific compensation claim issues into treatment settings, and it may greatly increase the potential for resentment of clinicians when adverse decisions occur. In the long run, the best compromise to avoid apparent conflicts of interest is for staff with specialized expertise to train claims examiners.

RESEARCH

Research in every aspect of PTSD is needed. Several practical problems must be faced in any inpatient treatment program where clinical research is carried out. First, because of the scarcity of appropriate treatment resources, it is difficult to establish control groups for the comparison of two supposedly effective approaches. Second, since effective treatment is multimodal, the problems in testing the efficacy of one treatment or all possible combinations of treatment are substantial. Finally, veterans are suspicious of being made guinea pigs.

GOALS

The goals of inpatient treatment should be established in advance, in some detail. When the program is initiated, sound and practical patient goals will be identified, including the following:

- An improved capacity for intimacy and responsible relating,
- An ability to sustain productive work and to find stable employment, and
- An appropriate exercise of control over aggression.

Observing first hand what qualities Viet Nam veterans can unfurl, the staff will see heightened sensitivity to life, pride of survivorship, watchful concern for government responsibility, and stewardship roles assumed in the community. For those who have sustained perhaps the deepest wounds of war, no goal is beyond reach if the effort is made (28, 51–57).

REFERENCES

1. Pokorny AD: Prediction of suicide in psychiatric patients: report of a prospective study. Arch Gen Psychiatry 40:249–257, 1983
2. Murphy GE: Clinical identification of suicidal risk. Arch Gen Psychiatry 27:356–359, 1972
3. Weisman AD, Worden JW: Risk-rescue rating in suicide assessment. Arch Gen Psychiatry 26:553–560, 1972
4. Farberow NL: Suicide prevention in the hospital. Hosp Community Psychiatry 32:99–104, 1981
5. Helzer JE, Robins LN, David DH: Depressive disorders in Vietnam returnees. J Nerv Ment Dis 163:177–185, 1976
6. Van Putten T, Emory WH: Traumatic neuroses in Vietnam returnees. Arch Gen Psychiatry 29:695–698, 1973
7. Bond TC: The why of fragging. Am J Psychiatry 133:1329–1331, 1976

8. Lehmann LS, Padilla M, Clark S, et al: Training personnel in the prevention and management of violent behavior. Hosp Community Psychiatry 34:40–43, 1983

9. Lehman AF, Strauss JS, Ritzler BA, et al: First-admission psychiatric ward milieu: treatment process and outcome. Arch Gen Psychiatry 39:1293–1298, 1982

10. Thomasma DC: Beyond medical paternalism and patient autonomy: a model of physician conscience for the physician-patient relationship. Ann Intern Med 98:243–248, 1983

11. Manasse G: Patient government: history, structure, and ethics. Am J Soc Psychiatry 1:9–16, 1981

12. Horowitz MJ, Wilner N, Kaltreider N, et al: Signs and symptoms of posttraumatic stress disorder. Arch Gen Psychiatry 37:85–92, 1980

13. Van der Kolk B: Psychopharmacological issues in posttraumatic stress disorder. Hosp Community Psychiatry 34:683–691, 1983

14. Horowitz MJ: Stress Response Syndromes. New York, Jason Aronson, 1976

15. Friedman MJ: Post-Vietnam syndrome: recognition and management Psychosomatics 22:931–943, 1981

16. Ware JC: Tricyclic antidepressants in the treatment of insomnia. J Clin Psychiatry 44:25–28, 1983

17. Blank AS: Apocalypse terminable and interminable: operation outreach for Vietnam veterans. Hosp Community Psychiatry 33:913–918, 1982

18. Lacoursiere RB, Godfrey KE, Ruby LM: Traumatic neurosis in the etiology of alcoholism: Vietnam combat and other trauma. Am J Psychiatry 137:966–968, 1980

19. Penk WE, Robinowitz R, Roberts WR, et al: Adjustment differences among male substance abusers varying in degree of combat experience in Vietnam. J Consult Clin Psychol 49:426–437, 1981

20. Johnson AW: Medical and psychiatric treatment policy and practice in Vietnam. Journal of Social Issues 31:49–65, 1975

21. Bey DR, Zecchinelli VA: Marijuana as a coping device in Vietnam. Milit Med 136:448–450, 1971

22. Manasse G: Patient government: history, structure and ethics. American Journal of Social Psychiatry 1:9–16, 1981

23. Horowitz MJ, Wilner N, Kaltreider N, et al: Signs and symptoms of posttraumatic stress disorder. Arch Gen Psychiatry 37:85–92, 1980

24. Akhtar S, Byrne JP: The concept of splitting and its clinical relevance. Am J Psychiatry 140:1013–1016, 1983

25. Berman S, Price S, Gusman F: An inpatient program for Vietnam combat veterans in a Veterans Administration Hospital. Hosp Community Psychiatry 33:919–922, 1982

26. Krystal H: Affect tolerance. Annals of Psychoanalysis 3:179–219, 1975

27. Krystal H: Trauma and affects. Psychoanal Study Child 33:81–116, 1978

28. Krystal H: The aging survivor of the holocaust: integration and self-healing in post-traumatic states. J Geriatr Psychiatry 14:165–189, 1981

29. Hendin H: Psychotherapy for Vietnam veterans with posttraumatic stress disorders. Am J Psychother 37:86–99, 1983

30. Walker JI, Nash JL: Group therapy in the treatment of Vietnam combat veterans. Int J Group Psychother 31:379–389, 1981

31. Progoff I: At a Journal Workshop. New York, Dialogue House, 1975

32. Hagben GL, Cornfield RB: Treatment of traumatic war neurosis with phenelzine. Arch Gen Psychiatry 38:440–445, 1981

33. Pettera RL, Johnson BM, Zimmer R: Psychiatric management of combat reactions with emphasis on a reaction unique to Vietnam. Milit Med 134:673–678, 1969

34. Goldsmith W, Cretekas C: Unhappy odysseys: psychiatric hospitalizations among Vietnam returnees. Arch Gen Psychiatry 20:78–83, 1969

35. Wilmer HA: Vietnam and madness: dreams of schizophrenic veterans. J Am Acad Psychoanal 10:47–65, 1982

36. Keane TM, Kaloupek DG: Imaginal flooding in the treatment of a posttraumatic stress disorder. J Consult Clin Psychol 50:138–140, 1982

37. Brene JO, Benedict BD: The Vietnam combat delayed stress response syndrome: hypnotherapy of "dissociative symptoms." Am J Clin Hypn 23:34–40, 1980

38. Kipper DA: Behavior therapy for fears brought on by war experiences. J Consult Clin Psychol 45:216–221, 1977

39. Geer JH, Silverman I: Treatment of a recurrent nightmare by behavior modification procedures: a case study. J Abnorm Psychol 72:188–190, 1967

40. Haynes SN, Mooney DK: Nightmares, etiological, theoretical, and behavioral treatment considerations. Psychology Record 25:225–236, 1975

41. Greenberg R, Pearlman CA, Gampel D: War neuroses and the adaptive function of REM sleep. Br J Med Psychol 45:27–33, 1972

42. Lavil P, Hefetz A, Halperin G, et al: Long-term effects of traumatic war-related events on sleep. Am J Psychiatry 136:175–178, 1979

43. Figley CR, Sprenkle DH: Delayed stress response syndrome: family therapy implications. Journal of Marriage and Family Counseling 6:53–59, 1978

44. Atkinson RM, Sparr LF, Sheff AG, et al: Diagnosis of posttraumatic stress disorder in Vietnam veterans: preliminary findings. Am J Psychiatry 141:694–696, 1984

45. Haley SA: When the patient reports atrocities: specific treatment considerations of the Vietnam veteran. Arch Gen Psychiatry 30:191–196, 1974

46. Frosch JP: The treatment of antisocial and borderline personality disorders. Hosp Community Psychiatry 34:243–348, 1983

47. Horowitz MJ: Self-righteous rage and the attribution of blame. Arch Gen Psychiatry 38:1233–1238, 1981

48. Lemre F: Psychotherapy of Vietnam veterans. JAMA 246:125, 1981

49. Sparr L, Pankratz LD: Factitious posttraumatic stress disorder. Am J Psychiatry 140:1016–1019, 1983

50. Atkinson RM, Henderson RG, Sparr LF, et al: Assessment of Vietnam veterans for posttraumatic stress disorder in Veterans Administration disability claims. Am J Psychiatry 139:1118–1121, 1982

51. Kardiner A: The Traumatic Neuroses of War. New York, Hoeber, 1941

52. Balson PM, Dempster CR: Treatment of war neuroses from Vietnam. Compr Psychiatry 21:167–176, 1980

53. Borus J: Reentry, III: Facilitating health readjustment in Vietnam veterans. Psychiatry 36:428–439, 1973

54. Archibald HC, Long DM, Miller C, et al: Gross stress reaction in combat: a 15-year followup. Am J Psychiatry 119:317–322, 1962

55. Grinker RR, Spiegel JP: Brief psychotherapy in war neuroses. Psychosom Med 6:123–131, 1944

56. Rado S: Pathodynamics and treatment of traumatic war neurosis (traumatophobia). Psychosom Med 42:363–368, 1942

57. Horowitz MJ, Kaltreider NB: Brief treatment of post-traumatic stress disorders. New Directions in Mental Health Services 6:67–79, 1980

13

A Guide to Obtaining a Military History from Viet Nam Veterans

Raymond Monsour Scurfield, D.S.W.
Arthur S. Blank, Jr., M.D.

13

During the past decade, the phenomena of delayed and chronic post-traumatic stress disorder and related postwar readjustment problems have been increasingly identified in Viet Nam veterans. However, assessment of veterans and diagnosis of PTSD remain confusing tasks for some clinicians. The principal focus of difficulty is usually a mutual inability of clinician and veteran to talk comprehensively about the actualities of the veteran's experiences during military duty. Probably no other war involving American military personnel, at least in this century, has so commonly produced such hesitation. The following guide provides both the clinician and the veteran with a way out of the silence which has prevented adequate diagnosis and treatment.

It is important to note several cautions in the utilization of this interview guide.

- It is a comprehensive catalog of questions. In actual practice, the clinician will wish to select certain questions for use and omit others.
- It addresses experiences about which the veteran or the mental health professional may be intensely ambivalent and conflicted.
- A treatment relationship may have to be established before the

Portions of this guide are excerpted from a series of questions prepared in 1980 by a Readjustment Counseling Service working committee for the videotape "The Vietnam Veteran Then and Now," which was produced in 1983 by the Veterans Administration St. Louis Learning Resource Service. The working committee included Tom Ambrose and Lee Crump (Cochairmen), Gary May, Joel Brende, Clarence Davis, Maria Aviles, Elaine Alvarez, Erwin Parson, and Gregory Piña. Other questions and structure are derived from "Everything You Wanted to Know About the War in Vietnam But Were Afraid to Ask Until Now," an unpublished manuscript by Arthur S. Blank, Jr., M.D.

Some of the guidelines to conducting the interview are derived from "Post-Traumatic Stress: Assessment and Treatment: Overview and Formulations," by Raymond M. Scurfield, D.S.W., which will appear in *Trauma and Its Wake* (Vol. 1), edited by Charles Figley (New York, Brunner/Mazel, in press).

veteran will be able or willing to remember or discuss traumatic experiences in the war.

- There may be fear on the part of both the veteran and clinician of losing control of powerful emotions, such as being unable to stop crying.
- The veteran may believe that he or she will not be understood or accepted, particularly by persons who are not Viet Nam veterans.
- The veteran may project rage towards the clinician or question the clinician's trustworthiness or capacity to understand war experiences.
- Some veterans with un-worked-through sequelae of wartime psychic trauma have highly complex stress disorder states, with multiple psychological relationships among combat events, pre- and post-war history, and current symptoms. As a result, detailed examination of the war history may be an imposing task.
- The clinician may be ambivalent about exploring or listening to graphic recounting of war trauma. Feelings of rage, horror, and sadness or impulses towards judgmental behavior may arise within the clinician. Any of these may lead the interviewer to ignore or become confused about essential dynamics within the veteran. Also, the clinician may have to deal with painful empathic responses.
- Frequently, it is helpful to chronologically talk through the military history, at whatever pace is comfortable to the veteran. However, if the veteran is talking very fast or skipping details, it may be useful to slow the pace down and be very concrete. The clinician may choose initially not to probe deeper at certain points where the veteran is not yet ready to go on, and return to such areas later. During a later session, the veteran may be "walked through" a particular piece of the history in more detail.
- It may be prudent to terminate, temporarily, the discussion of military history when the veteran has verbalized enough for one session and needs some time to digest what has been related.
- Strong feelings and emotions may well emerge which require immediate clinical interventions.
- Discussion of particular experiences in the military history may trigger feelings or thoughts about another event or experience that occurred prior to or following active duty. Clinical judgment will indicate whether to pursue such areas at that time or to continue with the chronological history.

The veteran needs to know that he or she is being accepted in human terms by the clinician; that events, actions, or feelings are not condemned; that the importance, validity, and potential usefulness of the Viet Nam experience is recognized; and that the clinician cares and knows enough to ask, and to listen.

It should be made clear to the veteran that the clinician seeks to understand the military history as one part of the veteran's life experience. The veteran can then consider the ways in which life events before, during, and after military service interact. The veteran can thus understand that life experiences influence one another, and that none can be ignored.

OUTLINE OF THE INTERVIEW GUIDE

The following is a listing of the key areas of inquiry that are included in the interview guide:

I. *IMMEDIATE PREMILITARY EXPERIENCES*
II. *ENTRY INTO MILITARY SERVICE*
III. *MILITARY TRAINING*
IV. *VIET NAM HISTORY*
    A. The News: Receipt of Orders to the Combat Zone
    B. Leaving for Viet Nam
    C. Arrival
    D. Major Role or Specialty
    E. Basic Itinerary and Chronology
    F. Rank
    G. Relationship with Authorities
    H. Combat Time
    I. If Not a Combat Veteran
    J. Major Offensives
    K. Noncombat Time
    L. Relationships with Vietnamese
    M. Changes in Attitudes or Behavior
    N. Responses to the Uniqueness of the War
    O. Stress and Conflict Unique to Minority Military Personnel
    P. Some Specific Traumatic Events
    Q. Positive Experiences in the War Zone
    R. Drugs
    S. R & R (Rest and Recreation)
    T. Happenings Back Home
    U. Moral and Value Conflicts Precipitated by the Unique Nature of the Viet Nam War and Their Effects on Viet Nam Combatants and Support Troops
    V. Getting Short (Close to Military Discharge)

W. Getting Ready for the Return Home
X. Freedom Bird (Up and Out)
V. *MILITARY DISCHARGE*
VI. *POST–VIET NAM READJUSTMENT*
    A. The Homecoming and the First Month After Return
    B. The Next Few Months
    C. The First Two or Three Years After Viet Nam
    D. Talking About Viet Nam Since the Homecoming Transition
    E. Prime Features of the Military-to-Civilian Transition
    F. Reviewing Possible Causes of Conflict
    G. Being Different After Viet Nam
    H. Your Identity as a Viet Nam Veteran
    I. Contact with Other Viet Nam Veterans and Their Families
    J. Successful Readjustment Resources, Coping Mechanisms, and Adjustment Options
    K. Readjustment Obstacles or Difficulties
    L. Counterproductive or Destructive Readjustment Coping Mechanisms
    M. Recognition You Received for Viet Nam Service
    N. Positive Results of Your Viet Nam Experience
    O. Souvenirs and Memorabilia

The Viet Nam Military History Interview Guide

I. *IMMEDIATE PREMILITARY EXPERIENCES*
    A. What was the status of your marriage (or other significant interpersonal relationships) at time of entry on active duty?
    B. Did you have children? How many? Describe your premilitary relationship with them.
    C. How did parents and other significant others (relatives, friends) feel about your going into the military? How did that affect you?
    D. Did you try to avoid the draft? What, if anything, did you do to make it harder for you to get drafted?
    E. When and how did you first begin to pay attention to and know about the war? Did you have a father (uncles, brothers) in the military? Did you have friends go to Viet Nam before you? What happened to them? What were your political views before you went, especially your views about the war?
    F. Before you went into the service, can you describe what your life was like and what kind of person you were?

    1. How did you see yourself fitting into the American dream?

    2. What did you feel was the social/political mood of the country and your community?

    3. What were your feelings about the war and the protests against it? What were the views of your friends and family?

  G. How did going in the military disrupt, upset, or help whatever was going on in your life at that time—relationships, education, career, etc.?

II. ENTRY INTO MILITARY SERVICE

  A. How old were you when you entered the service and what were your expectations and fears?

  B. Did you enlist or were you drafted; which of the following best describes your situation?

    1. Enlisted voluntarily.

    2. Enlisted to avoid draft.

    3. Enlisted as alternative to receiving a court sentence.

    4. Other reason(s) for enlisting.

    5. Drafted.

  C. Did you try to get out? If so, how? Did you think about it? If so, why did you decide not to?

  D. Why did you select or prefer the Army (or Air Force, Marines, Navy, or Coast Guard)?

  E. When were you inducted?

  F. What branch and unit did you go into?

  G. What were your active duty service dates? If more than one period of active duty, list each.

  H. List each duty assignment: location, dates, and job assignment.

III. MILITARY TRAINING

  A. What type of training did you go through and how did it prepare you for Viet Nam? If not, what did it not prepare you for, or how was it lacking?

  B. Did military training alter or change your values and beliefs in any way? Discuss the following:

    1. Basic training.

    2. AIT (Advanced Infantry Training).

    3. Other: Jungle, Ranger, Special Forces, Aviation, Jump School, etc.

  C. What was good about your training? What was bad or not

worthwhile (to others, to yourself)?

D. What happened during training, both positive and negative, that particlarly sticks out in your mind?

IV. *VIET NAM HISTORY*
   A. Getting The News: Receipt of orders to the combat zone.
      1. How was it that you got orders to Viet Nam? What was the nature of your orders?
         • Routine orders?
         • You volunteered? (Why?)
         • Orders "as punishment"? (For what?)
         • Other (explain)
      2. Where and how did you hear you were going to Viet Nam? Were you ordered with a unit or alone? What were your first reactions and thoughts about going? What did you think would happen there, what was the advance picture? Where did you get your shots? Did you make out a will at JAG (Judge Advocate General)? What dreams do you recall having just before leaving? Who did you say goodbye to? Who didn't you say goodbye to? Why?
      3. Overall, how did you feel about going: very positive, mixed, or very negative? Explain why.
      4. Do you remember any songs you focused on during your last weeks in the United States?
   B. Leaving for Viet Nam
      1. On what date did you leave the United States?
      2. How did you travel? By plane: from where to where, in what kind of aircraft? What do you remember that happened on the aircraft? By boat: How long was the trip, who was on the boat, what port did you leave from and arrive at? What do you remember that happened on the boat?
      3. Who did you most regret leaving behind in the United States? (Explain)
      4. What else did you leave that you felt good or bad about, or had mixed feelings about?
   C. Arrival in Viet Nam
      1. On what date did you arrive?
      2. What were your first impressions of the land, the climate, the people of Viet Nam? How did the land smell?
      3. What were your first impressions of the war? What were the initial sights and sounds?
      4. What were your first movements in Viet Nam? To where, then where, then where after that?

      5. Were you in replacement companies? For how long?

      6. What unit were you first assigned to? Where was it and how did you get there? What was happening there in the unit when you first arrived?

      7. What dreams did you have during the first weeks?

      8. How many weeks did it take you to acclimatize to the heat?

D. Major Role or Specialty

      1. What was your MOS (Military Occupational Specialty)? Army and Marines = MOS, Navy and Coast Guard = Rate and Primary NECs (Naval Enlisted Classifications), and Air Force = AFSC (Specialty Code).

      2. What did you actually do during most of your time in Viet Nam? What jobs did you have?

      3. Can you give me the sequence of your jobs, with rough dates?

      4. Was this what you had *thought* you would be doing? If not doing that, how did you feel about it? Did you try to accomplish a change in your assignment?

E. Basic Itinerary and Chronology

    Can you tell me in sequence the units you were in, the rough dates for each, and the reasons for going from one to the next? What were the locations? (How do you spell that? Can you show me that on the map?)

F. Rank

      1. Did you go up or down in rank? When and why?

      2. *Should* you have gone up or down in rank? Why? What are your feelings about the rank changes or lack of them?

      3. What was your highest rank while on active duty; what was your rank at discharge?

G. Relationship with Authorities

      1. How did you get along with military authorities (both officers and noncommissioned officers)?

      2. Did you have any hassles? Article 15s or nonjudicial punishments? Court-martials? Disagreements with superiors?

      3. Did you go AWOL while in Viet Nam; for how long, and to where? What did you do while AWOL?

      4. (To explain hassles) Did you feel singled out or picked on by anyone, or did you cause the hassles? How did that come about? Your feelings then? How did you handle it? Consequences?

H. Combat Time (Skip 1 and 2 if veteran was not an active combatant)

1. Describe your first and second experiences in combat. What did your unit do? Tell what you did or didn't do. How did your fellow soldiers treat you?

2. Describe your first kill; your second kill. Or, describe the first and second time when you felt at least partly responsible for the death of someone else: Who, what, where, when, and how? Your feelings then; a little later; after Viet Nam; now?

3. Could you tell me more about your combat experience, or your exposure to the effects of combat? What was it like for you and your unit?

   a. What kind of operations were you on, or what kind of activities were you engaged in?

   b. What were the types of combat, or exposure to combat effects, that you experienced?

   c. Can you describe a typical day? A typical bad day? A typical good day? (What percentage of days were each?)

   d. What were the worst things that happened to you? Incidents in which you were wounded, nearly killed, or in which you lost some of your friends or members of your unit?

   e. How did your unit get along; do you feel that you got close to the men (or women) you served with?

   f. Can you contrast your experience in a rear support area to combat?

      (1) Did you feel there was a cooperative relationship between those in the support groups and the troops in combat?

      (2) What did you do to relieve the boredom that was characteristic of the support areas?

   g. What were the most stressful things about combat or exposure to combat, and what effect did they have on you?

      (1) Did you feel that the climate, terrain, and physical environment were stressful?

      (2) Did you feel that the invisible enemy and the trouble telling friend from foe were particularly stressful? How? What was that like for you?

      (3) Did you feel stress from acts of terrorism (booby traps, mines, snipers, sappers, acts of sabotage)? Did you ever really feel safe in Viet Nam? Where?

      h. Did you ever feel betrayed or abandoned by buddies, other American military persons, or persons in leadership positions while you were in Viet Nam? Did you do anything about that, or did anyone else in your unit? Are you aware of any fraggings or did you observe any? How did you feel about the fraggings?

      i. Did you observe mutilations or atrocities committed by our side or the other side, involving either Vietnamese civilians or Americans?

  4. Who showed you the ropes and taught you how to survive? What happened to him or her?

      a. Did you have trouble getting weapons, grenades, etc.? Were there problems about weapons working?

      b. What kind of operations were you on—how long, where to, with whom? Wet or dry season? Conditions: what were they?

      c. What about the food?

      d. What kind of contact did you have with the other side: the North Vietnamese Army and the Vietcong? What fire were you exposed to: rifle, grenade, RPG (rocket propelled grenade), mortar, mines, booby traps? Did you use white phosphorus, napalm, call in air strikes? Did you order others to fire, or kill? Your feelings about doing this?

      e. Did you disobey orders very much? Openly or covertly? Why? What happened? How did you feel about doing that: then, later, now? Did you ever *wish* you had disobeyed orders? Explain.

      f. Losses: Who was killed whom you knew or were close to; what happened?

      g. What violence did you do? How and to whom, if you know?

      h. Were you wounded or injured? Where and how; what caused it?

      i. Were you medevac'd? To where? How long were you there; what was it like?

      j. Did your unit or buddies get zapped while you were in the hospital?

      k. Was the hospital attacked while you were there as a patient?

I. If Not a Combat Veteran

  1. What did you do mostly (if not clearly described earlier)?

2. How did you feel about *not* being a combat soldier: good, mixed, bad?

3. Did you do anything to avoid going into combat or to avoid combat assignment? What? How did you feel about that then? How do you feel about that now?

4. Was your job easier, just as hard, or harder than combat soldiers? (Explain)

5. What exposure did you have to the effects of combat (e.g., to the destruction, death, etc.)? Describe.

6. Could you have been stationed stateside and had the same experiences that you had in Viet Nam? If yes or no, explain.

7. If in a rear support role: what was the connection between what you were doing and what was going on in the bush? Was there a good cooperative relationship between support and combat roles?

8. Were you under attack at any time: Mortars, snipers, etc.? Were there any terrorist attacks nearby?

J. Major Offensives

1. What major U.S. or NLF or NVA offensives happened while you were in Viet Nam? Or that you just missed? Where were you at the time? What happened to you, to your buddies, or to your unit?

2. Were there any other major military operations or outcomes while you were there that directly affected you and your unit? Explain.

K. Noncombat Time

1. Describe your base camp: Where was it, how big, how many men and women were there, what did you do?

2. How often was it attacked? By mortars, snipers, or what? Did you go out on patrols? In hospitals, dust-off (medevac helicopters), or morgue duty, what did you see?

3. What experiences did you have with terrorism? Did you hear about any grenades in jeeps? Were you in or around any buildings that were blown up?

4. What did you do for fun and relaxation? With whom? Did anything particularly good or bad happen during these times?

5. What kinds of contact, if any, did you have with Americans or other non-Vietnamese who were civilians? Describe this contact.

L. Relationships with Vietnamese

1. Describe your contact with the Vietnamese: What kind,

how much, its nature and frequency? Was it military duty, social, business, etc.? Was it with ARVNs (Army of Republic of Viet Nam), with elderly, with women, with children, with Montagnards, with Vietcong, with North Vietnamese, with others?

2. How did you feel about the Vietnamese in general? Why? How did you feel about specific groups of Vietnamese (children, women, etc.)? Why?

3. Did you have any close relationships with any Vietnamese? Explain, if not explained above. What happened to these relationships during your tour? Afterwards? Do you ever think about them these days?

4. Did you agree with the way other Americans treated or related to the Vietnamese? What did you do about the way other Americans treated Vietnamese; how did it make you feel: then, later, and now?

5. Did you have sexual contacts with Vietnamese? Was it in client-prostitute contacts, or a girlfriend (boyfriend) relationship? Live-in? Was it your first (or an early) sexual experience? What happened to the relationship or relationships? Was anyone killed or maimed with whom you had had such a relationship? What were the circumstances surrounding this? (Repeat the same questions for other Vietnamese with whom the veteran had an ongoing relationship: child, elderly, ARVN, etc.)

6. Were you around Vietnamese who were in the hire of the United States (cleaning or construction crews, interpreters, etc.)? Did you see any prisoners? What happened to them? Did you see any dead Vietnamese? From which side? How old? Other details?

7. How often were you directly involved in the wounding or deaths of Vietnamese civilians? How often were you indirectly involved in (or observed) the wounding or death or remains of Vietnamese civilians?

8. How often did you feel at least partly responsible (through actions or inactions) for the wounding or deaths of Vietnamese? (Explain; specify age, relationship, etc.) How often did you observe mutilation of Vietnamese? Were you somehow involved in deaths or woundings that weren't really necessary? Were you directly or indirectly involved in mutilating any Vietnamese (cutting off body parts, etc.)?

9. Did you ever go "kill crazy" or were you in a situation in

which you "just went off" or were "getting back"? What set you off? How long did it last? Describe these experiences.

10. Did you have any other experiences with Vietnamese?

M. Changes in Attitudes or Behavior
   1. Was there a particular time in your tour in Viet Nam when your attitudes or behaviors about being there really seemed to change?
   2. When? What events caused these changes? Describe these changes: the changes in your attitudes and your behavior.

N. Responses to the Uniqueness of the War
   1. How did you feel about the social and political circumstances under which the war was fought: the unpopularity of the war at home and the lack of clear commitment by the U.S. government?
   2. How did you feel about the undeclared nature of the war, the policy of military restraint, and the absence of clear measures of victory or defeat? Were you bothered by commanders interfering with offensive action?
   3. Viet Nam was America's first guerilla war, there were no front lines, the enemy was everywhere. How did this affect you?
   4. How were you affected by the 12- or 13-month tour of duty in Viet Nam and the way in which you arrived and left?
   5. If you served for more than one tour of duty, describe similarities or differences in the tours.
   6. How did you feel about the war being televised at home? Did you ever watch it? How did it affect you?
   7. Were you aware of the antiwar protests back home while in Viet Nam? How did this affect you and your unit?
   8. What do you feel the United States accomplished in Viet Nam? What do you feel you personally accomplished?
   9. Do you think the United States should have become involved in the war or not?

O. Stress and Conflict Unique to Minority Military Personnel
   While the following questions apply specifically to minorities (as defined by race, culture, ethnicity, sex, etc.), a number of these questions (or a rephrasing of them) are important to ask all Viet Nam veterans, such as 1 and 3.
   1. Did you have problems or particularly close positive interactions with minority American military personnel?
   2. What was it like being a minority person in Viet Nam; did

you have any problems with communication, trust, racism, sexism, or others accepting your values or beliefs?

3. For some minority veterans, the experience was that there was no racism in the bush, but that there was at other times. What was your experience?

4. Did you have any language problems in Viet Nam, or other problems in understanding and being understood by others?

5. Did you feel that others accepted you and were you comfortable with others in your unit, including the NCOs and officers?

6. Did you feel that others in your unit appreciated or understood the way you talked, looked, and behaved?

7. Did the expression of things you grew up thinking and believing, or were important to you and your family, clash with the beliefs, etc., of others in your unit?

8. Were your values different from those of others so as to create problems for you?

9. Whom in Viet Nam did you trust and of whom were you suspicious? Why?

10. Were you ever betrayed by someone in your unit in Viet Nam?

11. Did you feel betrayed by the United States?

12. As a minority person from the United States, how did you feel about fighting against the Vietcong?

13. In your opinion, how extensive was racism in Viet Nam? Explain.

14. In your judgment, were you or others discriminated against because of your race, sex, or cultural background? In what ways?

15. How were women (both American and Vietnamese) treated by the male personnel in support units? How extensive was sexism? (For male veterans) Did you have contacts with American women? Describe these.

P. Some Specific Traumatic Events

1. Did you have any near misses? Where and how? What saved you? Were friends torn up? Were you pinned down, lost, isolated, or overcome with exhaustion or fear? Did you get very sick? With heat stroke, cerebral malaria, meningitis, plague, cholera, pneumonia? What experiences did you have with mines, booby traps, punji pits?

2. Did you seek or receive psychiatric, religious, or spiritual help? Did you wish that you had counseling from someone? Why?

3. What are the first and second worst scenes or events that you remember?

4. What was your most scary or frightening time in Viet Nam? What was your most bizarre or strange experience in Viet Nam? What was your most thrilling time?

5. What were you most ashamed of that happened in Viet Nam, or what did you have the most regrets about, that you wish hadn't happened?

6. What atrocity-type events did you see or hear about? Who did what to whom? Why did it happen?

7. Are there things that happened that you have never discussed or never wanted to discuss?

8. If you could do something over again, or do something different that happened, or didn't happen in Viet Nam, what would it be?

9. Is there anything that happened in Viet Nam that you just can't forgive others for? That you can't forgive yourself for?

Q. Positive Experiences in the War Zone

1. What were your most positive experiences in Viet Nam? Friendships? Accomplishments or actions you did? Other? How frequent were these? How did they compare to the frequency and extent of negative experiences?

2. What are you most proud of that you did in Viet Nam?

R. Drugs

1. How many people in your unit were using drugs or alcohol heavily?

2. How did you feel about other Americans who drank or used drugs heavily? Did it hurt or help them do their jobs?

3. How much did you drink, and when? *What* did you drink, usually? When did you start smoking marijuana? Usually with whom, and how often? What did it do for you? What effects? How did it affect the way you felt about your surroundings? Did you use heroin or opium? Where, when, with what effects? Overall, how did alcohol or drugs make it easier, or harder, for you to survive?

4. What was the "unit policy" on drugs and alcohol? Did the military or your unit commanders 1) punish or harass you or others for drug or alcohol usage, or 2) supply or make it easy to obtain and use?

S. R & R (Rest and Recreation)

1. How many R&Rs, if any, did you get out of Viet Nam? (Specify: where and when during tour; with whom did

you go; whom did you meet? What happened? Were you able to enjoy it? If not, why?)

2. How many incountry R&Rs did you get? Where? When during your tour? How were they? If you didn't go on any R&Rs, why not? What were your feelings about this?

3. What happened that was good, or not-so-good, in your unit or with buddies while you were on R&R?

4. How did R&R affect you when you got back to your unit? Were you changed from when you left for R&R? Was it easier or harder?

5. Any feelings then, or now, that you shouldn't have gone on R&R when or where you did? If so, why?

T. Happenings Back Home

1. What kind of communications did you have with people back home: the frequency, who initiated, tone and effect of communications on you and on the people back home? Was the news sent to you mostly good or bad or what? What did you tend to say?

2. What, if anything, was happening back home that you felt particularly good or bad about? Were there any bad happenings back home: "Dear John" letter, death of a family member or friend, parents get divorced, other family hardships, etc.? Could things have been any different if you had been back there at the time? Did you feel then or now that you were at least partly responsible for some things that happened back home while you were in Viet Nam? Were others back home blaming you at all for what was happening while you were away (in Viet Nam)?

U. Moral and Value Conflicts Precipitated by the Unique Nature of the Viet Nam War and Their Effects on Viet Nam Combatants and Support Troops

1. During your tour in Viet Nam, did you experience moral and value conflicts that were derived from such practices and realities as:

- The guerilla nature of the war?
- The inability of the ARVN to make a strong positive commitment to winning the war?
- Poor military leadership?
- Black market operations and political corruption?
- Body count and the technological nature of the war?
- Difficulty in determining who the enemy was?
- Meaningless death of friends?

- The brutality of the war?
- Atrocity-type events or needless killings?
- Fraggings?
- Peace demonstrations and lack of support at home?
- Racial problems?
- The use of drugs and alcohol?
- The language of the war ("Gooks," "Going back to the 'world,' " etc.)?

2. Did you ever recall killing (or thinking you may have killed) someone, or otherwise being involved in the deaths of others that you thought later was a mistake?

3. As opposed to the way you felt and believed before going into the service, did you feel that your experience in Viet Nam altered your values and beliefs? Your convictions? Your religious beliefs? While in Viet Nam, did you feel any "moral pain" over what others, or yourself, were doing in Viet Nam? If so, how did it change you? Positively? Negatively?

4. How did you feel about the methods and the necessity of killing? Did the following emotions and practices affect you as you were trying to survive in Viet Nam?

- Terrorism from the other side?
- Obedience to authority?
- Body count?
- The use of drugs and alcohol as a coping mechanism?
- Fraggings?
- Over-kill tactics by our side?
- The wide range of emotions experienced in combat; from fear, to exhilaration, to boredom?
- The functioning of automatic reflexes during crisis situations?
- Dehumanization of the Vietnamese?
- Lack of clear guidelines governing military operations?
- Detachment from feelings?
- Sometimes running and hiding or otherwise avoiding rather than aggressively seeking out the enemy?
- The use of patrols to draw fire?
- The wish to prove yourself?
- The fear of being killed, maimed, or crippled?
- The feeling of "kill or be killed"?

5. Did you experience guilt feelings (or other feelings about killing, atrocities, or even surviving)?

6. Do you ever recall feeling that you abandoned someone (perhaps to die) in Viet Nam? Or that someone abandoned you?

7. Were you proud of your service in Viet Nam? Please describe and explain.

8. If you felt proud of your service, have you been supported by others for having served?

V. Getting Short (Close to Military Discharge)

1. When did you start feeling that you were getting short?

2. What did you do when your time got short? Did you start getting lower (staying in and down more)? Any relief from your commander; how long before DEROS (date of expected return from overseas)?

3. Did you get sent on duty or missions that you *shouldn't* have been sent on while you were short? Why? What are and were your feelings about that?

4. Did anything particular happen while you were short that you have negative feelings about; anything you did or did not do?

5. What do you most remember about your last few weeks incountry?

W. Getting Ready for Your Return Home

1. What was it like getting ready to come home from Viet Nam?

2. While in Viet Nam, did you talk with anyone about returning to the world and what it might be like? What did you imagine your return would be like?

3. Did you come home with the rest of your unit, with any buddies, or alone? How long was it from the time you came in from the bush or from the time you left your unit, until you were back home?

4. Do you feel that you were adequately debriefed before returning home from Viet Nam or were you able to prepare yourself? How? Do you feel that you had problems that you had to work through by yourself before leaving Viet Nam, or that you were unable to help yourself to work through?

X. Freedom Bird (Up and Out)

1. If you flew from Viet Nam to the United States: Where did you fly out from, in what kind of craft? Who else was on the plane? What was the general mood on the plane in others, in you? Did you have any special feelings at about 1,000 feet? What stops on the way back, for how long? Where did you land in the United States? What did you

do when you first got out of the plane? Where did you go
to at first? What town, to what people did you go to and
how did you get there? What did they say and how did
you feel?

2. If you didn't fly from Viet Nam to the United States, how
   did you get back to "the world"? (Then repeat relevant
   probes listed above.)

3. If you were medevac'd out from Viet Nam, describe what
   you remember from the time you left your unit in Viet
   Nam until you arrived at a medical facility in the United
   States.

V. *MILITARY DISCHARGE*

A. What is the story of your discharge? How soon after leaving
   Viet Nam did it occur? Specify the type and conditions. If
   other than honorable, describe what type, the reasons why,
   and your feelings about it. Did your discharge involve an
   article 15, a court-martial, fighting with superiors or peers,
   going AWOL, drugs, or homosexuality? Did you want out
   badly? Why? How did you feel at the time about how you got
   out? How do you feel now?

B. If applicable, have you done anything about an upgrade of
   your discharge status? If not, why not?

C. Did you and do you have a service-connected condition or
   disability? If yes, what type, medical and/or psychiatric?
   What specific condition was or is involved? When was the
   claim awarded? What circumstances surrounded your
   claim? What disability benefits were you awarded? Did you
   file a claim and get turned down?

D. Do you feel that you *should be* granted service-connected
   status by the Veterans Administration for a medical or psychiatric condition, because it developed or was aggravated
   while you were in the military or because it occurred as a
   result of military service? If you have already been granted
   service-connected status, do you feel your disability percentage rating should be higher? If so, why?

E. Do you think that you were exposed to agent orange? How
   often, in what circumstances, to how much? Do you think
   you have physical conditions that are related to agent orange? How much do you think or worry about agent orange
   exposure? What are you doing, or have you done, about
   this?

VI. *POST–VIET NAM READJUSTMENT*

In this section, the interviewer may wish to refer to the specific individuals and questions listed in items A and B, while questioning under items C and D.

A. The Homecoming and the First Month After Return

I would now like to ask you some specific questions about your actual arrival in the States from Viet Nam, and your experiences during that first month back.

1. If you went directly to a medical facility in the United States following medical evacuation from Viet Nam, describe your stay there: where, when, for what condition, for how long, adequacy of treatment received, experiences with others who were hospitalized there, your psychological state, contact with Viet Nam buddies or folks back home, going out of the hospital for visits, your posthospital plans.

2. Describe your first in-person contact with whomever it was that you were coming home to meet: who, where, when, in what circumstances? What were the results?

3. Describe your first contacts with others whom you knew before Viet Nam, whom you met within the first several days back home.

4. Thinking about the following folks back home, would you say that they generally seemed prepared for your homecoming? Did anyone ever thank you for having gone to Viet Nam? Did anyone have a welcome home party for you? Were you blamed by the folks back home for anything? What sense of welcome, no welcome, or unwelcome did you receive from the following persons?

   - Strangers you encountered coming home
   - Spouse/girlfriend or boyfriend/live-in partner
   - Mother, father (or parent substitutes)
   - Brothers, sisters
   - Other close relatives
   - Close friends from before Viet Nam
   - Others you knew before Viet Nam
   - Others whom you had not known before Viet Nam

5. How were you feeling about yourself as a Viet Nam veteran just returned from Viet Nam, and what were you wanting or needing, if anything, from your folks back home, or from anyone else? Were you feeling proud or

guilty or ashamed about your role in Viet Nam? What effect did this have?

6. What were your reactions to the United States and being back in the States? What specifically did you do during the first month back?

7. Did part of you wish you were back in Viet Nam? How so? What were you missing, or what weren't you comfortable with or not liking here?

8. Did you want to talk about Viet Nam, or did you actually talk about it? With whom? What were the results? Did the fact that we weren't "winning" have any effect on your homecoming? Did folks hassle you because you were "a loser" or a "baby-killer"?

B. The Next Few Months

1. What was your itinerary: from where to where, for how long? What kind of psychological state were you in? Describe dreams, nightmares, trouble sleeping, increase or decrease in appetite, and how often you were drunk, stoned, or high on other substances. Describe any irritability, anxiety, paranoia, relief, euphoria, or joy.

2. How were you doing in the following relationships and activities?

- Spouse/girlfriend or boyfriend/live-in partner
- Father, mother (or parent substitutes)
- Brothers, sisters
- Other close relatives
- Close friends from before Viet Nam
- Others you knew before Viet Nam
- Interest or involvement in school, work, leisure time activities
- Interest in making, or ability to make, new friends

3. Did you want to talk about Viet Nam? Did others want you to? Who? What were the results?

4. (This section of questions applies only to Viet Nam veterans who returned to stateside military duty after the first month back, or who went back for a second tour or additional tours.)

   a. Where were you stationed? For how long? What was your position and job? How did you feel about being where you were and doing what you were doing?

   b. How did your Viet Nam experience affect your behaviors and attitudes at this next military duty assignment? How did it affect your ability to do your job and meet your responsibilities? How did it affect your ability to deal with military authorities and your buddies/military cohorts? How did it affect your relation to nonmilitary people? How did you feel as you were getting short (close to military discharge)? If you made a career of the military, how did your Viet Nam experiences affect your decision to stay in the military? What was its effect on promotions and career opportunities within the military? Were there any other effects on your functioning at this first post–Viet Nam duty station?

c. If you continued in the military beyond this first post–Viet Nam assignment, how did you do in later assignments and tours? Were you able to put your Viet Nam experience behind you? Did you want to? Did you have much interaction with other active-duty Viet Nam veterans? Did you seem to have much in common? Did you talk about Viet Nam with other active-duty military personnel? What were the results?

d. If you returned to Viet Nam for another tour or tours, what was happening that made you decide to return to Viet Nam? What were you missing that was in Viet Nam, or what were you hoping to accomplish there? Was anything going on back home that you weren't comfortable with or wanted to get away from? How did the news that you were going back affect your spouse or partner, other family, friends, etc.?

C. The First Two or Three Years After Viet Nam
(Repeat relevant questions from A and B.) Also, were you making changes or undergoing changes in relationships, activities, feelings about yourself, etc. that were different from the first few months back?

D. Talking About Viet Nam Since Homecoming Transition
1. Did you want to talk about Viet Nam? To whom? Did you try? Why or why not? What were the results?
2. Did others want to talk to you about Viet Nam? Did they want you to talk to them about Viet Nam? Who? When? What were the results?
3. Did you have any special or close interaction or connec-

tions with others over talking and sharing about Viet Nam? Did you have any bad scenes over you or someone else wanting you to talk about Viet Nam? Who? When? What were the results?

4. Have you ever been in counseling with a professional mental health person, clergy or other religious person, or other kind of counselor? Explain. Did Viet Nam ever come up in the talking? How? To what extent? Your feelings? What happened? If Viet Nam did not come up, why not?

E. Prime Features of the Military-to-Civilian Transition
What stands out in your mind (and describe why) during:

- The actual arrival and going home?
- The first few months back?
- The first few years back?
- After the first few years back?

F. Reviewing Possible Causes of Conflict
Did you have strong reactions after Viet Nam (or do you today) to any of the following events:

- Tet Offensive?
- Martin Luther King's assassination?
- Lyndon Johnson's decision not to seek reelection?
- The peace talks in Paris?
- Invasion of Cambodia?
- The POWs and Americans going to Hanoi?
- The truce of 1973?
- The pullout of 1975?
- The refugees?
- *Coming Home* and other motion pictures about Viet Nam?
- Television documentaries on the Viet Nam War?
- Hostage rescue attempt in Iran?
- Hero's welcome for returning Iranian hostages?
- Viet Nam Veterans Memorial in Washington, D.C.?
- National Salute to Viet Nam Veterans in 1982 and 1984?
- U.S. military activity in Central America?
- Travel of Amerasian children from Viet Nam to the United States?
- Presence of U.S. Marines in Lebanon, especially bombing of October 1983?
- Any other events concerning you or your family, close

friends, etc. that brought back memories or dreams about Viet Nam?

G. Being Different After Viet Nam
    1. Describe what was most different about you after the war (if anything) in contrast to before the war. Describe any changes, positive or negative, in your appearance, personality, attitudes, stability, temper, interest, relationships, etc.
    2. Did others say that you were different in ways you couldn't see? In what ways?
    3. What about your interest in, and feelings about, using weapons since Viet Nam? What weapons do you own? Describe where you keep and use them. Do you ever carry weapons with you? How often? Why?
    4. How are you still different today from before Viet Nam in ways that seem to be at least partly connected to the war or the military-to-civilian transition?

H. Your Identity as a Viet Nam Veteran
    1. Did you let many people know you were a Viet Nam veteran after you got back? When, how, who, with what results? If not, why not?
    2. Did you think of yourself as a Viet Nam veteran? What *are* your feelings about yourself as a Viet Nam veteran?
    3. Do you identify yourself to others as a Viet Nam veteran these days?
    4. If once you didn't feel like a Viet Nam veteran, but now you do, explain how and when that change occurred, and what the difference in feeling is.

I. Contact with Other Viet Nam Veterans and Their Families
    1. Did (do) you know, talk to, or attempt to locate any other Viet Nam veterans? When, where, who? Why or why not?
    2. What about buddies who left Viet Nam before or after you? What were the results?
    3. Did (do) you have contact with the families of buddies or other Viet Nam veterans who were killed? Why or why not? What were the results?

J. Successful Readjustment Resources, Coping Mechanisms, and Adjustment Options
    1. What has worked for you in helping you readjust? Have friends, family, and your career been important in helping you readjust? How do your spouse or partner and family relate to the war?

2. How have the following resources been helpful in your readjustment process:

- Your family and friends?
- Individual readjustment counseling?
- Family counseling?
- Viet Nam veteran rap groups? Other group therapy?
- Substance abuse treatment and counseling?
- Vocational and educational counseling, planning, and achievement?
- Involvement in volunteer social or human services activities?
- Reentry into the military or related career systems?
- The ability to develop long-term goals?
- The feeling of being a survivor?
- The Veterans Administration?
- Service organizations?
- Psychotherapy/psychoanalysis?
- Meditation?
- Other stress reduction techniques?
- Church or religion?
- Any other resources?

K. Readjustment Obstacles or Difficulties
  1. After returning from Viet Nam, what difficulties in readjustment from military-to-civilian status have you experienced?
     a. If you had a physical or psychological disability when you returned from Viet Nam, how has it affected your readjustment?
     b. If you received a less than honorable discharge, do you feel it was fair? How has it affected your readjustment?
     c. Did you attempt unsuccessfully, or were you reluctant to try, to get help for a particular physical problem, emotional difficulty, or other symptom after coming home?
     d. Have you not received G.I. Bill and other V.A. benefits that you felt you deserved, or received benefits that you felt were inadequate or less than you deserved?
     e. What has been your employment and economic situation since your return from Viet Nam? What was it like during the first several years after you came

home? Are you underemployed? Do you go after jobs that are beneath your abilities? Did Viet Nam improve your abilities as a worker?

f. Do you feel that the unpopularity of the war at home led to the negative stereotyping of Viet Nam veterans as "social misfits"? Has the negative image of Viet Nam veterans caused problems for you? Has it affected your feeling of self-worth?

g. How do you contrast yourself to those of your age group who did not go to Viet Nam and avoided military service? Does your contrast represent a difficulty for you?

h. Do you feel that the generation that participated in World War II and Korea has a lack of understanding or appreciation for what you went through in Viet Nam? Do you feel that their attitude has affected your readjustment?

i. Have you been affected by any symptoms of post-traumatic stress disorder: nightmares; flashbacks; startle reactions; feelings of guilt, betrayal, or rage; alienation; doubt about the ability to love and trust others; difficulty in concentrating or completing tasks; depression and anxiety; irritability; or aggressive and impulsive behavior? How have these symptoms affected your readjustment? (This area should be explored further in the clinical history.)

j. Do you feel used, abused, and discarded? Do you feel appreciated?

k. How do you see yourself fitting into American society, into the American dream? Is this vision a difficulty for you?

l. Does your time in Viet Nam sometimes feel like it was unreal? Describe this feeling.

L. Counterproductive or Destructive Readjustment Coping Mechanisms

1. After returning from Viet Nam, many veterans used severe forms of coping mechanisms that may have provided short-term relief but in the long run proved to be counterproductive. Which of the following short-term coping mechanisms have you used and how have they affected you?

• Drug and alcohol?

- Social withdrawal?
- Numbing or emotional withdrawal from people?
- Denial or minimalization of stress problems?
- Suppression of feelings of anxiety and depression?
- Rage spells or aggressive and impulsive behavior?
- Living on a day-to-day basis without any goals or plans for the future?

2. Do you sometimes think you should be punished for something you did in Viet Nam? In what ways, if any, have you tried to punish yourself?

M. Recognition You Received for Viet Nam Service
Do you think that you should be rewarded or recognized more for what you did in Viet Nam? In what ways? How were you recognized in or since Viet Nam? How have you tried to ask for rewards or recognition, or given them to yourself?

N. Positive Results of Your Viet Nam Experience
  1. How has your Viet Nam experience strengthened or helped you?
  2. Can you give specific examples: in work, in intimate (family, marital, partner) relationships, with friends?
  3. What are your feelings about yourself and your values about life as a result of your Viet Nam experience?
  4. Has your Viet Nam experience affected your ability to deal with stressful situations?
  5. Describe any other positive results of your Viet Nam experience.

O. Souvenirs and Memorabilia
(Certain concrete objects may provide a catalyst for exploration of war experiences.)
  1. What parts of your uniforms from Viet Nam do you still have? If you no longer have any, when and how did you dispose of your uniforms?
  2. When do you sometimes wear war-related clothing or accessories (fatigue jacket, hat, etc.)?
  3. Were you awarded any medals? Where are they?
  4. Did you bring back any clippings, books, souvenirs, or other objects from Viet Nam? Where are they?
  5. Do you have any photographs, drawings, or other pictures from Viet Nam? How many? What other people besides yourself have seen them?
  6. Were any letters you wrote from Viet Nam, or letters

written to you there, saved? Where are they now?

7. Do you have any weapons from Viet Nam? What? Where are they?

It is not realistic that most of the areas of inquiry identified above can be, or should be, adequately addressed in one session. Therefore, it is important to ensure that the veteran is not forced to open up or delve into more areas of inquiry than can be reasonably absorbed at one sitting. In addition, the veteran should be kept informed of the overall objectives of the interview process and the areas of exploration that will eventually be addressed, so that he or she has a sense of the military history assessment strategy.

Finally, it is highly likely that current concerns will be triggered by inquiries concerning the military history. Therefore, clinical judgment must be employed as to the appropriateness of addressing various areas of experience at the outset. A delay in such discussion may be appropriate and more supportive of subsequent therapeutic efforts. Indeed, clinical sensitivity to such dynamics during every phase of military history taking will enhance the development of effective therapeutic relationships with Viet Nam veterans.

14

The Unconscious Flashback to the War in Viet Nam Veterans: Clinical Mystery, Legal Defense, and Community Problem

Arthur S. Blank, Jr., M.D.

14

Remembering is worse than being there.
   —Viet Nam veteran, August 1980

For the past decade, every so often somewhere in the United States, a Viet Nam veteran, otherwise living peacefully, has suddenly engaged in explosive behavior in such a way as to involve others in family or community. These episodes rarely cause harm, but sometimes include hostage-taking, demands for treatment, or other threatening behavior. As well known by therapists who treat Viet Nam veterans, the episodes are associated with flashbacks, a sudden access into consciousness of dissociated war experiences and related affects, fantasies, and impulses. And along with the few veterans who engage in dramatic actions in response to flashbacks, there are many others who experience intrusive imagery of war events privately, without public notice.

The extreme public episodes are quite rare, given the total of approximately 3.5 million persons who served in Southeast Asia between 1964 and 1975 (1). However, they create havoc for the patient and others and occasionally lead to injury or death. Although they sometimes gain extensive media exposure, neither the public nor the private episodes have ever been elucidated in the clinical literature. A few writers have mentioned the phenomenon in passing (2–4). This absence of study of flashbacks is perhaps an example of our general national denial of war and its psychological consequences for participants.

The views expressed in this paper are solely those of the author and do not necessarily reflect those of the Veterans Administration.

I thank Sarah Haley, M.S.W., and John Russell Smith, M.A., for other clinical material that supports the findings in this chapter.

However, there is a special taboo about flashbacks. Even in clinical papers, the term is usually placed in quotes, notwithstanding its universal usage among veterans. In the news media, such comments as the following (from a Veterans Administration counselor) are common: "There's a strange syndrome where someone will go along for 10 or 12 years with apparently no trouble. . . .Then they begin to have nightmarish recollections. *I hate to use the term,* but they do describe them as flashback experiences" (5) (emphasis added). One may speculate that the phenomenon, especially when massive, is unconsciously perceived as a state of being possessed and therefore mobilizes primitive fears. Perhaps the phenomenon has been subject to intense disavowal precisely because it is a vivid and compelling return by a veteran to the perceptual reality of the Viet Nam War. Just as many Americans, including mental health professionals, have a strong aversion to remembering the war, so may they have an equally strong aversion to studying its vivid and forceful recall by some veterans.

However, since early 1979 probably a few hundred major legal cases have arisen in which flashbacks play a role, and the phenomenon is continuing to emerge in clinical contexts. It is therefore imperative to clarify the nature of flashbacks and their place in the legal assessment of responsibility.

TYPES OF FLASHBACKS

We may distinguish among four types of intrusive recall in post-traumatic stress disorder:

1. Vivid dreams and nightmares of combat events, as described for decades (2, 3, 6, 7).
2. Vivid dreams from which the dreamer awakens, then having difficulty shaking the sense of reality of the recollected war events and possibly showing motor behavior related to the dream content.
3. Conscious flashback experiences, in which the subject vividly experiences images of war events. The recall is intrusive and may consist of visual, auditory, or olfactory memories, with little loss of contact with present reality. Or there may also be ensuing dramatic behavior—climbing a tree and shouting that one is surrounded by Vietcong, for example—with loss of contact with present reality. The sensory recall may progress to great intensity and is then properly labeled a pseudohallucination (4). Even if contact with the present is temporarily lost, the veteran experiencing conscious flashbacks can later report what imagery has occurred and is aware, within a few

hours or days, of the separate realities of the present and the past. He or she knows that a flashback has occurred, and can say so. (In a variant of this phenomenon, there is partial or total amnesia for the content of the flashback, although not for the fact of its occurrence.) Such episodes are not peculiar to Viet Nam veterans, having been reported in survivors of Nazi concentration camps (8, 9) and in World War II aviation personnel by Grinker and Spiegel in their standard work, *Men Under Stress* (7). In their cases 56 through 59, termed "psychotic-like states," the patients had pseudohallucinations of being in combat, of women and children being killed, or of being pursued by Nazis. We should now note that in all of those cases, the aviator had either been lost for a time in enemy territory or (a psychological equivalent) was in a supposedly secure base camp which was invaded by German parachutists. This was analogous to the terrorized guerilla situation in Viet Nam, where also the fundamental sense of being in a place with a definable level of safety was often not present. The three patients whose cases are presented in this chapter similarly experienced intense, chronic, and pervasive loss of security of their immediate surroundings.

In recent years, a determination of conscious flashback with overwhelming intensity has been used in support of mitigation of punishment in a hostage incident (10), a homicide (11), and as a part of a successful insanity defense in an assault incident (12).

4. Unconscious flashbacks, our principal concern here, are episodes wherein the veteran has a sudden, discrete experience, leading to actions, where the manifest psychic content is only indirectly related to the war; in addition, the veteran does not have conscious awareness of reliving events in Viet Nam, neither at the time of the flashback nor later. However, with thorough interviewing, the episode unmistakably defines itself as a repetition of some event or events in the war. The individual's state of consciousness, outwardly observed, may or may not be altered. Memories, affects, and impulses that are pressing against profound and heretofore intact denial and repression come forth, but only in action, without conscious visual or other registration. The subject is thus in the situation of the main character in *The Manchurian Candidate* (13), carrying out complex integrated actions based on past experiences that are not consciously remembered, with no awareness that he is repeating anything. However, unlike the Manchurian Candidate, the preponderant motive of the veteran who is the victim of this phenomenon is usually not to hurt someone, but quite the opposite, as we shall see presently.

The structure of the unconscious flashback is like that of the dream, in having manifest and latent content. As in posthypnotic suggestion, the subject invents rationalizations for his or her behavior, which upon careful investigation can easily be seen as lacking in substance. Notwithstanding sometimes extreme behavior, unconscious flashbacks have gone undetected in clinical and forensic cases during the past decade, because both veterans and examiners have been unaware of this phenomenon and its direct linkages to war experiences. Treatment has been impeded and the management of legal cases has been marred; both can be corrected by accurate detection and exploration of the meaning of behavior.

CASE EXAMPLES

Three cases of this phenomenon will now be described. Identifying information has been altered to protect anonymity but to not affect the psychological accuracy of the description.

Case 1

Dr. N. is a 37-year-old general surgeon who was troubled for five years with periodic severe pain in the eyes, since his army discharge in 1977. In early 1982 he suddenly walked into a school classroom with a rifle and informed the students and teacher that they were hostages until the Mayor agreed to come and hear his complaints about not being able to obtain treatment for his symptom. In the ensuing crisis, SWAT team snipers set up posts from which to shoot Dr. N., and officials negotiated with him. The Mayor came and listened to Dr. N.'s complaints, which were laced with vague references to Viet Nam, and Dr. N. surrendered after about five hours. No injuries occurred, and he was placed in jail. Extensive press coverage included discussion of post-traumatic stress disorder. In jail, Dr. N. was compliant and quiet and said nothing about what had happened. Psychiatric evaluation did not clarify the episode, and Dr. N. remained in jail for a full 12 months. Professionals and authorities were puzzled as to what should be done with him.

When I interviewed this veteran, he was bland, anxious, depressed, and without psychosis or organicity. The early history was ordinary, with no psychiatric or mental problems in the family. In college his MCAT scores were high, and he joined the Army in return for financing of medical school. In 1967 he volunteered for Viet Nam believing it was his patriotic duty. For 10 months he worked at a large field hospital in the combat headquarters base. There was a steady stream of casualties incoming by helicopter, with many deaths at the hospital. Many patients were mutilated or paralyzed. He himself had several near misses from mortars, rockets, booby traps, or mines. The base camp included a Vietnamese village within the perimeter and was thus grossly insecure. After 10 months he was evacuated for a mysterious life-threatening disease and was diagnosed and cured only after a three-month hospitalization.

Dr. N. then finished his surgical residency and worked at several Army hospitals stateside. This included several months on the neurosurgery service: the patients were chiefly the wounded from Viet Nam—paraplegics, quadriplegics, amputees, and men with severe head wounds. He became attached to one particular patient, who had been shot through the head such that both eyes had been destroyed; this patient's face was disfigured, but he had no brain damage. The injured man's wife visited him upon his arrival from the combat zone and soon divorced him. Dr. N. visited the patient repeatedly and could not forget him. The patient was 20 years old. Several months later, Dr. N. first had episodic eye pain. He continued to work, but 18 months after being on the neurosurgery ward, he began to have a recurrent nightmare in which he was lying somewhere totally paralyzed, except for his head; he was alone and struggled to move. Several months later he became acutely anxious, depressed, and irritable for the first time, and he had rage spells. At this point, eight years after his duty in Viet Nam, military psychiatrists treated him with major tranquilizers and did not ask him about Viet Nam.

In 1977, Dr. N. terminated military service. The eye pain slowly worsened and gradually began to interfere with his work. The nightmare continued, but the anxiety and depression receded.

During extensive interviewing, the following facts emerged: 1) The school he invaded (which was next to his house) strikingly resembled a school next to his hospital in Viet Nam. 2) The recurring nightmare referred directly to an incident in the war in which two detached human heads, all that remained of two American soldiers, were brought in by medevac helicopter to the morgue tent next to his hospital. 3) In Viet Nam he had shot and killed a North Vietnamese Army prisoner brought in for treatment who was trying to escape. He expressed intense guilt that he, a noncombatant, would have done that. 4) He had a fixed pervasive amnesia for his tour in the war, which could be by-passed slightly during the interviews with the aid of my own personal knowledge of military medical operations in Viet Nam. 5) He had never talked with anyone about Viet Nam and his subsequent exposure to casualties. 6) The eye symptom had been mistakenly diagnosed as migraine, and he had been given medications for years by physicians with no effect. 7) When he burst into the school in

1982, he had had two things consciously in mind: either he would get help for his eyes or he would be killed by a sniper. He thought the latter acceptable because he could not stand to live any longer with the intractable eye symptom, now making his work very difficult. Finally, 8) fine details of the school incident revealed that it was an overdetermined re-creation of three incidents: a) his shooting the prisoner in Viet Nam, b) a scene in which a group of people were under siege in a similar building in Viet Nam, and c) an incident with a sniper which occurred on Dr. N.'s first day in Viet Nam.

It became clear that in the school episode Dr. N. was attempting to get himself shot in a war-like situation and thus take the place of the prisoner he himself had shot. In fact, subsequent investigation revealed several remarkable facts. At a moment when the snipers were close to shooting Dr. N. at the school in 1982, a senior state official arrived and took charge. He was a retired Army officer who had been a commander in Viet Nam during the same year as Dr. N. Stationed within 30 miles of Dr. N.'s field hospital, he was familiar with the layout of, and conditions in, Dr. N.'s base camp. The official, upon learning that Dr. N. had been in Viet Nam, made an accurate intuitive psychological diagnosis and gave orders to negotiate without any time limit. The patient's survival and the availability of this history may be due to this remarkable coincidence.

Six months after the school incident, Dr. N. had no conscious awareness of specific links between it and his Viet Nam War experiences. Furthermore, during a subsequent follow-up evaluation after a total of 12 months, he mentioned casually—as though it were of no importance—that over the years, during several severe episodes of eye pain, he had experienced total blindness.

Case 2

George L. is a 32-year-old man with two children, who was steadily employed. One day in the late 1970s he began drinking before noon with two friends in their small town in Oregon. They traveled from bar to bar, and at one point they visited a small ocean inlet. Beginning at a point during the return to his home, he has complete amnesia for subsequent events. The trio returned to George's house, where without provocation he attacked his wife. His buddies attempted to restrain him, and he beat them off with tremendous ferociousness, saying little. His friends say he "was like a string of firecrackers going off." George was usually nonviolent, had no criminal record, and had never drunk to the point of loss of control since returning from Viet Nam 10 years previously. George took out a shotgun, at which moment all others left the house. George began shooting at neighboring houses.

The police arrived. George gathered five rifles, the shotgun, and a pistol and barricaded himself on the second floor. He threw furniture downstairs, threw stereo equipment out the window, pushed a refrigerator across the room, and smashed up other objects. He threw a scythe at a neighbor who beat a hasty retreat, the scythe narrowly missing. He shot at a policeman who was standing less than 50 feet away and missed; he told another neighbor to get inside, then shot at his house. He put his hand through a window and spread blood around the room from a severe laceration on his arm. He then lost consciousness from blood loss, fainting, intoxication, or some combination of those factors. A friend gingerly entered and found George sitting on the floor, back against the wall, slumped amidst the rubble. Thus the episode ended with no injuries except George's laceration.

There was no precipitating stress for this event, although for the prior six months George had without awareness arranged his work schedule so that it corresponded to his daily routine in Viet Nam. Ever since the episode he has not drunk any alcohol, for fear of losing control. Concerned about his condition, several months after the episode he joined a rap group established by a nearby Viet Nam Vet Center, set up by the Veterans Administration (see Chapter 11). Prior to this time, he had not discussed his Viet Nam tour with anyone; now he began to do so at length, in this all–Viet Nam veterans environment. Interestingly, however, by the time of my evaluation several months after his joining the group, there had been little talk of the flashback episode. He was still mystified by it and afraid to drink any alcohol at all.

The interview revealed that in Viet Nam George was a machine gunner on supply trucks for seven months, making regular runs from a port on the South China Sea deep into hostile territory. Cargo frequently included ammunition and fuel. The trucks were often fired upon en route, and the base camp was subjected to rocket attacks. On one occasion his base was overrun and the Vietnamese National Liberation Front forces were beaten off only after fierce fighting. Other trucks hit mines on the road, although his did not. He and his mates drank every day, starting around noon. They drank just enough through the rest of the day, especially when on a supply run, to hold down fear and anxiety without too substantially impairing alertness.

One time in his barracks (which was well-appointed with a stereo, stove, refrigerator, etc.) George picked up some cans of soda and went outside to join his buddies for a drink. About 60 seconds after he left the barracks, a rocket hit. The rocket entered the barracks and exploded inside where George had just picked up the sodas. A lone soldier, two weeks incountry, was in the barracks and was killed immediately. George says, "There was not a cut on him—he was just turned into jelly," and he describes the dead man's position in detail as exactly the same as that in which he (George) was found at the end of the flashback episode. The furnishings in the barracks were thrown about and blown up. Detail by detail, George's explosive episode in 1978 repeated his experience 10 years previously in Viet Nam. It turned out that the rather bizarre scythe-throwing was linked to his custom of sleeping with a machete next to him in Viet Nam, in case of overrun by the National Liberation Front forces. This had made his buddies there wary of surprising him in any way while he was asleep.

When the isomorphism between his bewildering flashback episode and the events in Viet Nam was pointed out to George, he was only slightly curious and mostly indifferent. However, the next association was that for years he had also had *conscious* flashbacks, which were not previously mentioned in two hours of interviewing. Loud truck sounds at night caused him to wake up convinced he was being shelled, and sometimes that sense of reality lingered for a few hours. While deer hunting, he was sometimes overcome with memories of smells and sights from an episode in Viet Nam when he had to retrieve the remains of two men who had been killed when their helicopter crashed in a swamp. In addition, he went on to describe free-floating anxiety and a vague feeling that he had not gotten over his war experiences.

Case 3

Michael R. is a 35-year-old college graduate who works as an electrician. Since the end of his Viet Nam tour in 1971, his life had been stable, although there was intermittent use of marijuana and amphetamines. Early in 1982, after being divorced by his wife, losing a close friend who moved across the country, and experiencing the serious illness of his girlfriend, he armed himself with a pistol and set out at about 4:00 A.M. Michael, who had no prior criminal record, broke into a store which he frequented and knew to have an alarm system, with the idea of stealing money. A policeman soon drove up in response to the alarm signal. Michael fled to nearby woods. Watching the policeman through the thin cover of early spring, he was spotted because of unnecessary movement. Upon command, he came out of the woods with his hands up, but then suddenly tried to disarm the policeman. He succeeded, but a struggle ensued during which Michael was nearly shot. The policeman was much the larger of the two, but neither was clearly winning when Michael simply surrendered. At no time did he attempt to use his own pistol.

On interview, there was no history of family or prewar psychiatric disturbance. Michael enlisted in the Army in 1970, seeking excitement and considering it his patriotic duty. After five months of infantry duty, during which he was shot and hospitalized, he volunteered for long-range reconnaissance patrol. For six months, in a six-man team he stalked the soldiers of the National Liberation Front and the North Vietnamese Army in jungles and woods. The patrol spent considerable time hiding in the bush; the task was to completely avoid engaging the enemy and to gather intelligence on their movements. Often, as he sat or lay in hiding, fully camouflaged, the passing troops looked directly at where he was hiding. Michael and his comrades then waited, wondering if they had actually been seen; they prepared for the enemy to double back to attack. During the 12-month tour, he experienced the usual horrors. A buddy near him was blown apart when a grenade he was carrying on his chest accidentally exploded. Some combat soldiers cut off and collected ears of dead soldiers from the other side. A close friend was shot through the spinal cord and is permanently paraplegic. Another trooper near him bled to death when a neck artery was pierced by a piece of shrapnel. Another friend had his jaw blown away. While on patrols, the men were issued amphetamines to stay awake. Thus began his drug usage.

On his return to the United States, Michael had PTSD with irritability, nightmares, sleeping with a weapon, and other symptoms. With no psychiatric contact, the symptoms slowly abated, except for the nightmares which continue to the present. In the interviews, he eventually revealed that the central and most frequent nightmare, recurrent for 10 years, is as follows: He is hidden in the jungle and is spotted by a passing enemy soldier, who then begins to come after him. Michael is out of ammunition and in the dream thinks it is just a short time until he is captured or killed. The jungle cover in the dream has been blasted away by shelling and is sparse, like the thin cover in the woods near the store where he was found hiding by the policeman in early 1982.

Initially Michael was mystified by the store incident. He was tense and halting, and he said that he could make no sense of it. He had no conscious awareness that he had recreated in action his central war nightmare, present for 10 years. (Referral for psychiatric evaluation was by happenstance; a friend had seen a magazine piece about PTSD in Viet Nam veterans.) When it was pointed out to him that he had brought to life his nightmare, the immediate result was intense weeping and a flood of additional memories about war experiences.

The emergence of the nightmare and the details of his life in the war revealed why this man with no criminal record, an expert at combat and hiding in woods and jungle, for no substantial reason arranged to have himself confronted in a hapless burglary attempt, passed up an easy opportunity to escape from or shoot a lone policeman, got himself discovered, and then engaged in a senseless and life-threatening hand-to-hand struggle.

DISCUSSION

These cases illustrate the phenomenon of unconscious flashback to Viet Nam War experiences, to be differentiated from overpowering combat dreams and conscious flashbacks. The phenomenon is one example of intrusive recall—in action—as noted by writers on PTSD (14). However, at the same time such episodes are dynamically and structurally congruent with various action manifestations of hysterical dissociation, dreams, and posthypnotic suggestion. They share features with hysterical spells (*la grande hystérie* of Charcot): multiple identifications and the enactment of a complex drama (6).

There is in these cases an acting-out of complex unconscious conflicts, fantasies, and impulses. There is a seeking for abreaction and perhaps also an element of repetition in search of mastery. The incidents also have qualities of a waking dream, with manifest and latent content. And like the actions produced by posthypnotic suggestion, the patient produces rationalizations about their meaning.

There are here the typical efforts, as described by Fenichel for hysterical acting-out, "to get others to participate in the daydream," to return repressed material to reality, and to get rid of the trauma (6). When I pointed out to Michael (Case 3) that he had brought to life his central nightmare, he said, "Does this mean I won't have the nightmares anymore?"

One of these cases had total amnesia for at least as long as 18 months after the episode; the other two recall what happened, but are puzzled about the events and retain considerable affective distance. The wide cleft between these outbursts and the individuals' characteristic behavior, with massively dissociated material producing actions which are carried out with a fair degree of automaticity, suggests similarities also to both somnambulistic and hysterical fugue states.

Diagnostic and Forensic Considerations

In the large group of Viet Nam veterans with PTSD coming to V.A.

Medical Centers and the U.S. government's Viet Nam Vet Outreach Centers, the phenomenon of unconscious flashback is not uncommon. Until this time, however, the episodes have usually been regarded simply as outbursts of uncontrolled rage, and the clinical task has been defined as helping the patient with his supposed poor impulse control. With such a misdiagnosis, a valuable treatment opportunity is lost; recognizing the direct historical record contained in the veteran's behavior speeds a therapeutic unfolding of trauma, brings about clinical improvement, and is the only sure path to prevention of future outbursts.

Because of 1) the overpowering intensity of affects expressed; 2) the suddenness of the episodes; 3) the extreme discontinuity with characteristic behavior; 4) the presence of subsequent amnesia or confusion; 5) the direct linkages to highly traumatic experiences; and 6) the primal nature of the psychological issues—annihilation versus nonannihilation—in some cases the behavior may be significantly beyond conscious control. With loss of capacity for understanding the nature of one's actions or for "adhering to the right," therefore, there may be a basis for an insanity defense or a justification for mitigation of punishment. Judges and juries are so deciding (as in cases noted in references 10, 11, and 12). This manifestation of PTSD has gained a legal status similar to that of hysterical fugue states, hysterical dissociative episodes, severe acute stress reactions, and acute psychotic states. This, too, makes recognition of this clinical syndrome important.

The following criteria represent a first step toward recognition of the unconscious flashback phenomenon in Viet Nam veterans:

1. There is a retrievable history of one or more intensely traumatic events.

2. The flashback behavior is atypical for the individual.

3. The episode recreates the veteran's traumatic experiences in the war concretely and directly. Though manifest content may obscure latent content, upon careful scrutiny isomorphism is found between present behavior and its consequences and war events (perhaps with intervening condensations, displacements, etc.).

4. The patient may rationalize the episode and his motives, but the rationalizations lack substance and convincing application. They do not fit with expected motives and circumstances. (Case 3 here exemplifies this most strikingly. The patient said blandly that his purpose was to steal money, but he did not need to get money that way, and he did not show a pattern of thefts.)

5. There may be *la belle indifference*. This may be manifested directly or indirectly, such as by failure to seek psychiatric treatment, failure to

seek clearly indicated psychological evaluation as part of legal proceedings, or avoidance of the episode in psychotherapeutic treatment.
The patient may come to professional notice only through the intervention of a third person.

6. There may be amnesia for all or parts of the episode.

7. The episode may be isomorphic with a recurrent nightmare
about war events.

8. Physical environmental features of the episode may objectively
approximate conditions of the original experiences in Viet Nam, or,
more subtly, subjective perception of these links may be unwittingly
revealed by the patient when the episode is recounted in interviews.
Examples are climate (heat, high humidity, monsoon-like rain), a
particular type of intoxication (alcohol, amphetamine), or the surrounding terrain (mountains, woods/jungles, paddy/swamp, tree line
across an open space). Man-made structures in the present may resemble those in the original Viet Nam situation; a room in a house may be
like a bunker or a barracks, or buildings may be of the same shape or
style as they were in Viet Nam.

9. Multiple identifications can emerge during the episode. A patient may act like an exploding rocket, like the victim of the blast, or
like both. He may enact the role of a soldier in Viet Nam fighting the
other side or that of a prisoner or victim of torture.

10. The patient is mostly unaware of the specific ways he has
repeated and reenacted experiences in Viet Nam, although he may
vaguely connect the episode to the war.

11. The patient has, or has had, other symptoms of PTSD.

These criteria should be the subject of further clinical research,
which can also clarify the psychology of conscious flashbacks and other
behavior deriving from PTSD. Apostle (15) suggests that a legal
defense based on flashbacks is analogous to that for actions deriving
from febrile delerium, psychomotor epilepsy, acute cerebral concus-
sion, and involuntary intoxication. He holds that overwhelmingly
intense conscious flashbacks incur a similar incapacity for control of
one's actions. He argues, however, for a restrained and cautious use of
the legal defense, contingent on the availability of effective treatment
if incarceration is avoided. I concur with his position. This chapter
demonstrates how thorough diagnosis and detailed historical reconstruction of war experiences, and the drawing of careful distinctions
such as that between conscious and unconscious flashbacks, can facilitate treatment, forensic evaluation, and sophisticated treatment planning.

It must be kept in mind that the subject's reports are crucial in the diagnosis of PTSD and flashbacks. Fabrication might therefore be a problem, although it has apparently been present in only two of approximately 30 cases that I have reviewed with colleagues from 1980 to 1985. None of the three veteran patients whose cases were presented here had had any exposure to technical literature. However, mental health professionals are well advised to instruct persons in legal cases to avoid reading literature on post–Viet Nam problems until evaluation is complete. If the issue of fabrication arises in future cases, hypnosis or sodium amytal may prove useful. One may anticipate that fabrication of the subtle patterns of repetition found in these cases will be recognized by courts as exceedingly difficult.

Terror and Dissociation

In the cases reviewed here the veterans had spent long periods in enemy-held territory. In Grinker and Spiegel's four cases there had been hiding and evasion behind Nazi lines (or assault on a supposedly secure base camp) (7). The same experience—immersion in diffusely hostile territory—had happened to all five Viet Nam veterans with conscious flashbacks reported by Van Putten and Emory (4). Survivors of concentration camps have shown the same symptoms (8, 9). The hypothesis is therefore plausible that a diffusely terrorizing environment is influential in the development of large-scale dissociations which later emerge into perceptual consciousness, emerge as action, or both.

Veterans of guerilla war, or those immersed in an enemy milieu in ordinary war or concentration camps, have had to endure lengthy periods when primary distinctions between annihilating and nonannihilating objects were profoundly confused and difficult to maintain. Under such conditions, primitive distinctions (referable to the first year of life as regards the psychic structures involved) between good and bad objects are of immediate, continuous, live-saving importance and are constantly challenged. We may therefore speculate that in some individuals, archaic levels of ego development are activated, and infantile traumas from the time of first good-bad object differentiations are evoked, or that healthy psychic structures previously adequate for such differentiations in ordinary living are undermined.

REFERENCES

1. Fischer V, Boyle JM, Bucuvalas M, et al: Appendix D, in Myths and Realities: A Study of Attitudes Towards Vietnam Era Veterans. Washington, DC, Veterans Administration, 1980

2. Haley SA: Treatment implications of post-combat stress response syndromes for mental health professionals, in Stress Disorders Among Vietnam Veterans. Edited by Figley CR. New York, Brunner/Mazel, 1978

3. Shatan CF: Stress disorders among Vietnam veterans: the emotional content of combat continues, in Stress Disorders Among Vietnam Veterans. Edited by Figley CR. New York, Brunner/Mazel, 1978

4. Van Putten T, Emory WH: Traumatic neurosis in Vietnam returnees: a forgotten diagnosis? Arch Gen Psychiatry 29:695–698, 1973

5. Maurice J: State's Vietnam vets fare well. Daily Mail. Charleston, WV, October 23, 1979

6. Fenichel O: The Psychoanalytic Theory of Neurosis. New York, W. W. Norton, 1945

7. Grinker RR, Spiegel JP: Men Under Stress. New York, McGraw Hill, 1945

8. Niederland WG: Clinical observations on the "survivor syndrome." Int J Psychoanal 49:313–315, 1968

9. Jaffe R: Dissociative phenomenon in former concentration camp inmates. Int J Psychoanl 49:310–312, 1968

10. *State vs. Stephen Wyatt Gregory.* Circuit Court for Montgomery County, Maryland, Criminal Number 19205, February 1979

11. *Commonwealth of Pennsylvania vs. Michael J. Mulcahy.* Court of Common Pleas, Criminal Trial Division, Philadelphia, Pennsylvania, Number 460–464, December 1978

12. *People of the State of California vs. Charles W. Pettibone.* Superior Court of the State of California, County of Sonoma, Number 9632–C, February 1980

13. Condon R: The Manchurian Candidate. New York, McGraw Hill, 1959

14. Horowitz MJ: Stress Response Syndromes. New York, Jason Aronson, 1976

15. Apostle DT: The unconsciousness defense as applied to post-traumatic stress disorder in a Viet Nam veteran. Bull Acad Psychiatry Law 8:426–430, 1980

15

Women Viet Nam Veterans

Janet Ott, R.N., M.N.

15

Once upon a time there was a handsome, blonde soldier.
I grabbed at flesh
combing out bits of shrapnel and bits of bone
with bare fingers.

A virgin undressed men, touched them,
raped them in public.
By the time I bedded a man
who didn't smell like mud and burned flesh
He made love and I made jokes.

—Sharon Grant, Lt., A.N.C., Ret.

It has only recently been recognized that the term "Viet Nam veteran" includes thousands of women. Although complete demographic information is not available from the United States government, we do know that thousands of women served in Viet Nam, including at least 8,000 on active military duty, with the remainder serving as Red Cross and USO service workers, entertainers, journalists, and civilian medical personnel working with government agencies. Most military women who served were nurses, but some worked in communications, intelligence, supply, security, and clerical positions. Since my own personal and professional experience has been primarily with nurses, this chapter will focus on their problems while recognizing that other professional groups will have both similar and different clinical issues.

Until recently, women Viet Nam veterans were largely ignored by researchers. The only completed piece of research addressing women is Jenny Schnaier's study in 1982 entitled: "Women Vietnam Veterans and Mental Health Adjustment: A Study of Their Experiences and Post-Traumatic Stress" (1). This descriptive study examined problems of 87 self-selected women who served in military medical positions in Viet Nam. Although limited, her study offers us some interesting information about this population, and will be referred to throughout this chapter.

Because of the dearth of research material, this chapter will be based on my own personal and professional experiences. I was an emergency room and intensive care nurse in Viet Nam for 12 months, and as a psychiatric nurse clinician I have recently cofacilitated a 16-week therapy group for women Viet Nam veterans. I have also worked individually with several women veterans who have come forward.

WAR EXPERIENCE

Wilson has indicated that exposure to injury and death is one of the best predictors for post-traumatic stress disorder (2). Women in Viet Nam were certainly not spared this exposure. Hospitals were frequently the target of mortar and rocket attacks, as were planes and helicopters carrying nurses and other personnel. As in any guerilla war, we began to see anyone outside "the compound" as a potential threat and enemy, and hence developed an attitude of hyperalertness, suspicion, and distrust. Nurses were not assigned weapons, but some relate stories of having to use weapons in times of emergency. One nurse in our therapy group was finally able to talk about the time she used a machine gun on three Vietcong who were attempting to infiltrate her hospital.

Nurses worked a minimum of 12 hours a day, six days a week, under grueling medical conditions, often experiencing emotional and physical exhaustion. Large numbers of casualties could be brought to field hospitals within minutes of injury, and often their injuries were especially massive and mutilating. It was common to receive soldiers and other casualties with multiple traumatic amputations, total body burns, disfiguring head and facial wounds, and open chests and abdomens. Sometimes these casualties were friends, relatives, or coworkers of medical personnel.

Compounding the horror of the injuries was the fact that many of the nurses were young (often in the same age range as their patients), inexperienced, and ill-prepared in terms of the medical skills demanded of them. I remember my first night in the emergency room, being expected to insert intravenous lines in new casualties. Not only had I never started an intravenous line before, but I was confronted with boys who had no arms or legs to receive them.

The nature of war necessitates dealing with difficult emotional and ethical issues. Because of lack of personnel, facilities, and time, nurses were forced to practice triaging in the emergency room. Several times we had to put young men behind a curtained partition where they were left to die while we worked on those we believed we could save. We nurses were often the ones who had to tell patients that they had permanently lost limbs or vision. Due to shortages of supplies, we frequently had to decide which patient was going to get the last respirator, antibiotic, or pain medication. We cared for wounded Americans, mutilated children and adult civilians, and wounded prisoners of war. The latter were often patients on the same wards as Americans they had wounded. We often struggled for days or weeks to keep patients alive, only to lose them to massive infection or respiratory failure. The author of the following passage committed suicide several years after working as a nurse with wounded soldiers in a military hospital in Japan.

> How could I forget you? The faces you had and the faces you didn't have. Some of you came back so many times to haunt me with your faces blown off. For some of you there was so little we could do. . . . The despair and hopelessness I felt. . . . I remember changing your dressings and the roaches that came crawling out of the wounds of your stumps. The roaches that were eating you alive and you didn't know it. They were difficult days for me too. I remember your screams when they had to amputate your legs. I had compassion for you and cared about your recovery. I held your hand then, too. I cleaned the blood up in the operating room and then had to carry your amputated leg to the laboratory and prepare the room for the next case, all day and sometimes all night. There were so many of you. . . . (3)

Transitory relationships were another problem of Viet Nam. In-country transfers and staggered tours of duty meant short but often intense relationships with colleagues. Since most severely wounded men were evacuated quickly to Japan or the Philippines, medical personnel rarely knew what happened to patients they had helped to stabilize. This was particularly difficult for operating room personnel who rarely saw their patients conscious. Many women also had romantic encounters during the war, only to have the lover killed in action or discharged home to his wife and family.

For obvious reasons, women were in constant demand in Viet Nam, both socially and sexually. This was a source of conflict for some women, especially those who lacked adequate social or assertiveness skills. Some women had their first heterosexual or homosexual experience in Viet Nam. A war environment, with its danger and fear, fosters highly charged, intense, significant sexual and romantic encounters, which may negatively influence subsequent sexual expression. Additionally, some women engaged in what some may judge as "promiscuous" sexual behavior in order to be accepted and acknowledged in a predominantly male environment. Other women—especially those of enlisted rank—report having experienced sexual harassment, assault, or both.

The trauma of the abrupt transition from war zone to home was just as severe for female veterans as male veterans. Women tended to encounter even greater hostility and indifference from those at home than male veterans, since the concept of women participating in war violates sacred mythology concerning a woman's role. Women report that they were seen at home in stereotypic images of army women: prostitutes or lesbians. Professionally, their medical experience was discounted by civilian employers. After making life and death decisions for a full year, they now had to get a physician's order to give an aspirin to a patient. Today, many in our society still do not realize that women played an integral and indispensable role in the war; as a result, the woman veteran finds herself burying her war experience and discarding her identity as a competent, experienced veteran.

CLINICAL ISSUES

In my experience the most apparent clinical problems of women veterans are denial of their pain and difficulty in asking for help. I have spoken with several veterans who denied having any problems with Viet Nam, while their body language clearly indicated otherwise. The painful feelings engendered by the war experience had to be so vigorously suppressed during their tour of duty and for years afterwards that many women have effectively convinced themselves that their lives have been unaffected by the war. Nurses in general are notorious for seeing themselves as caregivers and nurturers who can take care of themselves without help. There is also the sometimes realistic fear that an admission of problems may jeopardize their jobs or professional reputations.

Although almost one-half of the 87 respondents in Schnaier's study had sought professional help for a mental health problem, less than one-half of those ever discussed in counseling their experiences in Viet Nam (1). Just as society discounted these women's Viet Nam experiences, so did many of these veterans themselves.

Many women veterans talk about how they have built walls to protect themselves from the pain of dealing on a daily basis with horror, suffering, and death. In Viet Nam, there was the fear that an unstifled cry would become a scream that would never stop. The military nurse's role demanded emotional control and constant attention to the patient, with no provisions for processing her experience. Pain went unexpressed, and energy became focused on professional tasks. For some, pain was numbed with drugs, alcohol, frenetic activity, and sleep.

Unfortunately, these coping patterns tend to continue in civilian life, with some women trying to recreate the intensity and drama of Viet Nam by working in intensive care and burn units or emergency rooms. Others engage in thrill-seeking, dangerous activities in their personal lives. Still others leave the medical profession altogether. Several women have mentioned continuing drug abuse problems, but in this area, too, we have no solid data.

Women will often seek help initially because of depression, nightmares, insomnia, or flashbacks precipitated by sounds (helicopters, fireworks) or smells. Once in group or individual therapy, they tend to focus on their anger toward the military, the Veterans Administration, the Vietnamese, and those in society who "don't understand": they complain bitterly about these institutions and individuals. They speak of inappropriate outbursts of anger and rage in their personal lives and in general demonstrate a low frustration tolerance.

Women talk about their self-imposed isolation—their belief that their experiences and feelings will not be validated by spouses, family, friends, or society. I have worked with women veterans who are married to Viet Nam veterans, and Viet Nam is often a forbidden topic in their homes. Some women veterans choose isolation because closeness always entails a potential loss. Most importantly, to allow intimacy would mean contacting and experiencing the pain they so diligently deny and defend against.

Shame is an issue that usually arises with women once they are willing to share their stories. Many experienced a painful shattering of an ideal self-image when they discovered that they were capable of violence, of participating in the torture of prisoners, of withholding pain medication, and of being cold and distant in a profession that is the epitome of care and warmth. I personally had to deal with the knowledge that I was not heroic in all situations—that consideration for my patients' welfare did not always come before my own. Finally, many had to live with the responsibility for our frequent life and death decisions.

I believe one of the most critical issues facing women veterans is the apparent meaninglessness of the entire war experience. Many went over very idealistically, with strong beliefs in God, in their country, and in their own purpose: to heal and comfort. Illusions were quickly stripped away as they found themselves participating in a meaningless "theatre of the absurd," where they healed boys in order to send them back to be killed; where they "saved" men from death so that they could live out their lives without arms, legs, penises, spinal cords, and faces; where they were confronted with the potential of their own meaningless deaths; and where there seemed to be no purpose to the wanton waste and destruction, brutality and horror. Their God appeared to have abandoned the scene, and their moral structures often crumbled.

All of these issues were raised by the respondents in Schnaier's study (1). She found that at least 25 percent of the women in her study recognized such feelings as anger, self-consciousness as a Viet Nam veteran, and a sense of meaninglessness in their lives, occurring 10 to 30 times a month. When asking about symptoms during the previous six months, Schnaier found that 27.6 percent reported having suicidal thoughts, 19.5 percent reported feeling alienated from other people, and 19.2 percent reported feeling depressed.

CLINICAL INTERVENTION

As with all Viet Nam veterans, the primary goal in intervention should be the establishment of an intimate relationship between the veteran, the therapist, and—in group therapy—the other group members. Through this method, the veteran can discover the patterns in her life that are keeping her from being fully alive physically, spiritually, and emotionally. Ultimately, the veteran should be able to integrate her Viet Nam experience and find increased enjoyment and meaning in her life.

The therapeutic process is not one of strategies and manipulations, but one of complete engagement with the client in a dialogue characterized by mutual vulnerability and sharing of the self. For this intimacy to occur, it is imperative that clinicians working with women veterans know and understand their own personal characteristics that might result in distancing themselves from their clients. These characteristics include biases and mistaken beliefs about the Viet Nam War, about women, and especially about women who serve in the military.

I want to briefly address the issue of group therapy. An all-women veteran support group is an attractive and safe prospect for many women and may result in more women coming for help. The reality, however, is that there are usually insufficient numbers of women Viet Nam veterans in some areas to make this type of group possible. I see no problem with women being included in male veteran groups, as long as their own particular needs are addressed and they are prevented from taking over the role of nurturing caretaker in the group. I would like to see someone explore group work with medical professionals who are Viet Nam veterans, since medics, physicians, and nurses all share many similar experiences.

Both Schnaier and I have found that women veterans will often seek counseling without disclosing their Viet Nam or military experience. This reflects either denial of its importance or fear of disapproval. Any intake interview with a woman of appropriate age should include the question, "Have you had any military experience?" If the answer is yes, a detailed military history should be taken, and the client should be encouraged to explore the meaning of that experience.

Our women's group found that books by and about women in Viet Nam can be a powerful and effective catalyst for getting women to share their experiences. Several women found that giving such a book to friends and relatives was a nonthreatening first step in sharing their own stories and a means of testing the other's acceptance and willingness to listen. Those interested in working with women veterans should read *Forever Sad the Heart* by Joan Walsh (4) and *Home Before Morning* by Linda Van DeVanter (5). The use of these books as tools to establish a common ground of knowledge with women veterans or among members of a therapy group, and to establish an atmosphere of acceptance and safety, is highly recommended. This technique is especially important if the therapist is not a veteran. Asking a woman to bring in photographs, slides, or other mementos of her war experience is also useful in helping her to share her story.

Feelings blocked and suppressed during the war experience need to be reexperienced and expressed in order to free one's energy for living more fully and deeply. In our group we discovered that veteran nurses had much unfinished business with their patients in Viet Nam, with whom they were not willing or able to share their feelings of grief, sadness, anger, or caring. They can start to achieve resolution by using the gestalt "empty chair" technique or by having male veterans who were patients in field hospitals attend a group session for mutual sharing.

"He made love and I made jokes." The ending of the poem that introduced this chapter is a poignant statement of the problems some women veterans have experienced with emotional and sexual intimacy. These problems often center around fears of emotional and sexual vulnerability and surrender, which may lead these veterans to maintain emotional distance in their personal relationships. Romantic and sexual encounters were both readily available and intense for women in Viet Nam, and it is imperative that the clinician obtain, in a nonjudgmental manner, a thorough sexual history that encompasses time periods before, during, and after the war. Women veterans should be encouraged to explore the meaning of their sexual experiences in Viet Nam. The exploration of the veteran's relationships with both men and women during the war may lead to greater understanding of current difficulties with intimacy.

As I mentioned earlier, many women will focus on their anger and bitterness toward society and government institutions. It is an easy trap to support the woman veteran's self-assessment as yet another victim of an ugly war and an insensitive government, especially if the clinician has negative feelings about the Viet Nam War. Politicizing anger is often an effective means of avoiding the underlying pain, fear, and despair. The clinician's focus should be that of facilitating the veteran's taking responsibility for her actions and feelings, staying with her anger long enough to encounter her fear and pain, and ultimately recognizing that the real issue is not society's forgiveness and acceptance, but the need to accept and forgive oneself.

When the client is willing to accept responsibility for her actions in the war, she must acknowledge her "dark side" and her possible betrayal of her personal value system. This often results in an intense feeling of shame and exposure and is unfortunately often quickly followed by self-condemnation, self-hatred, and guilt. This judgmental stance, in which one condemns oneself to punishment and remorse, results in a psychological process of contraction and withdrawal. Shame, however, can be a valuable experience in that it offers increased access to the self, with the possibility of greater self-knowledge and the freedom to make changes.

With shame one is vulnerable and open; in the sharing of one's shame with another there is the possibility of greater intimacy. Self-knowledge and insight thus gained allow one to reevaluate, choose, and create new personal standards and values.

Schnaier found that some women reported positive, growth-producing aspects of their war experiences. Areas of growth include a shift of priorities, increased self-awareness, and an increased sense of strength (1). I have found that the anguish that comes from knowing about tragedy, suffering, nonbeing, and meaninglessness can be transformed into a source of strength, purpose, and meaning. Meaning can be found by engaging actively in life and by making commitments to action and to the expression of one's self and one's creativity. This process begins with the veteran's experience of engagement and intimacy in the relationship with her therapist.

The veteran must first be willing to descend to the depths of her pain and despair and experience it fully, without judgment. Healing begins with the intimate sharing of this pain with someone who will acknowledge its reality and validity. The task of the therapist is to accompany the veteran on this journey and to discover, experience, and share his or her own pain in the process.

The therapist can then help the veteran discover that pain and sorrow can be a source of compassion, understanding, and empathy; that the veteran's knowledge of dehumanization and objectification can be the impetus to reject violence and depersonalization and to live fully in the awareness of one's connectedness to others. This understanding can ultimately enable the veteran to say *yes* to life, to go forth with courage and self-respect, and to accept herself in spite of knowledge of the "dark side" of human existence.

Finally, I want to emphasize the urgent need for further research on the issues confronting women veterans, especially because more and more women are involving themselves in the military as a career. We need information on how women experience, cope with, and react to war in ways different from men. Carol Gilligan has done fascinating research on female moral development and how it differs from the male experience (6). I would like to see her research taken a step further; the moral issues confronting male and female participants in a war situation must be studied. This will help in the management of professional stress and burn-out in future situations in which medical personnel, both men and women, confront unusual tragedy, suffering, and death.

REFERENCES

1. Schnaier JA: Women Viet Nam veterans and mental health adjustment: a study of their experiences and post traumatic stress. Master's thesis submitted at the University of Maryland, 1982

2. Wilson JP, Krauss GE: Predicting post traumatic stress syndromes among Viet Nam veterans. Paper presented at the 25th Neuropsychiatric Institute. Coatesville, Pa, VA Medical Center, 1982

3. Marron J: A woman veteran speaks. The Veteran November-December, 1982

4. Walsh P: Forever Sad the Heart. New York, Avon Books, 1982

5. Van DeVanter L: Home Before Morning. New York, Beaufort Books, 1983

6. Gilligan C: In a Different Voice: Psychological Theory and Women's Development. Cambridge, Mass, Harvard University Press, 1982

16

Viet Nam Veterans On Active Duty: Adjustment in a Supportive Environment

Harry C. Holloway, M.D.
Robert J. Ursano, M.D.

16

Shatan suggested that Special Forces troops who served in Viet Nam should be afforded the opportunity to be "rehumanized" (1). This suggestion indicates how far the reification of the concept "dehumanized" has progressed and how ideologically vigorous the discussion of Viet Nam veterans has become. For a few citizens, Viet Nam veterans are heroes who served out of an unambiguous sense of duty to their country. For others the important symbolic figure of the Viet Nam era is the antihero who steps forward to confess his guilt as a misled perpetrator of an atrocity. It seems likely that service people and veterans (even those who served in the Special Forces) are human and not inherently in need of rehumanization or treatment. It is the task of psychiatrists to use their humanistic and scientific capacities to understand how this war has impacted upon their patients.

In this chapter we focus on how the experience of war may become a powerful metaphor and organizing symbol in the communications of Viet Nam veterans. As a metaphor, these experiences tie together a foreground and a background meaning, a present and a past. This unique conjunction establishes a symbolic vehicle that is unique to the individual and that is influenced and constructed from his or her psychosocial matrix. The importance of current life events to the elicitation of this symbol and the psychological state it communicates is emphasized. Since the significance of a metaphor to an individual is determined by internalized cultural symbols and the unique life experiences of the individual, it states the obvious to emphasize that one must elicit a detailed report from the person who experienced a severe trauma (like battle) of the historical context in which the trauma was

The opinions expressed in this paper are those of the authors and do not necessarily represent the conclusions or opinions of the Department of Defense or the Uniformed Services University of the Health Sciences.

embedded, the traumatic events of the current life experiences, and of how the significance of traumatic events has changed over time. The psychosocial context of the veteran is critical to understanding the twin phenomena of psychosocial growth and symptom formation which may be the consequences of such severe trauma. For these reasons, the active duty veteran may demonstrate a very different recall of the significance of combat experiences from the non-active-duty veteran, and in both this recall can be seen to change with time. As humans who have experienced acculturation to the military and have been caught up in the Viet Nam War, Viet Nam veterans have experienced potentially moving, painful, poignant, boring, terrifying, loving, and rewarding events in a complex, ever changing era. As interacting beings they have undoubtedly been affected by this. The study of the active duty veteran provides the opportunity to assess the developmental impact of an especially supportive social system on the life of Viet Nam veterans.

THE NATURE OF WAR AND WAR EXPERIENCES

A few introductory comments on the nature of war itself are in order. Wars are, by their nature, complex events. Wars that are fought without achieving the most fragile of group phenomena—an enduring national consensus—are particularly difficult to characterize in one pithy phrase. Frequently such pithy characterizations may disguise the ambiguous nature of the war. Veterans who served in Viet Nam at various times during the war may recall and reexperience the war differently. This recall may be influenced by the nature of psychosocial supports provided in Viet Nam and at home, by the veterans' understanding of the expected outcome of their combat efforts, and by how the veterans' expectations were reinforced or destroyed upon return after their one-year tour in Viet Nam. In addition, the capacity to organize the emotional and cognitive experience of the trauma of combat in the immediate postcombat period is influenced by the individual's use of psychoactive substances. The use of antinauseants and potent antipsychotic agents like prochlorperazine (Compazine®) and chlorpromazine (Thorazine®) during combat may impair the capacity to integrate emotional experiences. These medications were commonly used for symptom control in combat troops with diarrhea and nausea. For some, the use of alcohol, marijuana, opioids, and other psychotropic agents for entertainment and anxiety relief was also a part of the Viet Nam experience.

War and military service as life experiences also confer important advantages or disadvantages unrelated to battle experiences per se (2). There may be social or employment advantages secondary to the acquisition of a skill in the military; there may be disadvantages, owing to the loss of an employment opportunity because an individual was removed from the civilian work force at a critical time. A new soldier is generally a young person, usually in late adolescence or early adulthood. His or her separation from home and living in a foreign culture may itself constitute an important and sometimes decisive developmental event. The individual veteran's experience must, therefore, be viewed as cognitively complex.

Some time ago, S. L. A. Marshall (3) noted that the experience of battle is muddled and its recall rapidly modified—only immediate debriefing of the entire surviving combat group (in those situations where there were sufficient survivors) could provide a reasonably detailed, accurate representation of what had happened. The psychological and neuropsychophysiologic demands of the combat situation are extreme (4). Accurate, comprehensive accounts are unattainable unless special effort is made to achieve them. As Marshall has documented, given the fragmentary experiences that an individual has of a battlefield and the constant changing of states of consciousness and arousal in very stressful environments, the combat veteran has no opportunity to register a clear mental record of what he did or how his action related to the behavior of significant others (buddies) during the combat. This problem of the recall of life events is not unique to combat (5).

The following clinical example shows how recall is influenced by the chaos of traumatic experience and how information available after the event may affect the psychological significance of its recall.

A bombardier parachuted from a burning plane during World War II. He reports not knowing whether he pulled a lever that released the hatch that would allow one of the gunners to exit the burning aircraft or whether he destroyed the secret equipment in his possession. The rush of events that accompanied the exiting of the aircraft were characterized by overwhelming arousal, terror, and action. In this situation the bombardier continued to recall events with guilt until it was confirmed months later (at the war's end) that he had saved his fellow crew member. With the information that he had thrown the right switches, his evaluation of himself and his performance changed.

Thus, cognitive experience of and affectual value assigned to battle or disaster can be based on the context provided after the event. Spontaneous recall is subject to "symbolic reorganization" so that experiential and symbolically relevant statements become intertwined with language reporting fragments of real events. Further, the recall of events is likely to vary with life circumstances, group membership, political commitments, and maturation. Recall will be overdetermined by the antecedent history of the veteran, his or her psychobiological endowments (character structure), current life events, and his or her view of the future. The kind of symbolic reorganization that Weinstein et al. (6) have described in brain injury, and disordered and overloaded peripheral nervous system input, appears to also go on in the context of battle.

The impact of the combat community on the individual veteran is frequently overlooked. Tischler (7) has described the development of a hedonistic pseudocommunity in Viet Nam. In this pseudocommunity sexual license, drunkenness, and drug use were sanctioned by groups of peers who found permission to ignore moral restriction in their separation from home and the symbolic (and sometimes real) threat of death provided by war. In this shabby world of earthly delight provided by the deployed army in combat, life presents the young person with experiences (enjoyable and frightening) of illicit sex, venereal disease, and drug abuse. Conscious and unconscious ambivalence about these experiences are the rule. Drug abuse and arrest can threaten personal integrity or become the basis of personal bonds between people trying to work out their collective and individual fate in a strange and lonely world. The conflict between inhibitions and desires can occasion the development of psychiatric symptoms and behavioral problems.

The rapid movement of young soldiers from unit to unit, and frequent changes of command secondary to short tours as commander, characterized military service during the 1960s and 1970s. During this period after 1969, the rapid withdrawal of troops produced rapid turnover within units and marked personnel turbulence. This turbulence disrupted the social support function of the unit and constituted a significant stress itself (8, 9). The new soldier in the military moved from basic training to advanced individual training, to a brief garrison assignment, and then to a tour with a combat unit where he might be rapidly promoted to noncommissioned officer rank, and then be returned to a small town in the Midwest as the lone veteran—all within the space of 24 months. The capacity of the individual soldier to develop meaningful mutual support and commitment within his unit was put to a severe test in this setting. The rapidly shifting demands of the changing social system may occasion intrapsychic conflicts as well as conflicts that arise from competing group loyalties.

What of the influence of the home front on the capacity of service personnel and prospective veterans to achieve an integrated experience of their military and combat service? Their expectations and idealization of significant others and the consequent effects of the social support or nonsupport provided by these others may decisively influence the opportunity of these individuals to remain symptom-free. Changes in support for the war in the United States and major shifts in U.S. policy may influence these individuals' experience of support or lack of it upon return home. The ways in which the larger social group and significant others articulate their expectations of returning veterans have important effects on the roles, behaviors, and supports available to veterans as well as on their recall of the military experience.

For example, the anticipation that veterans will be violence prone or "junkies" influences not only how a veteran may view himself, but also concretely influences the kind of job opportunities made available to him. To date, studies of nonpsychotic individuals suggest that an increased propensity to violence does not result as a consequence of war per se (10). Nonetheless, the question continues to persist resulting in a stigmatization of veterans as potentially violence prone. This view of veterans is not unique to Viet Nam era veterans; however, it influences the consequences of the war for those who served during it by defining a particular image and social role for these veterans.

Finally, in considering the relationship of combat to postcombat psychosocial problems and illness, Ewalt (11) reported that Viet Nam combat veterans had a much higher incidence of problems than did Viet Nam era veterans who had not seen combat. Similar observations have been made by Card (2). In the final version of the Veterans Administration's report, this effect of combat was not statistically significant in those who served in Viet Nam before 1968, although much heavy combat was present during this time (12). Possibly the problems suffered as a result of exposure to combat after 1968 were increased because of the disruption of unit integrity that accompanied the final phases of the war, or perhaps they increased because of the poor reception that veterans received when returning to the civilian community. Veterans who remained in the service may have been far less susceptible to these effects.

ACTIVE DUTY VIET NAM VETERANS

Studies of the adaptation of Viet Nam veterans who remained in military service provide a look at a select population of Viet Nam veterans pursuing careers in a social milieu which highly values service in Viet Nam. The military services have been concerned for some time about the consequences of service in Viet Nam for subsequent life adjustment both in and out of the military. Populations studied have included enlisted personnel (13–15), drug users, prisoners of war, and others (2, 11, 14–21). The literature from studies of veterans of other wars has already established the probable validity of chronic post-traumatic stress syndrome or some manner of persistent, recurrent, or delayed psychophysiological and psychological symptoms in those exposed to combat (22–27). This literature also suggests that, given a chance, most people who have been exposed to the extreme rigors of war and battle will adjust adequately (28, 29). It is not clear what conditions provide the context for the recurrence and maintenance of post-traumatic symptoms: the predisposing psychobiologic attributes, the antecedent life history, the amount of stress provided by the traumatic event and its circumstances, the effectiveness of social supports provided at the time of or after the traumatic event, or the current psychosocial conditions. Certainly all of these factors must play some part.

Studies of Viet Nam veterans still on active duty have demonstrated various impacts of Viet Nam. One of the first reports to note changes in returnees was by Strange and Brown (30). Borus' study (31) carried out in 1970 and 1971 was the first to prospectively examine the consequences for soldiers of return from Viet Nam. He found that soldiers assigned to a garrison post had the same rather high level (approximately one in five) of disciplinary and mental health problems, whether they had served in Viet Nam or not. The active duty veterans reported experiencing the loss of the closeness and group support which their combat unit in Viet Nam had provided. They had confidence in their leadership in Viet Nam, but no such confidence in their leadership in the United States. Both blacks and whites commented unfavorably on the loss of the opportunity to associate with members of the other race as "buddies." The veterans felt heavily put upon by the "spit and polish" philosophy of the garrison post. Several authors reported that many veterans experienced troubles or were troubled by the process of establishing relationships with loved ones (31, 32). These included problems that related to the idealized image of the loved one which had built up during separation, the wish of the wife to retain an independent status, and the difficulties in communicating to others about Viet Nam experiences. Thus, although Borus' work failed to document any statistically increased risk to psychosocial adaptation due to Viet Nam service, he did document a number of substantial issues related to the transition from combat to garrison duty. He felt that the problems were concentrated in the group of soldiers who lacked the capacity to manipulate the social hierarchy of the U.S. Army.

Shortly after the Borus study another group of Viet Nam returnees was studied by Ingraham (33). This interview study of heroin users documented the fragmentation of units in Viet Nam into groups of "heads and juicers" and "lifers and heads." The ideologies of drug use and race were having an impact on the nature of group support and on intraunit cohesion. The era of fragging, avoidance of battle, and increased disciplinary problems was at hand (34). This was, of course, the era during which My Lai was a major issue, the "heroin epidemic" was at its peak, and withdrawal from Viet Nam was in process. The motto of the troops was, "Don't be the last one killed."

Follow-up work by Ingraham and the work of others tend to indicate that the "heads and juicers," upon returning to the unit in the United States, merged into barracks and military work groups that mirrored the sort of social organization that was traditional in the peace time military. In a 1974 five-year study of social networks, Newby (35) examined the organization of a barracks work group in a U.S. Army garrison post. In that report, one member of the group was called "Bierman." A noncombat soldier, "Bierman" became addicted to heroin in Viet Nam but was not detected. Upon return to the United States, he kicked the heroin habit and began to consume a large quantity of beer—24 to 28 cans per day. He ended each day in an alcoholic coma and yet each morning was at work. "Bierman" had simply reintegrated himself into the routine endemic patterns of alcohol and illicit drug use found in soldiers living in the barracks. It should be noted that the drug use in Viet Nam was a part of the worldwide problem of drug abuse in the U.S. military services; Viet Nam was not its cause as some might think. In fact, none of the internal studies of drug abuse done within the U.S. Army has established Viet Nam service as a significant risk factor for drug and alcohol abuse.

Most of the early follow-up studies of veterans drew their sample from the final era of the Viet Nam War. These studies were frequently motivated by a desire to study drug abuse. Thus, Helzer et al. found evidence of increased depressive symptoms on follow-up at two years (18), only to find that the depressed symptoms had disappeared when reevaluated on further followup (19). The news from a larger study by Robins (21) was that there was a relatively low rate of continued heroin addiction in Viet Nam users after return home. The rate of alcoholism and other psychosocial disability on follow-up was a continuing matter of concern. Nace et al. (20) in Philadelphia found a high incidence of depressive symptoms and alcoholism in their follow-up group. Comparable samples of Viet Nam veterans have not been studied within the military.

A review by Figley of the various studies of the Viet Nam veteran noted that 1) the adjustment of veterans was related to pre- and postservice factors and 2) that the adjustment of Viet Nam veterans was the same as other veterans as long as combat was not controlled for (36). The experience of combat per se had a critical impact on adjustment outcome. As far as it goes, this summary is most helpful. However, it fails to note that these studies failed to control for the social stress of the veteran at the time of follow-up and failed to consider the time when the service in Viet Nam occurred.

Panzarella et al. (37) found that their Viet Nam and non–Viet Nam sample of U.S. Army personnel in Germany in 1973 were equally symptomatic. This may reflect their use of a population selected from a military treatment clinic, a group already maximally stressed by difficulties in their current social-military setting. The social setting of both groups in the Panzarella study (and the earlier Borus study) were, therefore, characterized by marked personnel turbulence. The European Army in 1973 was in a very distressing situation as the draft ended and an all-volunteer Army began. It is quite possible that the lack of statistically significant effects attributable to Viet Nam service was due to the very stressful intraservice environment, causing both groups to look equally disturbed. The acute stress of these environments may have swamped any effects due to the Viet Nam experience.

One special group of Viet Nam veterans that has been followed since the end of the conflict are former prisoners of war (POWs). In general, the most impressive finding concerning these individuals has been their successful readaptation. Nonetheless, work with U.S. Air Force POWs has documented that the most stressed group of POWs (those imprisoned before 1970), who were exposed to the most torture, the poorest treatment, and the longest imprisonment, did show more adaptational problems and more marked indicators of psychopathology on the MMPI (16). In addition, it is clear that the impact of the severe stress of the POW experience may be perceived as benefitting the individual (17), and in some cases appears to help an individual to organize his life goals more effectively than prior to his POW experience. Studies indicate the absence of a clear relationship between psychopathology prior to imprisonment and problems after imprisonment (15). The data on U.S. Air Force POWs illustrate that severe stress has long-term impacts, that—in this highly selected population—the majority have coped successfully with their POW experience, and that some may have used their POW experience in a way that has facilitated personal psychological growth.

A questionnaire study carried out by Stretch (38) at the Walter Reed Army Institute of Research examined the prevalence of PTSD symptoms in Viet Nam veterans who were currently on active duty (N =

238; response rate, 53 percent), members of the reserve ($N = 667$; response rate, 73 percent), and civilians ($N = 499$; response rate, 50 percent). In addition, the prevalence of PTSD was examined for these active duty military, reservists, and civilians. For chronic and delayed PTSD, the active duty sample reported 5.1 percent, reservists reported 10.9 percent, and civilian Viet Nam veterans reported 32 percent. The reported prevalence was significantly higher in the civilian veterans than in the other two groups, which did not differ significantly from each other. Civilian veterans reported significantly more intense combat histories and poorer social supports during the first year back from Viet Nam. In the overall population and in the subpopulations, these two variables predicted most of the assessed variance in the rate of delayed and chronic PTSD (17 percent for the intensity of combat and 12 percent for the social support during the first year back). It should be noted that there may be sources of bias in this study: for example, the civilian veterans reported an average of seven years of active duty, while other data indicate that average active duty time for most veterans was much briefer. Given the important populations studied in this programmatic research, this work raises a number of methodological, conceptual, and epidemiological issues pertinent to understanding the multifactorial causation and assessment of PTSD (38). Unfortunately, as further follow-up studies are done, the period since the initial Viet Nam tour becomes longer, and the possibility increases that intercurrent variables are confounding the results of the study.

Since the end of the Viet Nam deployment, mental health practitioners in the service have occasionally seen cases in which a traumatic Viet Nam experience played a role. No large number of cases, however, has been noted. The cases of chronic PTSD have generally been noted in association with other stressors, with requests for disability, the diagnosis of chronic alcoholism, and conditions in which PTSD provided an explanation for an otherwise difficult to explain set of symptoms. As the standards for diagnosis have become appreciated and more Viet Nam veterans are approaching retirement age, more cases of PTSD are being recognized.

THE VIET NAM EXPERIENCE AS METAPHOR

The occurrence of late onset PTSD requires close attention to the meaning—the metaphorical use—of the Viet Nam experience rather than an assumption of a simple causative relationship. In one rather dramatic case which illustrates the point, a mental health professional described his patient's recurrent reexperiencing of Viet Nam trauma. The veteran reported recurrent dissociative episodes during which he found himself acting the role of an assassin, "just as he had in Viet Nam." He was similarly bedeviled by dreams and intrusive thoughts about himself being a killer. This individual was stationed with a finance unit in Viet Nam, and his reported "reexperience of Viet Nam" could not be documented and, in fact, was extremely unlikely. However, these symptoms served to provide him with a heroic past as an explanation for his anxiety and reported dissociative episodes. His father was a highly decorated Marine, and the patient was trying to make up for his lack of heroic achievement by the creation of a combat role for himself. This man was discharged from service with a psychiatric disability after a work up in which his reported role in Viet Nam as "the killer" was not documented. The case illustrates that psychological factors having to do with failure to achieve certain fantasized goals may be responsible for the development of pseudo-PTSD. Failure to perceive the meaning of the complaints unfortunately resulted in reinforcement by the provision of secondary gain.

Recurrent "traumatic" memory may also offer a bridge in the present between ambivalent feelings of anxiety and hope. This is illustrated by another patient in his late 40s who had completed three tours in Viet Nam with the Special Forces. Following the diagnosis of metastatic adenocarcinoma and the institution of chemotherapy, he began to experience severe anxiety before treatments and during the episodes of nausea, retching, and vomiting that accompanied treatments. He became concerned about loss of control and feared that he would publicly display anxiety. He received chemotherapy on a Tuesday afternoon once a month. Anxiety attacks with nausea began to occur spontaneously in his office at 3:00 P.M. on Tuesdays. At night he began to have an old combat dream about an instance in which he was ambushed by three Vietnamese in the jungle. The dream had occurred occasionally over the years since the real incident. In the dream he was able to best them in hand-to-hand combat and survive. The dream and intrusive thoughts increased as symptoms from his chemotherapy increased, and his tumor, although stable, did not go away. His doctor requested some help in managing the stress symptoms. Attempts at using relaxation procedures were partially successful, but hypnotic imaging was of no help. An antianxiety, antinausea regimen of high doses of promethazine hydrochloride (Phenergan®) resulted in control of the acute symptoms during chemotherapy. Gradually, as the chemotherapy progressed, the patient's conditioned anxiety and nausea cleared. His dream became less frequent and was accompanied by a thought he had recalled following the real event: "This is a hell of a way for a lieutenant colonel to earn a living." This thought seemed both humorous and reassuring to the patient. He changed his job to realistically take his illness into account and supported his wife in the development of her career, "since she's going to need the support." In this case, traumatic recall symbolized both the patient's current dilemma and a way out of it. It did not prevent him from taking appropriate steps to respond to the likely foreshortening of life.

In fact, a number of Viet Nam veterans receiving cancer chemotherapy have reported the recurrence of combat dreams. In every veteran who has experienced intense combat, one of us (H.C.H.) has been able to elicit the history of such a dream. In situations in which the dream could be followed as an active part of a therapeutic intervention, the dream changed as the illness progressed or regressed, or as coping capacities and achievements changed. The dream seemed in most of these cases to be a rich, complex symbol which the patient used as a way of encapsulating currently stressful situations. At times it helped the patient in coping; at other times it was used as justification for excessive alcohol use.

The importance of the metaphorical use of the Viet Nam experience can also be seen in less dire stress situations. In a senior enlisted man who had served as a helicopter gunner, the onset of intrusive thoughts about combat, combat dreams, startle reactions, dissociative episodes, and sleep disturbance coincided with his wife's becoming pregnant for the first time, four years after Viet Nam. He was very ambivalent about this event and was envious and furious at the unborn child. His father had always treasured his son's wife. "It's the only good thing you've ever done," the father said at the time of the marriage. "Don't fuck it up." The symbolism matches the oedipal and performance anxiety frequently seen in patients in clinical practice. In this case, the Viet Nam experience was the metaphor for this new trauma, a metaphor which persisted for four years and abated only when the disturbance in the marital relationship was addressed.

No one will pass through combat, disasters, or conditions of imprisonment unchanged; the degree of change may vary from individual to individual, and within individuals over time. The symbolic recall of the traumatic event will contain elements, conscious and unconscious, that represent issues—past, present, and future—that are related to both primary and secondary gain. Like the dream, the psychological meaning of recalled trauma must be understood in terms of its context and associations. Recall is always a state-dependent phenomenon, whether that be recall of a specific event or the reconstruction of the past which occurs in psychoanalysis (6). The report of trauma is insufficient to an understanding of the symbolic meaning being carried by what may seem to be a factual recollection. As in all metaphors, there is both a vehicle and a cargo. The meaning of a metaphor is never one or the other but the unique combination of the hidden and the expressed (39). For late onset symptoms of PTSD, this means that both the described combat trauma and its present day meaning must be sought, understood, and interrelated.

CONCLUSION

The experience of war is a complex, confusing, varying biopsychosocial phenomenon. PTSD is well documented after traumas of all kinds, from rape and industrial accidents to natural disasters and wars. However, a glib assumption concerning the causal relationship between the trauma and the biopsychosocial result does not reflect our knowledge or understanding of the phenomenon. The veteran's reported experiences in Viet Nam are only one aspect of analysis.

In order to fully understand the impact of the Viet Nam War on veterans, a broad perspective is necessary. In this chapter we have emphasized the following factors:

1. The importance of understanding the social system, both macro (country, army, community, and unit) and micro (buddies, wives, family, and personal history). In its final phase, the Viet Nam War itself contributed markedly to the decreased cohesion and psychosocial support provided by the primary social group—the military. Clearly, the process of rapidly rotating commanding officers and the rotating of personnel into and out of battle decreased the capacity of people to withstand the trauma of combat and the socially stressful situations of overseas service in the military. The drug abuse epidemic and other social disorders of the final stages of Viet Nam clearly made the experience more difficult for individual veterans and society to integrate. Veterans who remained in the services are a special group. The organization of the military unit and career reinforce this specialness. The military clearly feels that service in Viet Nam is an advantage in qualification for advancement. Many problems related to the lack of social acceptance of Viet Nam service may be mitigated by continued service in the military. Understanding such social factors is important to understanding how war disadvantages people.

2. The importance of understanding the time course of events— both the time of Viet Nam service and the time of onset of symptoms. The Viet Nam War was in many ways several wars to its participants, depending on when the veteran was there. Late onset responses to the

Viet Nam experience should be distinguished from acute responses.

3. The importance of understanding the role of metaphor. In order to describe anxiety-producing events, regardless of their causal relations to Viet Nam, veterans select symbols which are appropriate to their individual experience and acceptable to the community and society in which they live. Remote recall of traumatic events springs from the entire dynamic structure created by active generative recall and current interactions with the human environment. The importance of our symbolizing function must be remembered in order to understand the recall of trauma.

Several preventive programs are suggested by these factors as being useful in helping soldiers develop coherent integrated accounts of their traumatic life experiences and military service:

1. People should be rotated into and out of combat areas in units that live, fight, and sometimes die together. The problem of replacements for casualties is difficult but not impossible.
2. Commanders and noncommissioned officers should not be frequently rotated. Again, casualties will create a problem.
3. Whenever possible, debriefing using Marshall's methods (3) should be instituted immediately after combat action for the instrumental reason of developing cognitively comprehensive accounts of what happened. The debrief can also accomplish some of the necessary psychological work of dealing cognitively with the trauma involved.
4. Psychiatric consultations should continue to occur as soon after the battle as possible.
5. The length of exposure to combat should be limited.
6. No one should ever assume that combat does not change participants. However, the direction of that change depends on what life experiences and societal response came before and after the battle, as well as what happened during it.

As time passes, it appears that active duty personnel are most likely to begin to manifest PTSD symptomatology during periods of transitions and life crises—that is, during periods when the supportive environment breaks down under a potentially deadly illness, the approach of retirement, or the disruption of important interpersonal relationships. The recall of combat trauma appears to epitomize for veterans a reexperiencing of overwhelming helplessness, of horror, or of unexpected success in a seemingly impossible situation. In fact, various aspects of the same combat experience may be used to express various of these aspects of symbolization. Providing veterans with a supportive environment may promote an integrated recall of trauma, its antecedent and consequent context, and its meaning within the current life situation. Such integration allows veterans to use experiences that have been haunting them to understand how they are adjusting in the world. Active duty veterans are often in such a supportive environment.

REFERENCES

1. Shatan C (ltr to ed): Veterans' problems. Psychiatric News, April 17, 1981
2. Card JJ: Lives After Viet Nam. Lexington, Mass, Lexington Books, 1983
3. Marshall SLA: Inland Victory. Washington, DC, U.S. Infantry Journal Press, 1944
4. Jenkins CD, Hurst MW, Rose RM: Life changes, do people really remember? Arch Gen Psychiatry 36:379–384, 1979
5. Novey S: The Second Look: The Reconstruction of Personal History in Psychiatry and Psychoanalysis. Baltimore, The Johns Hopkins Press, 1967
6. Weinstein E, Kahn RL: Symbolic reorganization in brain injury, in American Handbook of Psychiatry, 2nd ed, vol 1. Edited by Arieti S. New York, Basic Books, 1974
7. Tischler GL: Patterns of psychiatric attrition and behavior in a combat zone, in The Psychology and Physiology of Stress. Edited by Bourne PG. New York, Academic Press, 1969
8. Bey DR: Group dynamics and the 'F.N.G.' in Viet Nam: a potential focus of stress. Int J Group Psychother 22:22–30, 1972
9. Bey DR: Change of command in combat: locus of stress. Am J Psychiatry 129:698–702, 1972
10. Archer D, Garther R: Violent acts and violent times: a comparative approach to postwar homicide rates. Am Sociol Rev 41:937–964, 1976
11. Ewalt JR: What about the Viet Nam veteran? Milit Med 146:165–167, 1981
12. Egendorf A, Kadushin C, Laufer R, et al: Legacies of Viet Nam: Comparative Adjustment of Veterans and Their Peers. Washington, DC, U.S. Government Printing Office, 1981
13. Strayer R, Ellenhorn L: Viet Nam veterans: a study exploring adjustment patterns and attitudes. J Soc Issues 31:81–94, 1975
14. Hunter EJ: The Viet Nam POW veteran: immediate and long-term effects of captivity, in Stress Disorders Among Viet Nam Veterans. Edited by Figley CR. New York, Brunner/Mazel, 1978
15. Ursano RJ: The Viet Nam era prisoner of war: precaptivity, personality, and the development of psychiatric illness. Am J Psychiatry 138:315–318, 1981

16. Ursano RJ, Boydstun JA, Wheatley RD: Psychiatric illness in U.S. Air Force Viet Nam prisoners of war: a five-year follow-up. Am J Psychiatry 138:310–314, 1981

17. Sledge WH, Boydstun JA, Rabe AJ: Self concept changes related to war captivity. Arch Gen Psychiatry 37:430–443, 1980

18. Helzer JE, Robins LN, Davis DH: Depressive disorders in Viet Nam returnees. J Nerv Ment Dis 163:177–185, 1976

19. Helzer JE, Robins LN, Wish E, et al: Depression in Viet Nam veterans and civilian controls. Am J Psychiatry 136:526–529, 1979

20. Nace EP, Meyers AL, O'Brien CP, et al: Depression in veterans two years after Viet Nam. Am J Psychiatry 134:167–170, 1977

21. Robins LN: A Follow-Up of Viet Nam Drug Users. Social Action Office Monograph, Series A, No. 1. Washington, DC, U.S. Government Printing Office, 1973

22. Grinker RR, Spiegel JP: War neuroses in flying personnel overseas and after return to the USA. Am J Psychiatry 101:619–624, 1945

23. Futterman S, Pumpian-Mindlin E: Traumatic war neuroses five years later. Am J Psychiatry 108:401–408, 1951

24. Mayfield DG, Fowler DR: Combat plus twenty years: the effect of previous combat experience on psychiatry patients. Milit Med 134:1348–1354, 1969

25. Miller CW Jr: Delayed combat reactions in Air Force personnel. War Medicine 8:253–257, 1945

26. Lavie P, Hefetz A, Halperin G, et al: Long-term effects of traumatic war related events on sleep. Am J Psychiatry 136:175–178, 1979

27. Dobbs D, Wilson WP: Observations on persistence of war neurosis. Dis Nerv Syst 21:686–691, 1960

28. Brill NQ, Beebe GW: A Follow-Up Study of War Neuroses. V.A. Medical Monograph Series. Washington, DC, U.S. Government Printing Office, 1955

29. Singer MT: Viet Nam prisoners of war, stress and personal resiliency. Am J Psychiatry 138:345–346, 1981

30. Strange RE, Brown DE: Home from the war: a study of psychiatric problems in Viet Nam returnees. Am J Psychiatry 127:130–134, 1970

31. Borus JF: Incidence of maladjustment in Viet Nam returnees. Arch Gen Psychiatry 30:554–557, 1974

32. Bey DR, Lange J: Waiting wives: women under stress. Am J Psychiatry 131:283–286, 1974

33. Ingraham LH: 'The Nam' and 'the world.' Psychiatry 37:114–128, 1974

34. Lewy G: The American Experience in Viet Nam, in Combat Effectiveness: Cohesion, Stress, and the Volunteer Military. Beverly Hills, Calif, Sage Publications, 1980

35. Newby JH: Small group dynamics and drug abuse in an army setting: a case study. Int J Addict 12:287–300, 1977

36. Figley CR (ed): Psychological adjustments among Viet Nam veterans: an overview of the research, in Stress Disorders Among Viet Nam Veterans. New York, Brunner/Mazel, 1978

37. Panzarella RF, Mantell DM, Bridenbaugh RH: Psychiatric syndromes, self-concepts and Viet Nam veterans, in Stress Disorders Among Viet Nam Veterans. Edited by Figley CR. New York, Brunner/Mazel, 1978

38. Stretch RH: Post-traumatic stress disorder among Vietnam and Vietnam-era veterans. Unpublished manuscript. Washington, DC, Walter Reed Army Institute of Research, 1984

39. Richards IA: The Philosophy of Rhetoric. New York, Oxford University Press, 1965

17

Viet Nam Era Prisoners of War: Studies of U.S. Air Force Prisoners of War

Robert J. Ursano, M.D.

17

Prisoners of war (POWs) have been studied following all major conflicts with the expectation that severe trauma leads to a higher incidence of medical and psychiatric illness. Nearly 100,000 former U.S. POWs are presently living. Although long-term follow-up studies have produced a paucity of data, what data are available lead to the conclusion that the extraordinary stresses of war captivity are related to an increased vulnerability to physical and psychological illness (1–4). Beebe (2) reported high rates of psychiatric impairment for World War II and Korean War POWs. Keehn (3) documented long-term increases in morbidity and mortality for World War II (Pacific) and Korean War POWs. Investigators differ in their interpretation of the role of preexisting personality structure in the development of psychiatric illness following captivity (4–7).

In the survivors of concentration camp experiences, Eitinger (8) identified depression, anxiety, and a neurasthenic-like illness (the KZ syndrome), which he attributed to an organic brain syndrome secondary to extreme starvation. The concentration camp victims may, however, represent a unique level of psychic traumatization. Studies on World War II soldiers and Korean POWs have emphasized the development of an apathy syndrome (9, 10) following extreme stress. A similar process of "psychic numbing" has been noted following other trauma, such as those experienced by the survivors of Hiroshima (11), the Coconut Grove fire (12), and the Hungarian Revolution of 1956

The opinions expressed in this chapter are those of the author and do not necessarily reflect the opinions of the Uniformed Services University of the Health Sciences or the Department of Defense.

Much of the research on U.S. Air Force POWs referred to in this chapter was done in collaboration with Richard Wheatley, Ph.D.; James Boydstun, M.D.; William Sledge, M.D.; Alton Rahe, M.S.; and Erin Carlson, Ph.D. I thank Diane T. Ursano for her editorial assistance in the preparation of this chapter.

(13). Greenson's study of the apathy syndrome in World War II (10) focuses on the loss of hope and the experience of helplessness which culminates in the withdrawal of libido from external objects. Strassman et al. (9) identified a similar syndrome in Korean War POWs immediately after repatriation. They related the syndrome to the chronic repression of aggression and the adaptational demands of captivity. Studies of groups isolated in the Antarctic (14, 15) have suggested a similar personality style, introversion, as adaptive to that isolated, monotonous environment. Bundzen (16), in fact, has demonstrated an increase in introversion and neuroticism in individuals wintering over in the Antarctic, which he attributes to the interaction of personality and environment.

A total of 5,353 American fliers were downed over Southeast Asia from 1961 to 1973. Many were rescued, some died, and some became POWs. Capture, torture, and solitary confinement were the three most important stresses to face the group of POWs (17). In the prison camps of North Viet Nam prior to October 1969, solitary confinement for months to years, maltreatment, torture, deprivation, and complete separation from the outside world were the norm for incarcerated POWs. In July 1966, the POWs were threatened with punishment for war crimes. The Vietnamese used leg and wrist irons, ropes, and other forms of torture to try to obtain information. Injuries were manipulated and medical treatment was denied, as part of the torture process. Being "broken" by such torture was a traumatic, guilt-inducing experience for POWs, which was relieved only when a POW could make contact with a comrade and hear of a similar experience. Ingenious methods for communicating between POWs were developed. Many hours, days, or months of solitary confinement were coped with by reviewing one's personal history or constructing in fantasy a dreamed-of house, one brick at a time.

After 1969, conditions improved somewhat, with torture dropping off considerably. As a result of the Son Tay raid in November 1970, the POWs began to be placed in large groups. They developed an organized military command, learned of current events from new arrivals, and taught each other languages and mathematics. Concerns of the later arriving POWs centered on separation from family and loved ones rather than survival, torture, and their captors (18). The POWs began receiving more food, and in 1970 a list of POWs was released by the North Vietnamese.

By 1973, when the vast majority of the 766 American POWs were repatriated, some captured aircrew had spent up to eight years in North Vietnamese prisons. Of this group, 332 were U.S. Air Force (USAF) personnel, nearly all pilots and navigators. A total of 226 had been captured prior to 1969 and 106 after. In general, the USAF POW was in his early 30s at the time he was shot down. He was married, a pilot (75 percent) or navigator, and a First Lieutenant or Captain, and he spent from eight years to 40 days as a POW (mean, 4.3 years). Most USAF POWs were college educated; all had been screened for psychopathology and had demonstrated ability in coping with the stressful aspects of flight training and operations.

POST-STRESS ILLNESS: THE DEGREE OF STRESS, SOCIAL SUPPORTS, AND COPING STYLES

Upon repatriation in 1973, all USAF POWs underwent extensive psychiatric evaluation. A voluntary five-year follow-up program was maintained through the USAF School of Aerospace Medicine. Results of this follow-up were analyzed both in terms of psychiatric diagnoses and MMPI measurements (19, 20). The pre-1969 maximum stress group was compared to the post-1969 high but submaximum stress group. Overall, the most striking finding was how well most POWs did. However, although these two groups were very similar in socio-demographic variables, the pre-1969 group did show a greater frequency of psychiatric diagnosis and more abnormal deviations on MMPI scales. The MMPI profile for this group was generally more elevated than that of the post-1969 group and did not return to normal as rapidly as did that of the post-1969 group. Most psychiatric disturbances following repatriation were in the area of adjustment reactions (interpersonal, marital, and occupational).

Interestingly, rank, rating (pilot versus navigator versus gunner/observer), and education correlated with risk of psychiatric disturbance in the post-1969 group: individuals with lower rank and rating and less education were at higher risk. In contrast, no sociodemographic variables were significantly related to the presence of psychiatric disorders in the pre-1969 group. It would appear that under maximum stress, no social buffering role can be identified in the POW experience. In less dire circumstances, group cohesion and social integration as reflected by these sociodemographic variables may be an important protector from POW stress. The protective role of social supports in this population must, therefore, be considered a function of the degree of stress.

These results support the importance of the severity of stress rather than predisposing personality factors in the development of post-stress psychiatric disturbances. The USAF POW was a highly screened flyer who was free of psychiatric disease, educated, intelligent, successful, motivated, and patriotic. As a group, the POWs would thus be expected to have a reasonably uniform and low predisposition to developing psychiatric illness. Yet the pre-1969 group had more indicators of psychiatric disturbance than did the post-1969 group. It is important to remember that in order to determine whether the degree of stress relates to psychiatric disease, one would want exactly such a group—uniform and with little predisposition to disease.

Further studies of these repatriated POWs (RPWs) have compared coping strategies to the rate of psychiatric disease (R. Ursano, R. Wheatley, W. Sledge, A. Rahe, and E. Carlson, unpublished observations). Each RPW was classified in three categories: high resister/other resister, marginal coper/other coper, and benefitted/nonbenefitted. High resisters (HR) and other resisters (OR) were identified by having spent time in a punishment camp, over a year in solitary confinement, or time in solitary after 1969, or by having received one of the highest decorations at repatriation. All high resisters were in the pre-1969 group. Marginal copers (MC) and other copers (OC) were selected based on peer evaluations and lack of decorations. The third grouping was identified by Sledge et al. (18): those RPWs who thought they had benefitted (B) from their POW experience versus those who felt they had not been benefitted (NB). The first two groupings (HR/OR and MC/OC) describe coping styles used during the captivity experience. The last grouping (B/NB) is a description of how the experience was integrated into the RPW's life after repatriation. In general, neither of the coping styles (HR/OR or MC/OR) was related to the development of psychiatric illness after the POW experience. For the B/NB groups, there was also no firm evidence of a relationship to psychiatric disease. However, this grouping appears to be complexly related to the time since repatriation and the degree of stress experienced. This B/NB grouping may measure factors similar to studies on the role of denial after major stress such as myocardial infarction, where those with high levels of denial are initially at less risk for disease but later in time may be at increased risk.

The KZ (concentration camp) syndrome described by Danish investigators (8) was of particular concern in the evaluation of the RPWs. Eitinger felt that this syndrome was the result of long-term physical trauma. He required at least five of a possible 11 symptoms to make the diagnosis: increased fatigue, memory impairment, dysphoria, emotional instability, sleep disturbance, feelings of insufficiency, loss of drive, nervousness, vertigo, vegetative lability, and headache. Of Eitinger's sample, 85 percent were diagnosed as having KZ syndrome. The strongest correlation with the development of the KZ syndrome in concentration camp victims was serious physical disease (encephalitis, typhus, loss of greater than 30 percent of weight) during captivity. Thus, there is good reason to construe the KZ syndrome as a manifestation of an organic brain syndrome. Because of concerns about the KZ syndrome, Wheatley (21) carefully and specifically looked at neuropsychological function in USAF RPWs. He examined the WAIS, Haltstead-Reitan battery, Hooper visual organization test, and Benton visual retention test of representative samples of the pre- and post-1969 RPWs. Results indicated that the RPWs as a group were comparable to other operational USAF aircrew. Pre- and post-1969 groups also showed no significant differences. Thus, no evidence of the KZ syndrome was found.

THE ROLE OF PREDISPOSITION

In addressing the issue of personality change, Freud aptly warned:

> So long as we trace the development of a mental process backward, the connection appears continuous and we feel we have gained an insight which is completely satisfactory and even exhaustive. But if we proceed the reverse way, if we start from the premise inferred from the analysis and try to follow up the final result, then we no longer get the impression of an inevitable sequence of events, which could not have been otherwise determined. We notice at once that there might be another result, and that we might have been just as well able to understand and explain the latter. (22)

The issues of personality change in POWs and the role of predispositions to illness are caught in a similar bind. The retrospective construction of the precaptivity personality is prone to error and leads to a perception of the POWs' present personality as an "inevitable" outcome. Using retrospective data, Hunter (7) has shown a higher rate of preexisting psychiatric symptoms retrospectively diagnosed in Viet Nam era POWs. Koranyi (5, 23), in contrast, has suggested that the lack of preexisting pathology in POWs with a survivor syndrome requires a reevaluation of the psychiatric theory of adult neuroses. This disagreement on the role of adult trauma and preexisting personality in the production of illness has continued in more recent publications (24–26) and is clearly made more difficult by the use of retrospective data.

After 1973, a five-year voluntary medical and psychiatric follow-up was maintained for RPWs of the military services. These were performed at the U.S. Naval Center for Prisoner of War Studies and the USAF School of Aerospace Medicine. In order to investigate the role

Table 1. Precaptivity Psychiatric Assessment

Case No.	Marital Status[1]	Reason for Evaluation	Psychiatric Evaluation	Psychological Testing	Other
1	M	Special project volunteer	+	+[2]	...
2	M	Special project volunteer	+	+[2]	+
3	S	Special project volunteer	+	+[2]	...
4	S	Seizure secondary to alcohol withdrawal	+	+[3]	...
5	M	Dizziness—history of anxiety	+	+[4]	...
6	M	Psychophysiologic gastrointestinal reaction	+	+[5]	...

[1]M = married; S = single.

[2]Rorschach, TAT, Draw-A-Person, Bender, WAIS, Miller Analogies, Minnesota Engineering Analogies Test, Doppelt Mathematical Reasoning Test, Gordon Personal Profile, and Edwards Personal Preference Schedule.

[3]MMPI and Sentence Completion.

[4]Rorschach, TAT, Draw-A-Person, Bender, and WAIS.

[5]WAIS, MMPI, Babcock Paragraph Recall, Rotter Incomplete Sentence Test, Guilford Zimmerman Temperament Survey, Adjective Checklist, Rorschach, and TAT.

of the pretrauma personality in the POW experience, a small number of cases with precaptivity psychiatric evaluations were examined. Of the individuals who were POWs, 12 had been coincidentally seen at the USAF School of Aerospace Medicine prior to being shot down. Of these 12, eight had had a psychiatric evaluation. For two of this group of eight, sufficient data were not available to warrant analysis. For the remaining six individuals, detailed case histories were compiled from their initial and subsequent evaluations. These were examined for predispositions to psychiatric illness, psychiatric diagnoses and personality change. A summary of these six cases is presented in Table 1. All individuals were officers in their late 20s to middle 30s when first evaluated. Four of the cases were first evaluated in the early to middle 1960s, and one in the early 1970s. Four of the six are college graduates. All are pilots or navigators.

Cases 1, 2, and 3 were evaluated at the USAF School of Aerospace Medicine as part of their evaluation as highly select volunteers for special projects involving actual or experimental duties related to flying. These individuals underwent the extensive psychiatric and psychological assessment designed for the space program. Evaluation was directed toward psychiatric illness, predispositions to psychiatric illness, and the ability to cope under stress. The thoroughness of this procedure has been described elsewhere (27). The psychiatric evaluations required 10 hours; the comprehensiveness of the psychological test battery is shown in Table 1. The "other" data available on case 3 were observations made during the special project. No psychiatric illness and no factors predisposing to psychiatric illness were found. All three individuals were approved for their special projects.

Cases 4, 5, and 6 were referred for the symptoms noted in Table 1. Case 4 was diagnosed after evaluation as having had a single seizure secondary to alcohol withdrawal without evidence of alcoholism. He was grounded from flying duties for one year and subsequently re-evaluated on two further occasions. He had totally abstained from alcohol during the interim, and no other psychopathology was evident. He was recommended for return to flying duties. Case 5 was evaluated for dizziness and anxiety symptoms which appeared during a stressful phase of training. On evaluation, he was considered to have a past history indicating a tendency to respond to stress with mild anxiety. Although no diagnosable psychopathology was present, he was described as an intense individual who might use his job to work off anger in a self-punishing manner. He was noted to have good resources but underutilized his own abilities and manifested strong support needs and a chronic underlying anger.

Case 6 was referred to the USAF School of Aerospace Medicine for evaluation with a history of nausea, cramping, and diarrhea which had its onset after flying in a combat area. He was evaluated independently by two psychiatrists and received psychometrics. Similar symptoms were noted 10 years prior to this evaluation with an asymptomatic period intervening. He was diagnosed as having had a psychophysiologic gastrointestinal reaction. He was described as being a somewhat rigid, tense, and driven individual who conformed to the rules of propriety, lacked playfulness and spontaneity, and was highly motivated to perform in his career field. After resolution of his symptoms, he was recommended for return to flying.

Five of the six cases were shot down and captured prior to 1969 (Table 2). These averaged 6.0 years in captivity, of which 1.4 years were spent in solitary confinement. They lost an average of 20.8 kilograms in weight during captivity. Case 5 was captured after 1969 with significantly less time in prison, time in solitary, and weight loss.

At repatriation in 1973, the six cases were 35 to 45 years of age (Table 3). Each was seen in follow-up on a yearly or biyearly basis from 1973 to 1978. Case 1 manifested mild depression and obsessive-compulsive traits at the time of repatriation. By 1974, these symptoms had

Table 2. Captivity Experience

Case No.	Date of Capture	Months in Captivity	Days in Solitary	Weight Loss (kg)
1	Before 1969	66	570	20
2	Before 1969	81	210	41
3	Before 1969	63	1,080	8
4	After 1969	18	12	3
5	Before 1969	75	540	15
6	Before 1969	76	210	20

resolved with good readaptation despite difficult situational events. He was described then as cheerful, enthusiastic, and outgoing with a superficial but adept social manner. Case 2 had been divorced since he was first evaluated. He showed only mild nondiagnostic traits of rigidity and need to control when first seen in 1973. However, later that year and continuing through 1976, he was diagnosed as having a situational adjustment reaction of adulthood related to difficulties in his role as a father and husband following his marriage to a widow with three children. He was described as being mildly depressed, controlling, intrusive, and suspicious of his children and wife.

Case 3 was noted to have an obsessive-compulsive personality and high achievement needs. Over the course of his evaluations, his obsessive-compulsive traits reached diagnostic levels. He was described as intense, ambivalent, and compulsively involved with his work to the exclusion of personal relationships with his wife and family. He was operating at an intense pace in pursuit of his career goals but excluding personal involvement away from work. In 1975, he was described as brilliant, bitter, depressed, and lonesome, yet compulsively compelled to maintain a life-style perpetuating these feelings.

Cases 4 and 6 showed no evidence of psychopathology on repatriation or later in the follow-up period. Case 4 had no problems with alcohol after repatriation. He made significant career decisions and pursued his goals with a determination not noted in his precaptivity evaluations. He attributed these decisions to what he had learned from other POWs while in prison. Case 6 had no symptoms of his psychophysiological disorder during or after captivity, and his wife believed that he had "mellowed" as a result of his experience.

Case 5 showed no diagnosable psychopathology at repatriation but was noted to be "making up for lost time" with a strong desire to be "first" and a questionable fatalism in his outlook on life. He felt little attachment to his wife. His evaluation in 1975 also noted his "moving

Table 3. Postcaptivity Psychiatric Assessment

Case No.	Marital Status at Repatriation	Date of Evaluation	Psychiatric Evaluation	Psycho-logical Testing	Standardized Mental Status	Diagnosis or Symptoms (+)
1	Married	1973	+	+	+	Mild depression and obsessive-compulsive personality disorder
		1974	+	+	...	0
		1975	+	+	...	0
		1977	+	+	...	0
2	Divorced	1973	+	...	+	+
		1973	+	+	...	Situational adjustment reaction of adulthood
		1974	+	+	...	Situational adjustment reaction of adulthood
		1975	...	+	...	
		1976	+	+	...	Situational adjustment reaction of adulthood
3	Married	1973	+	...	+	Obsessive-compulsive personality disorder
		1974	+	+	+	Mild depressive reaction and mild marital maladjustment reaction
		1975	+	+	+	Depressive neurosis, obsessive-compulsive personality disorder, and marital maladjustment
		1976	+	...	+	Depressive neurosis, obsessive-compulsive personality disorder, and marital maladjustment
4	Single	1973	+	+	+	...
		1975	+	+	...	...
		1977	+	+	...	...
5	Married	1973	+	+	+	...
		1973	+	+	...	+
		1975	+	+	...	...
		1978	+	+	...	Depressive neurosis
6	Married	1973	+	+	+	...
		1974	+	+	...	...
		1977	+	+	...	...

very fast." In 1977, he was again described as "in a hurry." He had recently changed jobs and had decreased libido, crying spells, and recurrent thoughts of his deceased grandfather with whom he had been very close. He received a diagnosis of depressive neurosis.

These six POW cases are unique in the quality of data available which describes their personality and psychiatric status prior to the captivity experience. Although the data are primarily clinical, it is clinical with objective support and far from the retrospective and anecdotal data usually available in such cases. The small number of cases does not allow for statistical conclusions but can provide results in line with the single case method which addresses the necessary and sufficient causes of psychopathology following the POW experience.

From this perspective, analysis of the six cases allows for two conclusions. First, the presence of antecedent psychiatric disturbances or symptoms usually thought to represent a predisposition to illness is not necessary to the development of psychiatric illness after long-term trauma (e.g., cases 1, 2, and 3). In fact, despite thorough evaluations with no detectable psychiatric illness or predispositions, socially advantaged, mature adults previously selected for psychological health and coping abilities developed diagnosable illness following their POW experience. Second, the presence of antecedent psychiatric disturbance is not sufficient for the development of post-traumatic illness. As evidenced in cases 4 and 6, although one might suspect a maladaptive precaptivity personality (in case 4 dependent and case 6 obsessive-compulsive), no postcaptivity psychopathology was present. The MMPI in case 6 continued to show him as an individual prone to psychophysiological symptoms.

PERSONALITY CHANGE OTHER THAN ILLNESS

Are the effects of captivity generalizable in some way? To consider this question, one must not only look toward what pathology develops after captivity but also consider the possibility that no personality change may occur. In addition, one must consider that certain alterations in personality caused by the POW experience may structurally alter a pathological personality to a healthier one or lead to only an alteration in predominant personality style. Koranyi (5, 23) has used this perspective to focus on the personality changing aspects of the POW situation rather than the necessity of pathological outcome.

Observations from the six cases presented above, particularly cases 1, 2, and 3 in which the precaptivity personality was considered normal, lead to the view that captivity supported the development of a decreased level of interpersonal relatedness associated with an increased rigidity of character. Such rigidity was manifested in isolation of affect and increased unifocal determination. An increased drive to master and achieve, accompanied by an experience of time pressure (e.g., effortful, driven, making up for lost time), was also experienced in these cases. The changes in personality are evidenced in cases 1, 2, 3, and 5. Case 4 may represent a move supported by the captivity experience toward a healthier independence and freedom from a passive orientation to life. Case 6 is difficult to interpret from this perspective but may have benefitted more from the decrease in interpersonal tension, while showing no change in character, which was described as rigid and driven prior to captivity.

This is not the apathy response found by Strassman et al. (9) after the Korean War, which was characterized by withdrawal and lack of energy. These alterations of personality style as seen in the USAF POW sample are neither pathological nor beneficial in and of themselves but depend upon the starting point of the personality structure. What may produce an obsessive-compulsive style in normal individuals may lead a basically dependent individual with little self-motivation to a more productive personality style.

This view of POW captivity as leading to personality change which may or may not be pathological is consistent with the MMPI findings on USAF POWs (19). Significant MMPI alterations were noted, but they were of variable clinical significance. The presence of marital maladjustment as the major diagnosis in both Navy (7) and Air Force (20) POWs may also indicate changes in personality unrelated to pathology per se.

To understand such personality change involves adaptational and intrapsychic perspectives on the POWs and their environment. Theories relating trauma and personality draw heavily on Freud's concept of a "stimulus barrier" which may be ruptured under too much stress (28). The Southeast Asian POWs, however, not only underwent trauma but also "strain," a term used by Sandler for a chronic high level of stress (29).

Levin (30) has identified loss, attack, restraint, and threats as the external factors capable of inducing psychological stress by drive defusion. This state may lead to psychopathology or increased development and adaptation. In their loneliness, isolation, degradation, deprivation, and maltreatment, the POWs were subjected to these factors in their extreme. The result can be intrapsychically depicted as creating a frustration of heightened aggressive drives and a loss of libidinally cathected objects. These factors have been discussed from the adaptational perspective in the apathy syndrome (9, 10) and conceived of as an adaptive withdrawal in the face of conflict over the expression of aggression and longing created by the forces of traumatic deprivation, torture, confinement, and threats.

The Viet Nam era pilot or navigator POW is different from the foot soldier POW of previous wars in education, background, and personality style. The effects of the POW experience as mediated by these variables and the coping styles adopted by the POWs would, therefore, be expected to be different. In the cases presented here, the character rigidity manifested in isolation of affect, a stubborn determination, and decreased interpersonal relatedness is an adaptive response to the captivity environment. This coping style protects the individual from the internal experience of fear, loss, and rage and denies the presence of interpersonal needs. Similarly, the individual is able to carry out the repetitive, monotonous tasks necessary to survive years of imprisonment, much of which was spent in social isolation. This adaptive style is similar to but less profound than the withdrawal component of the apathy syndrome.

From the intrapsychic perspective, one can also address the issue of structural alterations in personality attributable to the psychological stress of captivity. What changes in the components of the personality, in particular in ego and superego functions, may be attributable to the captivity experience? The structural theory of Freud has been built on the concept of intrapsychic conflict between the systems of the personality: ego, id, and superego. Hartman (31) was first to raise the issue of intrasystemic conflict in his discussion of the ego. Rangell (32, 33) elaborated this concept by identifying intrasystemic conflict as the conflict of choice between alternatives, as decision making rather than the opposition of forces which characterizes intersystemic conflict. Intrasystemic conflict exists within the ego and to some extent within the superego as a result of its need for order and consistency. Such conflict is nearly always accompanied by intersystemic conflict. The long-term POW personality alterations identified here can be conceptualized as intrasystemic superego alterations, born out of intrasystemic conflict during captivity and caused by the resultant changes in the relationship between the demanding, moralistic elements of the superego and the capacity for ambition of the ego ideal. Secondarily, what was observed can be conceptualized as intrasystemic conflict between the superego as a whole and the ego.

Aggressive drives are related to the ability to survive (24) and to master, cope with, and overcome the environment. Discharge of aggression can also be a defense against the experience of shame when under conditions of criticism, ridicule, scorn, or abandonment (34). The POW was in a constant struggle to survive and to daily withstand the shame associated with maltreatment, his living conditions, and the recognition of personal limitation despite goals or ideals. Aggression could not be relieved overtly, and even its sublimated release in activity was restricted.

Such constraint on aggressive drive discharge leads to an increased cathexis of the superego and an increase in the demands of the ego ideal (35, 36). The distinctive functioning of those two elements can be equated to the difference in roles between Simon Legree with the power of the overseer's whip in demanding compliance and the alluring call of Circe, a siren of the night who effects her power by the promises and seduction of hope and expectation (37).

The apathy syndrome may then be conceptualized as the product of the punitive superego's victory in the intrasystemic conflict. In contrast, the driven, mastery-oriented individual reflects the stronger position of the ego ideal in the intrasuperego conflict. Heightened aggressive drives can then be discharged in the pursuit of the now vociferous ego ideal.

The loss of object cathexes experienced during prison exacerbates the importance to the individual of meeting the ambitions of the ego ideal. In addition, when object cathexes are lost, self-cathexis occurs. Hartman has related this to the development of grandiosity (31). Short of this extreme, it may produce an increased investment in the self's goals and wishes at the expense of external objects. The ego ideal participates in adaptation by the maintenance of narcissistic equilibrium through idealization and the definition of perfection (38). In its origins, the ego ideal is an agency of wish fulfillment to provide pleasure and to undo the pain caused by frustration. To deal with situations of unpleasure which threaten self-esteem (narcissistic equilibrium), fantasies of grandeur in the child and norms, ethics, and ideals in the adult support the ego and the self (39, 40).

In the POWs presented here, the ego ideal is the image of the successful, powerful, first-in-all-things aircrew member who has not lost six years of experience, training, and family relations. These POWs ignored deficits and, at the expense of interpersonal relations, pursued Circe's call, leading to a "striving after perfection" relatively independent of objects (40). In cases 1, 2, 3, and 5, this resulted in psychopathology. In case 4, a healthy move to increased independence was facilitated. This same mechanism may be operative in the high percentage of the most seriously stressed POWs who saw themselves as benefitted from their captivity experience (18).

The personality changes discussed here were made possible by mental activity during incarceration. The study of such long-term "strain" effects requires a detailed look at the nature of the environmental and intrapsychic stresses and the potential responses of the mental apparatus. The adaptational demands of the POW environment and the intrapsychic shifts in drive and structure are helpful perspectives in explaining the personality changes observed in the

POWs. Why the styles of intrasuperego conflict resolution are different in the Korean War POWs compared to Viet Nam era POWs is unclear. Differences in the type of captivity stresses and precaptivity personality styles appear to be partial explanations. In addition, the apathy syndrome of the Korean experience was most prominent during the first two weeks after repatriation. The cases discussed here were examined longitudinally for several years after captivity and are described from that perspective.

CONCLUSION

Repatriated POWs have been studied following each armed conflict with results generally indicating an increased vulnerability to psychiatric illness. The role of preexisting personality structure in the development of psychiatric illness following captivity has been unclear. Results of the studies of Viet Nam era USAF POWs indicate that most USAF POWs have done well. However, those POWs subjected to the highest levels of stress are at increased risk to develop psychiatric disturbances after repatriation. Data support the importance of the severity of stress rather than predisposing personality factors in the development of post-stress illness in this population. Identified captivity coping strategies were not related to subsequent psychiatric disturbance.

The POW case studies are unique in the quality and amount of precaptivity psychiatric data available, thus avoiding the use of retrospective anecdotal reconstruction. Conclusions of the strength associated with a controlled experiment are not possible. Such data can never be expected for a study of the effect of the POW environment. Conclusions related to necessary and sufficient conditions for the development of psychopathology can be reached based on our present abilities to identify psychiatric illness and predispositions.

The analysis of the six POWs indicates that the presence of psychiatric illness or predispositions to psychiatric illness are neither necessary nor sufficient for the development of psychiatric illness after the extreme stress of the prisoner of war experience. This supports the view that neurotic illness can develop under unusually stressful conditions in individuals with no predispositions to psychiatric illness. The perspective of personality change unrelated to the development of psychopathology is necessary to explain the data. Personality change secondary to environmental factors may lead to psychiatric illness, psychiatric health, or merely a shift in a predominant style.

Personality change unrelated to pathology per se appears to be dependent upon the precaptivity personality style and the degree of plasticity of the personality structure. Plasticity is difficult to measure but is recognized as critical to personality change in clinical work. Indeed, plasticity is a function of personality structure and developmental stage. Rangell (41) has commented on the importance of the interaction between the developmental stage of the individual and the nature of the trauma. The developmental stage characterizes the area of personality which is both most vulnerable and most malleable at any given time. For most POWs, the captivity experience occurred during Erikson's psychosocial stage of intimacy and generativity. One might expect, therefore, the stresses of captivity to have their major impact in these same areas. In fact, this is what is seen in the case studies.

The mechanisms of personality change in the POWs described here are understandable from both the adaptational and the intrapsychic structural perspectives. In contrast to the apathy syndrome identified in the Korean War POWs, the present cases show a predominance of a heightened drive to achieve, character rigidity, and decreased interpersonal relatedness. This reflects both adaptation to the captivity environment and the impact of the ego ideal over that of the punitive elements of the superego in drive discharge. Personality structure after POW experiences is the result of the interplay of the environmental stress, the precaptivity personality conformation, and the degree of personality plasticity. Elucidation of the mechanisms of personality change in such environments requires a detailed look at environmental and intrapsychic stresses and the potential responses of the mental apparatus.

REFERENCES

1. Stenger CA: American prisoners of war in WWI, WWII, Korea and Vietnam. Proceedings of the 5th Joint Meeting on POW/MIA Matters. Brooks Air Force Base, Texas, 1978

2. Beebe GW: Follow-up studies of World War II and Korean war prisoners, II: morbidity, disability and maladjustments. Am J Epidemiol 101:400–421, 1975

3. Keehn RJ: Follow-up studies of World War II and Korean conflict prisoners. Am J Epidemiol 106:194–211, 1980

4. Segal J: Long-Term Psychological and Physical Effects of the POW Experience: A Review of the Literature (report no. 74-2). Naval Health Research Center, Department of the Navy, Washington, DC, 1974

5. Koranyi E: A theoretical review of the survivor syndrome. Diseases of the Nervous System 30:115–118, 1969

6. Saul L, Lyons J: Acute neurotic reactions, in Dynamic Psychiatry. Edited by Alexander F, Ross H. Chicago, University of Chicago Press, 1952

7. Hunter E: The Vietnam POW veterans, in Stress Disorders Among Vietnam Veterans. Edited by Figley CR. New York, Brunner/Mazel, 1978

8. Eitinger L: Preliminary notes on a study of concentration camp survivors in Norway. Israel Annals of Psychiatry 1:59–67, 1963

9. Strassman HP, Thaler MB, Schein EH: A prisoner of war syndrome: apathy as a reaction to severe stress. Am J Psychiatry 112:998–1003, 1956

10. Greenson R: The psychology of apathy. Psychoanal Q 18:290–302, 1949

11. Lifton FJ: Death in Life. New York, Random House, 1967

12. Lindemann E: Symptomatology and management of acute grief. Am J Psychiatry 101:141–148, 1944

13. Bene E: Anxiety and emotional impoverishment in men under stress. Br J Med Psychol 34:281–289, 1964

14. Palmai G: Psychological observations on an isolated group in Antarctica. Br J Psychiatry 109:364–370, 1963

15. Paterson RAH: Personality profile in a group of Antarctic men. International Review of Applied Psychology 27:33–37, 1978

16. Bundzen PV: Urgent tasks of psychophysiological studies in the Antarctic, in Medical Research on Arctic and Antarctic Expeditions. Edited by Matusov L. Leningrad, Gidrometeorologicheskve Izdatel' rov, 1971

17. Vohden RA: Stress and the Vietnam POW (student research report no. 091). Washington, DC, College of the Armed Forces, March 1974

18. Sledge WH, Boydstun JA, Rahe AJ: Self-concept changes related to war captivity. Arch Gen Psychiatry 37:430–443, 1980

19. Wheatley R, Ursano R: Serial personality evaluations of repatriated U.S. Air Force Southeast Asia POWs. Aviat Space Environ Med 53:251–257, 1982

20. Ursano R, Boydstun JA, Wheatley R: Psychiatric illness in USAF Viet Nam POWs: five-year follow-up. Am J Psychiatry 138:310–314, 1981

21. Wheatley R: Intellectual, neuropsychological, and visuomotor assessments of repatriated Air Force SEA POWs. Scientific Proceedings of the Aerospace Medical Association Annual Meeting, San Antonio, Tex, 1981

22. Freud S: Collected Papers, vol 2. Edited by Jones E. London, Hogarth Press, 1950

23. Koranyi E: Psychodynamic theories of the survivor syndrome. Canadian Psychiatric Association Journal 14:165–174, 1969

24. Geerts AE, Rechardt E: Colloquium on trauma. Int J Psychoanal 59:365–375, 1978

25. Moses R: Adult psychic trauma: the question of early predisposition and some detailed mechanisms. Int J Psychoanal 59:353–363, 1978

26. Furst S: The stimulus barrier and the pathogenicity of trauma. Int J Psychoanal 59:345–352, 1978

27. Perry C: Psychiatric support for man in space. International Psychiatric Clinic 4:197–221, 1967

28. Freud S (1920–1922): Beyond the Pleasure Principle, in Complete Psychological Works, standard ed, vol 18. London, Hogarth Press, 1955

29. Sandler J: Trauma, strain, and development, in Psychic Trauma. Edited by Furst S. New York, Basic Books, 1967

30. Levin S: Toward a classification of external factors capable of inducing psychological stress. Int J Psychoanal 47:546–551, 1966

31. Hartman H: Comments on the psychoanalytic theory of the ego. Psychoanal Study Child 5:74–96, 1950

32. Rangell L: The scope of intrapsychic conflict. Psychoanal Study Child 18:75–102, 1963

33. Rangell L: Structural problems in intrapsychic conflict. Psychoanal Study Child 18:103–138, 1963

34. Levin S: The psychoanalysis of shame. Int J Psychoanal 52:355–362, 1971

35. Hartman H, Kris E, Loewenstein R: Notes on the theory of aggression. Psychoanal Study Child 314:9–36, 1949

36. Freud S (1923–1925): The Ego and the Id, in Complete Psychological Works, standard ed, vol 19. London, Hogarth Press, 1961

37. Murray JM: Narcissism and the ego ideal. J Am Psychoanal Assoc 12:477–511, 1964

38. Laufer M: Ego-ideal and the pseudo-ego-ideal in adolescence. Psychoanal Study Child 19:196–221, 1964

39. Lampe deGroot J: Ego-ideal and superego. Psychoanal Study Child 17:94–106, 1962

40. Hartman H, Loewenstein R: Notes on the superego. Psychoanal Study Child 17:42–81, 1962

41. Rangell L: The metapsychology of the psychic trauma, in Psychic Trauma. Edited by Furst S. New York, Basic Books, 1967

18

The Intercultural Setting: Encountering Black Viet Nam Veterans

Erwin Randolph Parson, Ph.D.

18

While most persons seeking help for mental, interpersonal, and social problems present a complex array of needs and issues, the readjustment needs presented by black Viet Nam veterans are often even more complex. This is because the history and current life of black veterans in America reflect the usual ethnic minority problems, along with additional suffering related to stress reactions or war. I refer to the readjustment problems of black Viet Nam veterans as a "tripartite adaptational dilemma." By this I mean that the readjustment struggles of black veterans consist of three areas which care providers and counselors must assess in their (often cross-cultural) efforts to provide these veterans with meaningful readjustment help. The areas which comprise the tripartite adaptational dilemma specific to black veterans are listed below:

1. Surviving the potentially fragmenting "tug of war" of an acquired dual identity: being both African by heritage and white American by sociopsychologic conditioning (the "bicultural identity" or "bicultural ego" factor);
2. Surviving as a member of a kinship of men and women who are despised and discriminated against by American society for being descendants of African-American slaves (the "racialism/racism" factor); and
3. Surviving Viet Nam combat trauma and reacting to it (the "residual stress" factor).

As "triple-survivors," a role held by few others in society today, black Viet Nam veterans can be expected to mobilize a number of specific

I thank Linda McCarthy for her assistance with the various phases of this manuscript.

"survivor coping behaviors" during any kind of treatment encounter, especially with therapists and counselors who are not themselves black. Facilitating readjustment in black veterans requires that clinicians be knowledgeable in two highly specialized areas: 1) the psychosocial impact of slavery and racism; their interactive effects with the African heritage of black Americans; and how these cultural parameters converge to define normal, abnormal, and "survivor behaviors" in black Americans; and 2) the impact of insurgency and counterinsurgency Third World guerrilla warfare, along with an indifferent and hostile reception of Viet Nam veterans by the American people. Competency in the first area is referred to here as transracial competency, while competency in the second area is referred to as transexperiential competency.

Though there are many facets to the readjustment of black Viet Nam veterans (including health, employment benefits, agent orange screenings, compensation, legal problems, education, etc.), the focus of this chapter is on treating black Viet Nam veterans in cross-cultural psychotherapy and counseling. The term *intercultural setting* as used in this chapter refers to the ideas, emotions, and behavior that occur in a biracial psychotherapy setting. A flow of interpersonal elements between client and therapist characterizes any useful treatment venture, but the setting is here more complicated.

BLACK VIET NAM VETERANS IN CONTEMPORARY SOCIETY

The Sociopolitical Climate of the War Years

There are several issues the therapist working with black veterans must understand. These issues are intrinsic to the lives of black veterans—to their health and adaptation, as well as to their problems.

During the 1960s the social and political transformation of our culture resulted in a radical reexamination of American values and institutions. Many young people viewed society as profoundly sick. The prevailing middle-class ethic was challenged in an unprecedented fashion. No aspect of society was spared unsettling scrutiny. The war years of the 1960s contrasted with the war years of a quarter century before, in which national and international support for a war gave the period its special character of cohesiveness and national *amour propre*. The Viet Nam War was the heart of this new age; it highlighted societal and political ills that became intolerable to American youth.

The psychology of black veterans of the Viet Nam era is embedded in this historical context, and in the psychohistorical roots of the black experience in America. The call for change and examination of values forced the system to confront and modify its racist policies toward black Americans, and to examine basically shabby and uncaring attitudes toward the poor.

Leaders in the black community spoke out against institutional racism and pointed out the paradoxes in the American system. Black leaders were aware of the illustrious history of military service by blacks beginning before the Revolutionary War. They were aware that the first person to fire a fatal shot at the British in that war was a black man, Crispus Attucks, a sailor who had escaped from his slave-holder master in 1750. He was later killed in the Boston Massacre and given a hero's burial along with two white soldiers.

They were also aware that Crispus Attucks had given up his life to secure a freedom that he himself had not been granted. Indeed, the "full desserts of democracy" (1) had not been his to enjoy, nor had these ever been fully available to black Americans in the United States. If blacks during the Viet Nam era were without activism, they knew that the status quo would remain, just as it did after World War II, when "After helping to defeat the 'racist' regime of Adolf Hitler, the black veteran returned to find the racist regime of the United States unvanquished" (2, p. 60). Whereas in past wars blacks fought eagerly to prove themselves as worthy citizens, soldiers of the Viet Nam era knew that serving in the U.S. Armed Forces would not guarantee the benefits of full citizenship.

In a statement reflecting inherent American contradictions and ironies regarding the Negro, Dr. Martin Luther King, Jr., pointed out:

> Of the good things in life he [the Negro] had approximately one-half those of whites, of the bad he has twice those of whites. Thus, half of all Negroes live in sub-standard housing, and Negroes have half the income of whites. When we turn to the negative experience of life, the Negro has a double share. There are twice as many unemployed. The rate of infant mortality . . . among Negroes is double that of whites. The equation pursues Negroes even into war. There are twice as many Negroes as whites in combat in Vietnam at the beginning of 1967, and twice as many Negro soldiers died in action (20.6 percent) in proportion to their number in the population. (3, pp. 7–8)

Dr. King's statement captured the general feelings of frustration, disappointment, and reactive rage in black Americans and in black soldiers in Vietnam. These feelings boiled over when reports revealed that blacks were overrepresented in combat units in Viet Nam, and that they suffered a higher rate of casualties and deaths compared to white soldiers. For example, in 1966 a report in *U.S. News and World Report* revealed that although blacks represented only 11 percent of the 19- to 20-year-olds in this country, they sustained 25 percent of the losses in Viet Nam (4).

Black Soldiers in Viet Nam

As Binkin and Eitelberg (5) note,

> In contrast to the two World Wars and the early days of Korea when Blacks had to "fight for the right to fight," the advent of the Vietnam War brought charges that Blacks were doing more than their share of the fighting. And . . . many Black leaders and others now questioned the "special efforts" and methods that *favored* the recruitment of Blacks over whites." (p. 32)

The "special effort" to recruit blacks and other disadvantaged groups of Americans became a part of the Great Society's War on Poverty of the 1960s. Project 100,000 was thus conceived and implemented to give high school drop-outs, indigents, and unskilled American youths—a group that in the past were typically rejected for military service—a chance to enter military service and receive the benefits of education, training, and presumably a better life after discharge. Project 100,000 appeared to have been motivated by noble and humane ideals; its implementation, however, proved harmful and even inhumane to minorities—and to indigent white Americans as well. Low-income recruits under the Project were primarily given combat-related MOSs (military occupational specialties). Thus, over one-half of the servicemen who joined the Marine Corps and the Army under this program were sent to Viet Nam (6, 7). The Department of Defense revealed that blacks were overrepresented in both combat duty and in casualties, in relation to their proportions among American personnel in Viet Nam (8).

The military system was fully integrated for the first time in American history. The perceptions, attitudes, values, and beliefs which had been shaped over 300 years in an American racist society did not disappear merely because selected military initiatives toward integration had occurred. Blacks in Viet Nam were also aware of the irony that, although they fought alongside white soldiers against the common "enemy," they could not live in the same communities with whites in America, nor sit together in certain public places.

In a recent article titled "The Black Veteran," Harold Bryant, a black Viet Nam veteran who served with the First Cavalry Division (Airmobile), quotes a pertinent statement by Dr. Martin Luther King, Jr., made in April 1967:

> We are taking the young Black men who have been crippled by our society and sending them 8,000 miles away to guarantee liberties in Southeast Asia which they had not found in Southwest Georgia and East Harlem. So we have been repeatedly faced with the cruel irony of watching Negro and White boys on TV screens as they kill and die together for a nation that has been unable to seat them together at the same school. So, we watch them in brutal solidarity burning the huts of a poor village, but we realize that they could never live on the same block in Detroit. (9, p. 5)

In general, race relations in Viet Nam were better than in America. However, this deteriorated in noncombat units (in the "rear") and became worse everywhere after the murder of Dr. Martin Luther King, Jr. That year, 1968, also marked the turning point of the war: there were heightened stresses in the field resulting from responsive actions to the Tet offensive.

In Viet Nam, both black and white soldiers were subject to the same stresses of war. They fought together, walked through the booby-trapped and disease-infested jungles together, and died together. Soldiers of both races were capable of genuine mutual empathic response. Both black and white soldiers, moreover, were subject to the same confusion, chaos, disorganization, and futility of war. And both suffered the adverse effects of pervasive terror and the vicissitudes of a psychotic reality that characterized the Viet Nam War environment.

"Gook" Identification and the "Gook" Syndrome

Black soldiers could not forget what they had left behind in America: poverty, squalor, discrimination, segregation, and other ills associated with racism. They were mindful of the similarity between their exclusion in America and the basic plight of Vietnamese nationals, who were suffering and surviving in poverty. Blacks perceived the Vietnamese as an unusual breed of survivors: their homes and villages had for 30 years been constantly overrun by war. Black soldiers also viewed themselves as survivors: they had survived years of beatings, lynchings, home and church bombings, discrimination, and exclusion. Like the Vietnamese people, moreover, blacks were of the Third World, and for the first time in American history, whites found themselves fighting where they were the minority, just as black soldiers in Viet Nam were in the majority. The psychological implications of this racial dynamic for both blacks and whites were immense.

The powerful psychological identification of blacks with the Vietnamese has been referred to as the "gook" identification (10). This is the conscious and unconscious emotional identification by black soldiers with the devalued, maligned, abused, and helpless aspects of the Vietnamese people. In the psychological sense, such identification with Vietnamese civilians resonated within black soldiers in the form of personal pain, anguish, and guilt, especially when black soldiers killed Vietnamese people. As one black veteran put it, "It's like killing off a part of yourself." David DuBose, a black combat veteran who is now a Veteran Outreach Counselor in the Veterans Administration's Vet Center Program, highlights this intrapsychic conflict in black soldiers.

> In 1966, while in a Vietnamese village, I received a clipping from my home newspaper wherein there was a notice of a riot in my community. Tear gas had been thrown into the buildings where my family, my wife, two daughters, and in-laws were living. Upon reading the article, I broke down and cried. I became detached from my surroundings. . . . I questioned myself, "What am I doing here?" "I should be back home, protecting my family." Yet, I knew that I was helpless and trapped within a life and death situation. At this time, all my experiences supported the realization [that] *the very people I was commissioned to kill looked more like me than the ones who had been given orders to gas my family and gun my Asian kinsman.*" (11, p. 6; italics added)

During this period in Viet Nam, race consciousness rose to a crescendo among black soldiers. To make matters worse, during 1968, as Leventman and Camacho (12) observed, the "gook syndrome" rose within the American forces. This resulted in a conceptual separation of the allied fighting forces into "the Americans" (blacks and whites) and "the Vietnamese" (the "gooks"). At the same time black Americans, motivated by their gook identification with Vietnamese nationals, had psychologically divided the fighting forces into "the Americans" (white soldiers) and "the Third World Fighters for Freedom" (blacks, other minorities, and the Vietnamese). The Pentagon thus observed, "It is paradoxical that the Negro citizen in uniform has frequently been made to feel more at home overseas than in his hometown" (5).

Finally, the service of black troops in Viet Nam had put to rest the historically unsubstantiated prejudice that the battlefield abilities of black soldiers were inferior. According to Wallace Terry (13), General William Westmoreland and President Johnson, among others, concurred on the peerless soldiering abilities that characterized black troop performance in Viet Nam (see also "How Negro Americans Perform in Vietnam" [4]).

Black Veterans Return Home

Returning black veterans came home to a country that had changed in many ways, but not in its basic exclusion of black Americans. Now, however, not only was the exclusion based on their racial heritage, but black veterans were also discriminated against because they had served in Viet Nam. Additionally, unemployment was even higher than when they left for Viet Nam, and work was hard to find. Many black veterans withdrew in silence and bitterness after futile attempts to find employment. Poor or substandard housing remained a problem. The lofty promises of the Great Society and its War On Poverty did not shield these veterans from the despair of poverty. Department of Defense studies of 1969 and 1970 revealed that, compared to whites, black army veterans were more than twice as likely to be unemployed, and when working lagged behind in earnings (14, 15). The most comprehensive study to date on the readjustment of Viet Nam veterans revealed that having served in Viet Nam had a pernicious effect on occupational and educational attainment (16). Along these lines, to the question "Are blacks making it in civilian life?" Fendrich's research (17) answered *no*. He found that black veterans were disillusioned and highly alienated, with high rates of unemployment and underemployment.

In the wake of social and political turmoil across the nation, many whites feared that the rage and general discontent of black combat veterans would lead to the formation of urban guerrilla groups (13, 18). This fear surfaced more recently when unsubstantiated evidence by white law enforcement officials charged that black Viet Nam veterans instigated the first urban riots in Miami, in May 1980 (19, 20).

Yet another obstacle faced by returning black veterans attempting to readjust and reintegrate was the less-than-honorable discharge (or "bad paper"). Estimates indicate that black veterans received 45 percent of the half-million "bad paper" discharges given during the Viet Nam years (7). A large number of these discharges were given to blacks as a means of controlling civil rights activism within the military. Commenting on the adverse psychological impact of these discharges, the General Accounting Office stated in its 1980 Report to Congress that "The bad discharge is a constant reinforcement [to the recipient] of a negative self-image, a reminder that the individual is unsuitable, unfit, and undesirable in the eyes of his country" (21).

Post-Traumatic Stress Disorder Among Black Viet Nam Veterans

Recent developments in the understanding and diagnosis of psychic reactions to stressful life events resulted in a new official diagnostic entity, post-traumatic stress disorder, in 1980 (22). Symptoms found in Viet Nam veterans as a direct consequence of their Viet Nam and post–Viet Nam traumatic experiences include, but are not limited to, impaired self-esteem, concentration, memory, and attention; intrusive thoughts, feelings, and actions; recurrent dreams and nightmares; guilt; feelings of rage and abandonment; withdrawal; difficulty with intimacy; problems with authority; "settling for dullness" and choosing a "wandering life-style" (23); mistrust and alienation (in response to social and political injustice); and permanence of the affective residue of the traumatizing event. Like other survivors of psychic trauma, Viet Nam veterans who are symptomatic experience tension and pervasive anxiety. To achieve relief from these tensions and anxieties, many Viet Nam veterans utilize a variety of coping strategies (including alcohol and drug use) that paradoxically obstruct, rather than facilitate, the working-through of their stress response syndromes.

The stress reactions and symptoms observed clinically in Viet Nam veterans are also seen in others who have suffered a catastrophic event, and there is evidence that symptomatology is more a reflection of overwhelming trauma than personality predisposition (24). For example, many of the symptoms described above are found in those who experienced the horrors of the Holocaust (25), the Hiroshima nuclear blast (26), severe head injuries (27), rape (28), industrial accidents (29), or a variety of other personal injuries (30). Additionally, stress symptoms are observed in women having suffered a miscarriage (31); hostages taken in prison (32); repatriated prisoners of war (24, 33, 34); survivors of combat in the Yom Kippur War (35); and veterans of World War II, Korea (36), and the Viet Nam War (37–39).

In 1978, the Washington Urban League published research findings which found that a "mental disorder" was the most problematic readjustment disability in black veterans (40). A subsequent study mandated by Congress and reported in 1981, which was based on an unbiased sample of almost 1,400 veterans and nonveterans, substantiates this observation. This investigation, *Legacies of Vietnam: Comparative Adjustment of Veterans and Their Peers* (henceforth referred to as *Legacies*) concluded that those who served in Viet Nam have more problems than their peers—in education, in employment, in a higher incidence of arrests, in drug use, and in more medical and psychological complaints (16). *Legacies* also found that black Viet Nam veterans suffered significantly more readjustment problems than did white veterans—in psychic, social, vocational, and academic functioning. The following research findings are relevant:

1. Blacks and Chicanos have suffered more stress disturbances than do their white counterparts.
2. Though being in heavy combat was the most crucial factor correlated with the development of severe forms of post-traumatic stress reactions and symptoms, for black veterans merely being in the theater of war was sufficient to produce stress-related problems.
3. Almost 70 percent of black and Chicano veterans in heavy combat suffer stress disorders; 40 percent of the entire sample of black veterans suffer stress today, as compared with 20 percent of the entire sample of white veterans.
4. Black veterans who suffered stress reactions immediately following their war experience were more likely to suffer the effects of stress today than a comparable group of white Viet Nam veterans.

In the interest of easy reference and clarity, I will refer to the first and third items as the *comparative factor* (C factor), the second item as the *theater-presence factor* (T-P factor), and the fourth item as the *residuum factor* (R factor).

The C factor indicates that black veterans have more post-combat stress reactions and disorders than do white veterans; that these persist for a longer period of time is indicated by the R factor, and the T-P factor tells us that all this occurs, regardless of the degree of combat exposure. The question may be asked, "What features of the Viet Nam experience or of the general climate of the war might account for blacks' susceptibility to stress reactions during and after Viet Nam?" One hypothesis bears on black combatants' perceptions of and emotional reactions to their role in Viet Nam vis-à-vis the Vietnamese people. As noted earlier, black soldiers often held ambivalent feelings toward fighting and killing Third World people. The strong identification with Vietnamese civilians and even with Vietcong (the "gook" identification) may have contributed to subsequent stress reactions and disorders in black veterans. I first made this hypothesis based on clinical observations in 1980. It has since been substantiated in a recent report that reanalyzes the *Legacies* data (41). Additional clinical research is needed to further elucidate the inner dynamics of blacks vis-à-vis the Vietnamese: the psychic consequences of blacks fighting and killing in a Third World country—the unconscious equivalent of "killing oneself in one's own land"—are indeed complicated.

Clinical research is needed also to clarify issues involving the R factor. According to *Legacies*, stress reactions in white veterans tended to evaporate over time, but for blacks these reactions tend more to persist to the present. The reasons for this remain unknown. In what I have called a "stress recuperative phenomenon," the mind of the survivor typically moves toward resolution of post-traumatic responses through a series of normal and predictable phases. Thus, stress reactions do tend toward evaporation. When this normal process is unsuccessful, the sufferer enters into a phase of residual stress disorder, which in *DSM-III* (22) is classified as "chronic" (duration of symptoms six months or longer). Clinical evidence concerning black Viet Nam veterans with significant residual readjustment problems reveals that they suffer emotional turmoil related to 1) their "gook" identification with the Vietnamese; 2) their perceptions of sociopolitical changes of the war years; 3) their experience of racism; and 4) their feelings about the lower educational achievement, lower income, and poorer employment histories among blacks. All of these areas of turmoil may be causally linked to "higher levels of stress, especially among combat veterans," which—according to Kadushin et al. (42)—may explain the black-white difference in the incidence of post-traumatic stress disorder.

ACQUIRING TRANSRACIAL COMPETENCY WITH AFRICAN-AMERICANS

Since "different cultures tend to shape different kinds of psychopathology, and may respond to and define mental health and mental illness in divergent ways" (43), it becomes essential for therapists who treat transculturally to become personally and professionally prepared for this task. Such therapists must learn that "white, middle-class criteria" for mental health, when applied to minority group members (44) and indigent whites, may be inaccurate or even unethical.

Transculturally effective therapists should actively move away from rigid theoretical and technical postures of culturocentric limitation to a stance which reflects an increasing capacity for multiple-culturocentric awareness. In transracial psychotherapy or counseling, the helpers should be well-grounded in a variety of theories of personality and in a number of therapies and techniques. They should be aware that Western methods of psychotherapy do not work well in all cultures. It is necessary for them to study the psychohistorical and sociological roots of the black experience in America. Some suggested sources for review and study are listed below:

- "We Wear the Mask" from *Lyrics of Lowly Life* (1897) by Paul Laurence Dunbar (45);
- *Life and Times of Frederick Douglass* (1982) (46);
- *The Souls of Black Folks* (W.E.B. Du Bois, 1903) (47);
- *Negro Builders and Heroes* (Brawley, 1937) (48);
- *Notes from a Native Son* (Baldwin, 1955) (49);
- *The Seventh Son: The Thought and Writings of W.E.B. Du Bois* (50).

Also recommended is the poetry of Phyllis Wheatley, Francis Ellen Watkins Harper, James Weldon Johnson, Langston Hughes, Arna Botemps, Effie Lee Newsome, and Countee Cullen. As Derald Sue points out, "Black history should not be taken for granted or ignored in counseling. . . ." (51, p. 142).

Transracially adept therapists must constantly confront themselves with their feelings and values about race differences. They must become aware that the maligning stereotypes of black Americans held by white scientists in America (52), as well as the distorting influences of such stereotypes on realistic understanding of black patients, are destructive impediments to therapeutic work. Such therapists should attend specialized workshops and training programs, like those discussed in Brislin and Pedersen's book *Cross-Cultural Orientation Programs* (53), to enhance their sensitivity, while helping overcome their own ethnocentricity. Finally, the therapist should secure supervision with a professional and/or peer-group in the area of cross-cultural treatment. Other specific recommendations to therapists are discussed elsewhere (54).

DEVELOPING TRANSEXPERIENTIAL COMPETENCY WITH VIET NAM VETERANS

Therapists who have not been in combat in Viet Nam but who treat Viet Nam veterans are actually crossing over into an experiential domain that is "foreign" to their own psychological lives and experiences. Hence, I use the term transexperiential, which I have applied specifically to the situation in which there is an experiential imbalance in the therapeutic dyad. How does one meet the transexperiential challenge that confronts therapists who treat Viet Nam veterans? Just as in transcultural treatment—where therapists are called upon to study, ponder, and understand the nature of the black experience—so should transexperiential therapists study every facet of the individual veteran's Viet Nam experience and readjustment struggle. Specifically, therapists are offered the following principles and recommendations in developing competency with Viet Nam veterans and other survivors of traumatopsychic experiences:

1. Therapists should study the Viet Nam era and the effects of combat and their problematic reentry on the psychological growth, development, and general well-being of Viet Nam veterans. A good survey should include the following sources: Adler (55), Archibald and Tuddenham (36), Blank (37, 56), Bourne (57), Brende and Parson (58), Bryant (59), Caputo (60), Harris and Associates (61), Egendorf et al. (16), Fairbank et al. (62), Figley (38), Figley and Leventman (63), Finman et al. (64), Fendrich (17), Goff and Sanders (65), Herr (66), Kovic (67), Lifton (26), Parson (39, 54), Santoli (68), Young (1), and Webb (69).
2. Personal reflection and self-inventory about the Viet Nam period is essential. Therapists need to retrospectively locate themselves during the war years and be honest about buried feelings related to the war and the persons who fought it. Therapists and counselors must also honestly confront their own motivations for working with Viet Nam veterans, so that feelings that are beyond the reach of awareness do not interfere with treatment.
3. Many therapists need special consultation and supervision with a colleague who is experienced in psychotherapy or counseling with survivors of psychic trauma in general or with Viet Nam veterans in particular. Peer-oriented supervision has also proven very useful to therapists.
4. Therapists should focus on specific and pertinent clinical studies such as the following: Blank (70), Brende (71, 72), DeFazio (73), Fox (74, 75), Fairbank and Keane (76), Figley (38), Kardiner (77), Haley (78), Keane and Kaloupek (79), Kipper (80), Parson (10, 39, 54), Shatan (81), Williams (82), and Wilson (83).
5. Therapists should attend workshops on stress disorders that incorporate ethnocultural issues and that utilize small group experiences about ethnicity. This activity can expand therapists' awareness and cross-ethnic competency.

CLINICAL ASSESSMENT OF BLACK VETERANS

Clinical experience with Viet Nam veterans reveals that assessment often results in misdiagnoses (39, 84, 85). Victor DeFazio (73) summarizes the observations of several authors that:

The contraction of ego functioning often resembles schizophrenic deterioration while the phobic elaboration that the world is a hostile enemy-infested place is often mistaken for a psychotic persecutory delusion. Not infrequently they suffer from compulsive memories of an almost hallucinatory type which may be set off by the sight of one oriental face, a low flying plane, or other stimulus associated with the war. (p. 38)

As already indicated, a disproportionate number of black Viet Nam veterans suffer more severe symptoms of stress disorder for longer periods of time than do their white counterparts. It would seem plausible, then, that if white professionals frequently misdiagnose white Viet Nam veterans, these clinicians would probably run an even greater risk of misdiagnosis with black veterans, because of a number of culture-specific variables related to the picture presented by these black men and women.

Understanding the behavior of black Viet Nam veterans is difficult because of the emotional, social, and cultural elements of the veterans' bicultural identity (African-American) *and* their stress symptomatology. All this is often complicated by countertransference feelings. It is my belief that a personal synthesis in the therapist of transracial and transexperiental issues is the only way nonblack, nonveteran clinicians can recognize the interpersonal and intercultural distance between themselves and members of this patient group.

Being a black American and a Viet Nam veteran represents a triple frame of reference that shapes the veterans' reality. This shaping process determines the following:

1. How veterans view their symptoms;
2. What they define as a symptom;
3. The veterans' experiences of their own stress-related problems vis-à-vis the Viet Nam experience;
4. Their attitudes about sharing their problems with therapists and other helpers;
5. Their personal experience of pain;
6. The expected type of treatment they believe will meet their needs; and
7. How they understand the causes of their difficulties (whether caused by financial, sociopolitical, or psychological factors; by Viet Nam or post–Viet Nam veteran experiences; or by some combination of these).

As has already been indicated, without an adequate understanding of the cultural roots of black veterans, it is virtually impossible to diagnose or treat them. Regarding diagnosis, Adebimpe (86) discusses the high incidence of misdiagnosis of black psychiatric patients, and elsewhere I have added,

> Some of the reasons for these misdiagnoses are due to racist practices in mental health systems; however, others are due to the clinician's inability to understand the nature of verbal and nonverbal communication of the black patient, as well as the patient's symptoms and their meanings in the total psychic economy of black persons' experiences. (87, p. 5)

An example of how knowledge of black culture is crucial concerns the diagnosis of clinical depression among blacks. Carter (88) maintains that most white clinicians are not sufficiently knowledgeable to make adequate assessments of either the presence or severity of depression among blacks. This is in large part due to the manner in which blacks express depressive affect. Most white Americans show depression with dysphoric affect. For blacks, depression is typically accompanied by multiple somatic complaints such as headaches, gastrointestinal discomfort, painful joints, backaches, etc. In general, blacks tend to somatize emotional turmoil; when not understood by clinicians, this leads to a mistaken physical diagnosis.

Frequent Sources of Diagnostic Error

Though *DSM-III* aims at increasing diagnostic accuracy, its implicit assumption that all diagnostic criteria are equally valid with all cultural or ethnic groups is erroneous. Experience shows that among blacks many anxiety-driven symptoms of stress disorder, including intrusive ideation and numbing of affect, are expressed differently. This is in part due to the observation that blacks show less affect than do whites (86) and that blacks have developed what I have called a trained capacity for interior-exterior incongruity. Thus, "blacks are so proficient in wearing a 'mask' that psychiatric impairment can be very difficult to ascertain" (86, p. 282). Clinicians have observed that the facial expressions of blacks are misunderstood and result in misdiagnosis in the direction of more, rather than fewer, serious conditions. Another problem for the evaluator is a culturally determined hypervigilance in black patients: what may be "a healthy cultural suspiciousness and adaptive response to the experience of racism" (86, p. 282), may be misassessed as paranoid pathology.

Masked self-presentation, which is the name I have given to the phenomenon of black masking affect, is of great clinical importance. Such masking not only involves hiding one's true inner feelings from professional helpers (and others) through facial, bodily, gestural, verbal, and nonverbal communications, but is also a means of regulating perception of one's own feelings, in this case the affects associated with intrusive ideation related to Viet Nam. Kardiner and Ovesey (89, p. 22) state, "It is a consistent feature of the human personality that it tends to become organized about the main problem of adaptation, and this main problem tends to polarize all other aspects of adaptation toward itself" (p. 372). Halpern (90) believes that the main problem of adaptation for black people "was to hide from the white man the extent and intensity of their feeling of frustration and [the] anger that went along with this" (p. 126). As I see it, the main problem of adaptation for many Viet Nam veterans with stress disorders is to ward off intrusive thoughts, and they do this by employing counterintrusion defenses, including the use of the process of somatization. Masked self-presentation in black veterans, then, is a counterintrusion defense that reinforces and is reinforced by emotional numbing. These veterans are often described as alienated, withdrawn, unmotivated, emotionally aloof, and as having a flat or inappropriate affect.

Toward Increased Diagnostic Accuracy

The need for increased accuracy in diagnosing black persons is a serious clinical problem (86, 91–93). Thus, systematic description and validation of diagnosis is essential. The following are aids in the diagnostic process:

1. Performing a structured mental status examination. This offers a wealth of information on the patient's life and problems (86).
2. Developing transracial awareness (discussed earlier).
3. Overcoming white stereotypes of black psychopathology.
4. Acquiring transexperiential competency with Viet Nam veterans (discussed earlier).
5. Understanding the cultural meaning accorded by black veterans to their symptoms.
6. Taking into consideration race and ethnicity when evaluating data derived from psychiatric and psychological scales (such as MMPI, Rorschach, Wechsler scales, etc).
7. Using self-report questionnaires to avoid the difficulties often encountered at the initial interview. Such difficulties result in limited vital information on black clients (91).
8. Using the computer as a diagnostic aid. Adebimpe (92, p. 69) suggests that "actuarial diagnoses by computer, consisting of the assignment of a diagnosis by comparing the index patient with

thousands of other patients would avoid basing diagnostic statements in data which are more valid for Whites" (see also Hedlund et al. [94]).

9. Using behavioral approaches to assessment (such as those in Turner and Jones [95]). This facilitates interventions on specific symptoms rather than syndromes and avoids the potential problem of focusing on too large a cluster of symptoms or complex syndromes.

IMPLICATIONS OF CROSS-CULTURAL PSYCHOTHERAPY RESEARCH FOR BLACK VIET NAM VETERANS

Recent psychotherapy research with black and low-income Americans has yielded data of relevance to black Viet Nam veterans. Research findings fall into six categories, as listed below:

1. Expectational variables (96),
2. Patient variables (97–100),
3. Therapist variables (100, 101),
4. Therapist-patient similarity (102–104),
5. Process variables (105–107), and
6. Outcome variables (51, 100, 103, 108).

Based on these research efforts, the following assertions can be made:

1. Black Viet Nam veterans bring their own psychic and social reality to treatment.
2. Traditional approaches to therapy are not congruent with the cultural and experiential (Viet Nam) needs of black Viet Nam veterans, especially during the early phases of intervention.
3. Black Viet Nam veterans in therapy believe that they need problem-solving advice and goal-directed interventions, rather than an experience of insight or reflection.
4. Veterans' perceptions of their needs may differ substantially from the therapist's view.
5. Black Viet Nam veterans are best able to benefit from psychotherapy when these services are offered by a therapist who is transculturally and transexperientially competent.
6. If a black or white Viet Nam veteran therapist or counselor is not available to a black Viet Nam veteran, a woman therapist of either race may be the next choice.

7. Most black Viet Nam veterans would seem to prefer a black therapist. However, a white therapist from a culturally marginal background may also be successful with this population.

THE INTERCULTURAL TREATMENT SETTING: CRITICAL INGREDIENTS OF A USEFUL PSYCHOTHERAPY

Imparting a Sense of Personal Power

The treatment of black Viet Nam veterans is conceptualized as a bipersonal process involving therapist and client. From my own experience, it is a technical error for the therapist to maintain a passive, "blank screen" posture and analyze transference and unconscious derivatives. The clinician should instead adhere to the here-and-now dynamics described by Lewin's (109) formula, $B = f(P, E)$ (that is, behavior is a function of the person *and* the environment). If this is done and the clinician is fully sensitized and aware—both transculturally (race) and transexperientially (effects of Viet Nam)—he or she will be able to engage the veteran in a therapy leading to restoration of morale and confidence.

The therapist's aim should be to assist black veterans in discovering, gaining, and maintaining a sense of self-generated power as they attempt to deal with their thoughts, feelings, and environment. This sense of power helps the veteran transcend the impediments of racism. For black Americans the issue of power is an emotionally charged, ever-present concern that must be addressed in treatment. This is as important for black Viet Nam veterans as is the understanding and integration of their Viet Nam and post–Viet Nam experiences.

I have conceptualized the complex task facing the therapist and black patients as a process of empowerment. Successful treatment leads black veterans to develop a sense of power, a feeling that they deserve the good things of life, and a belief that they are competent to live in the real world.

The Tridimensional Treatment Plan: A Model of Care

The tridimensional approach to the treatment of black Viet Nam veterans aims to provide patients with 1) a solid understanding of their problems, their expectations for treatment, and the expectations of the therapist; 2) satisfaction of their immediate psychosocial needs (such as career counseling and development or help with housing and in obtaining food stamps); and 3) exploration of their intrapsychic conflicts.

Roger is a 33-year-old black Viet Nam veteran who saw heavy combat during the Tet Offensive of 1968. He spent almost eight months in the bush and vividly remembers mutilated bodies, killings, terror, and despair. During the initial interview Roger was reluctant to discuss many aspects of his experience in Viet Nam and was generally unclear about the nature of his current problems. He did say that he had spent some 10 years after Viet Nam underemployed and had now been unemployed for several months. Roger is married for the second time and has four children—two from each marriage. He was also reluctant to discuss his previous marital difficulties and only vaguely mentioned that two of his children were learning disabled.

Roger had dropped out of high school at age 16 and had attempted to earn an equivalency diploma. However, he had been unable to do this because of concentration problems. Roger was the oldest of four children, in an intact family. His father died when he was 16 years of age, and the reason he left high school was to work and support the family. He was drafted into the Army at age 18 and was sent to fight in South Viet Nam.

In Viet Nam, Roger was on a search-and-destroy mission during which eight civilians, among them women and children, were killed. He then began to drink heavily. His drinking persisted for eight years after Viet Nam; he says he drank to "deal with my 'nervousness' because I was never the same when I came back." He complained also of somatic problems including headaches, joint pain, and stomach upset.

Roger avoided direct eye contact with the therapist. Initially, he did not seem as interested in exploring "the why" of his current problems as he was intent upon "the how" in solving them. He focused on solving his economic problems so that he could "take better care of my family and get myself together." Finally, he added "I think my problems are medical, aren't they?"

Focus I: Orienting Veterans to Treatment.   Experience with black Viet Nam veterans suggests that, because of their unique cultural and war experiences, they are often distrustful of mental health service providers. Often they are not aware of what to expect from treatment or what treatment requires of them. The first phase of treatment, which I call the orienting phase, helps to acquaint veterans with the treatment process and the realities of its limitations. Seeking mental health services is alien to black and low-income Americans. Black family members take pride in having been able to survive these many years without such services. They often feel that anyone seeking psychotherapy is weak or defective. Thus, an important part of the orienting phase involves helping patients abandon these prejudices. This will permit therapy to begin in earnest.

This phase also provides an overview of therapeutic issues, problems, and challenges. Cross-cultural issues are explored, sometimes employing visual aids and role induction techniques. A brief overview is given concerning Viet Nam, the nature of stress disorder, and the relationship of these to the veterans' current life difficulties.

The orienting phase for black Viet Nam veterans has the effect of reducing their anxiety and laying the foundation for a therapeutic relationship characterized by their commitment and trust.

This orientation period was very useful to Roger because in it he dealt with his concerns about therapy, Viet Nam, and his current life. He learned assertive skills during this period, which made it easier for him to work effectively in therapy; he also developed realistic therapeutic expectations. This latter occurrence was facilitated because the therapist detailed and constructed a forecast of what Roger should expect as he passed through the treatment. Because Roger's strengths and resources were identified, he developed a sense of optimism and could negotiate his treatment goals in behavioral terms.

Focus II: Psychoecological Therapy. This aspect of the trifocal approach focuses on the immediate environmental problems of the veteran. For Roger, this meant assisting him in contacting his children's school and arranging for an appropriate remedial program, securing his veterans benefits, entering an educational program to earn his high school diploma, securing his military records, and working toward improving his employment status. Intervention on the psychoecological level helped give Roger confidence in the therapeutic process. He felt that he was being helped in a manner that reduced life stress. Research and clinical evidence indicate that such social intervention meets the therapeutic expectations of blacks, other minorities, and low-income white Americans and is necessary for success of psychological treatment (51, 108, 110).

Focus III: Psychotherapy. This aspect of treatment must operate simultaneously with ecological intervention. In psychotherapy the therapist invites the veteran to explore his inner life in a well-focused, direct, and time-limited fashion. In the case of Roger, he was seen for six sessions in which limited therapeutic goals were identified and met. This number of visits approximates the national average for patients seen in both public and private settings (111).

At the outset Roger expressed relief that he would not have to remain in therapy for a long time. He was informed that after the six visits a reevaluation of his needs would be made, and that if he and his therapist agreed that further sessions were needed, the number could be extended. Most black veterans coming for assistance with their mental and social woes view psychotherapy as a treatment for "crazy folks"; by limiting the initial contact to six sessions the veteran is spared the feeling of being "mentally ill."

In therapy attentiveness to nonverbal communication is especially important with black veterans, since black Americans place great importance on nonverbal behavior (51). In fact, blacks trust nonverbal behavior more than talk and view nonverbal cues and actions as an accurate indicator of people's feelings and motives (112). Though it is generally believed that rapport is built by verbal means, cross-cultural therapists or counselors will have to depend on nonverbal indicators of trust on the part of black veterans and will have to develop the ability to convey their own helping attitude nonverbally.

During psychotherapy, it was at first extremely difficult for Roger to disclose details of his personal life. His white therapist, being trans-racially aware, was able to understand this problem of self-disclosure. While many white middle-class therapists become impatient with black veteran clients, Roger's did not. Though Journard (113) may be correct that mental health is often related to one's ability or willingness to self-disclose, in a cross-racial context with black clients this is not an accurate generalization. Black families communicate to the younger generations the historical necessity for "wearing the mask"—for hiding one's only unalterable possession, one's inner life. Clearly, during the days of slavery one's inner feelings, thoughts, and beliefs were the only things that white men could not take from their chattel. Therefore, for many blacks sharing too much too soon with a therapist is not only culturally impossible, but is an indicator of a failure of family tradition, as well as a sign of mental disease. In my experience this point is important for most Third World clients. For many black Viet Nam veterans, sharing of oneself is even more problematic: it has been complicated by the additional mental burden of shame over having killed Third World brothers and sisters in the war.

In his therapeutic work, as trust in his therapist developed, Roger had the opportunity to express his feelings of guilt over the deaths of the eight civilians. Gently and sensitively, his therapist inquired whether other persons close to him had died. A gush of tears came to Roger's eyes. He recalled his pain and agony when, at age 16, his father died and left him. He had never been able to reflect on his pain and loss. Experiencing the therapist as "safe," empathic, sensitive, and transculturally informed, Roger then shared a number of other emotional crises in his current life, involving his wife and children. Roger later told the therapist that this was the first time he had someone to talk to who would not condemn him for his black English, his mannerisms, and "just my style."

Because social interventions were moving along smoothly, and because the therapist's whiteness had been explored from the start, Roger now felt that he was really being helped and that he had the personal power to make a difference in his own life and in the lives of his wife and children. Ego-building techniques that focused on Roger's positive accomplishments, and his psychological and social strengths, proved extremely useful in expanding this man's self-awareness and increasing his self-esteem.

The use of visual and other psychoimagery techniques (114) is therapeutically effective with black Viet Nam veterans. These approaches seem congruent with the cognitive orientation of many black Americans: they are relatively independent of verbal communication. In his psychoimagery therapy, Roger experienced a sense of inner power and control over his mind and found a fruitful avenue to self-exploration, disclosure, and insight. These techniques, then, were of great importance in what was a successful therapeutic outcome. Indeed, Roger and his therapist agreed that by the close of this experience he was functioning as a husband, father, and wage earner.

Finally, it should be stressed again that Third World and lower-class clients have found behavioral methods to be congruent with their life-styles. According to Goldstein (115), the active, directive nature of behavior therapy meets the expectations of black and white poor and working class clients. Insight-oriented approaches are useful with black veterans, as they are with white veterans, but as with Roger, immediate social and environmental needs have to be addressed first. In the long run black veterans, as "triple survivors," must find through treatment a sense of self-affirmation and the capacity to consolidate their identity. As they build a cohesive self-organization, they will develop the ability to find new meaning in their lives (39).

REFERENCES

1. Young W: The black veteran: when Negroes in Viet Nam come home, in The Vietnam Veteran in Contemporary Society. Washington, DC, Veterans Administration Central Office, 1972

2. Mullen R: Blacks in America's Wars. New York, Delacorte, 1974

3. King ML Jr: Where Do We Go From Here: Chaos or Community? New York, Harper & Row, 1967

4. How Negro Americans perform in Vietnam. U.S. News and World Report, August 15, 1966, pp. 60–63

5. Binkin M, Eitelberg M: Blacks and the Military. Washington, DC, The Brookings Institution, 1982

6. Project One Hundred Thousand: Characteristics and Performance of the "New Standards" Men. Washington, DC, Office of the Assistant Secretary of Defense for Manpower and Reserve Affairs, 1969

7. Baskir LM, Strauss WA: Chance and Circumstance: The Draft, the War and the Viet Nam Generation. New York, Knopf, 1978

8. Sloan L, Phoenix H: The quality of race relations in the Viet Nam era military. Paper presented at the Annual Meeting of the Society for the Study of Social Problems. Boston, August 1979

9. Bryant H: The black veteran. Stars and Stripes—The National Tribune 105:5, June 1983

10. Parson E: The "gook" identification: its role in stress pathology in minority Viet Nam veterans. Paper presented at the First National Conference on Post-Viet Nam Stress Syndrome. Cincinnati, Ohio, October 1982

11. DuBose D: The minority Viet Nam veteran: delayed stress syndrome and dual character. Unpublished paper, 1981

12. Leventman S, Camacho P: The "Gook" syndrome: the Viet Nam War as a racial encounter, in Strangers at Home: Viet Nam Veterans Since the War. Edited by Figley CR, Leventman S. New York, Praeger, 1980

13. Terry W: Angry GIs "fed up" with the white man's war. Florida Times, June 21, 1970, p. 3

14. Department of Defense: Post-service earnings among men who separated from the army July 1968 through June 1969. Manpower Research Reports, Series MA-70-2, December 1970

15. Department of Defense: Post-service educational training and vocational status of army men separated July to September 1968. Manpower Research Reports, Series MA-70-1, October 1969

16. Egendorf A, Kadushin C, Laufer R, et al: Legacies of Viet Nam, vol 1–5. Washington DC, U.S. Government Printing Office, 1981

17. Fendrich J: The returning black Viet Nam era veteran. Paper presented at the 16th Annual Conference of the VA Cooperative Studies in Psychiatry, St. Louis, Mo, April 1971

18. Killian L: The Impossible Revolution? New York, Random House, 1968

19. Wrong people blamed again: black vets targeted for oppression. The Eclipse 4:2, Summer 1980

20. "Urban guerrilla force" of black vets behind Miami revolt: police. The Eclipse 4:2, Summer 1980

21. Military Discharge Policies and Practices Result in Wide Disparities: Congressional Review Is Needed. Government Accounting Report to Congress. Washington, DC, January 15, 1980

22. American Psychiatric Association: Diagnostic and Statistical Manual of Mental Disorders, Third Edition. Washington, DC, American Psychiatric Association, 1980

23. Lipkin J, Blank AS Jr, Parson E, et al: Viet Nam veterans and post-traumatic stress disorder. Hosp Community Psychiatry 33:908–912, 1982

24. Ursano R, Boydstrum J, Wheatley R: Psychiatric illness in U.S. Air Force Vietnam prisoners of war: a five-year follow-up. Am J Psychiatry 138:310–314, 1981

25. Krystal H: Massive Psychic Trauma. New York, International Universities Press, 1968

26. Lifton R: Death in Life: Survivors of Hiroshima. New York, Random House, 1968

27. Ader A: Mental symptoms following head injury. Archives of Neurology and Psychiatry 53:34–43, 1945

28. Forman B: Psychotherapy with rape victims. Psychotherapy: Theory, Research, and Practice 17:62–71, 1980

29. Bloch G, Bloch N: Analytic group psychotherapy of post-traumatic psychoses. Int J Group Psychother 26:47–57, 1976

30. Horowitz M, Wilner N, Kaltreider N, et al: Signs and symptoms of post-traumatic stress disorder. Arch Gen Psychiatry 35:85–92, 1980

31. Friedman R, Cohen K: The peer support group: a model for dealing with the emotional aspects of miscarriage. Group 4:42–48, 1980

32. Wolk R: Group psychotherapy process in the treatment of hostages taken in prison. Group 5:31–36, 1981

33. Corcoran J: The concentration camp syndrome and USAF Viet Nam prisoners of war. Psychiatric Annals 12:991–994, 1982

34. Ursano R: The Viet Nam era prisoner of war: precaptivity personality and the development of psychiatric illness. Am J Psychiatry 138:315–318, 1981

35. Moses R, Bargel D, Calev J, et al: A rear unit for the treatment of combat reactions in the wake of the Yom Kippur War. Psychiatry 39:153–168, 1976

36. Archibald H, Tuddenham R: Persistent stress reaction after combat. Arch Gen Psychiatry 12:475–481, 1965

37. Blank AS Jr: First Training Conference Papers on Viet Nam Veterans: Operation Outreach. St. Louis, Mo, Veterans Administration, September 1979

38. Figley C (ed): Stress Disorders Among Viet Nam Veterans. New York, Brunner/Mazel, 1978

39. Parson E: The reparation of the self: clinical and theoretical dimensions in the treatment of Viet Nam combat veterans. J Contemp Psychother 14, 4–56, 1984

40. Washington Urban League, National Urban League Disabled Veterans Employment Project: Who Says I Can't Work? (Pamphlet) Washington, DC, The Urban League, 1978

41. Yager T, Laufer R, Gallops M: Some problems associated with war in men of the Vietnam generation. Arch Gen Psychiatry 41:327–333, 1984

42. Kadushin C, Boulanger G, Martin J: Some causes, consequences, and naturally occurring support systems, in Legacies of Viet Nam, vol 4. Washington, DC, U.S. Government Printing Office, 1981

43. Parson E: NYSCP's commitment to minority psychologists and patients.

The New York Society of Clinical Psychologists Newsletter. Summer, 1980, pp 14–19

44. Korman M: National conference on levels and patterns of professional training in psychology. Am Psychol 29:441–449, 1974

45. Dunbar P: We wear the mask, in Lyrics of Lonely Life. New York, Dodd, Mead, 1897

46. Douglass F: The Life and Times of Frederick Douglass. Boston, De-Wolfe, Koske, 1982

47. Du Bois W (ed): The Soul of Black Folks. Chicago, McClurg, 1903

48. Brawley B: Negro Builders and Heroes. University of North Carolina Press, Chapel Hill, NC, 1937

49. Baldwin J: Notes from a Native Son. Boston, Beacon, 1955

50. Lester J (ed): The Seventh Son: The Thoughts and Writings of W.E.B. Du Bois, vol 1 and 2. New York, Doubleday, 1971

51. Sue D: Counseling the Culturally Different. New York, John Wiley & Sons, 1981

52. Thomas A, Sillen S: Racism and Psychiatry. New York, Brunner/Mazel, 1972

53. Brislin RW, Pedersen P: Cross-Cultural Orientation Programs. New York, Krieger, 1976

54. Parson E: The black Viet Nam veteran: his representational world in post-traumatic stress disorder, in Postraumatic Stress Disorders and the War Veteran Patient. Edited by Kelly W. New York, Brunner/Mazel, in press

55. Ader B: Letters From Viet Nam. New York, Dutton, 1977

56. Blank AS Jr: Apocalypse terminable and interminable: operation outreach for Viet Nam veterans. Hosp Community Psychiatry 33:913–918, 1982

57. Bourne P: Men, Stress, and Viet Nam. Boston, Little, Brown, 1970

58. Brende JO, Parson ER: Viet Nam Veterans: The Road to Recovery. New York, Plenum Press, 1985

59. Bryant C: Friendly Fire. New York, Putnam, 1976

60. Caputo P: A Rumor of War. New York, Holt, Rinehart & Winston, 1977

61. Harris and Associates: Myths and Realities: A Study of Attitudes Toward Viet Nam Era Veterans. Washington, DC, Harris and Associates, 1980

62. Fairbank J, Langley K, Jariri G, et al: A selected bibliography on post-traumatic stress disorders in Viet Nam veterans. Professional Psychology 12:578–586, 1981

63. Figley C, Leventman S (eds): Strangers At Home: Vietnam Veterans Since the War. New York, Praeger Press, 1980

64. Finman B, Borus J, Stanton M: Black-white and American-Vietnamese relations among soldiers in Viet Nam. Journal of Social Issues 31:39–48, 1975

65. Goff S, Sanders R: Brothers: Black Soldiers in the Nam. New York, Presidio, 1982

66. Herr M: Dispatches. New York, Knopf, 1977

67. Kovic R: Born on the Fourth of July. New York, McGraw-Hill, 1976

68. Santoli A: Everything We Had: An Oral History of the Viet Nam War as Told by 33 American Soldiers Who Fought It. New York, Random House, 1981

69. Webb J: Fields of Fire. New York, Bantam Press, 1979

70. Blank AS Jr: Unconscious flashback to the war in Viet Nam. Paper presented at the Annual Meeting of the American Psychological Association, Montreal, Quebec, September 1980, revised 1981 and 1983

71. Brende JO: Combined individual and group therapy for Vietnam veterans. Int J Group Psychother 31:367–378, 1981

72. Brende J: A psychodynamic view of character pathology in Viet Nam combat veterans. Bull Menninger Clin 47:193–216, 1983

73. DeFazio V: Dynamic perspectives on the nature and effects of combat stress, in Stress Disorders in Viet Nam Veterans. Edited by Figley CR. New York, Brunner/Mazel, 1978

74. Fox R: Post-combat adaptation problems. Compr Psychiatry 13:435–443, 1972

75. Fox R: Narcissistic rage and the problems of combat aggression. Arch Gen Psychiatry 31:807–811, 1974

76. Fairbank J, Keane T: Flooding for combat-related stress disorders: assessment of anxiety reduction across traumatic memories. Behavior Therapy 13:499–510, 1982

77. Kardiner A: The Traumatic Neurosis of War (Psychosomatic Medical Monograph). New York, Paul Hoebel, 1941

78. Haley S: When the patient reports atrocities. Arch Gen Psychiatry 30:191–196, 1977

79. Keane T, Kaloupek D: Imaginal flooding in the treatment of a post-traumatic stress disorder. J Consult Clin Psychol 50:138–140, 1982

80. Kipper DA: Behavior therapy for fears brought on by war experiences. J Consult Clin Psychol 45:216–221, 1977

81. Shatan C: The tattered ego of the survivor. Psychiatric Annals 12:1031–1038, 1982

82. Williams T (ed): Post-Traumatic Stress Disorders of the Viet Nam Veteran. Cincinnati, Disabled American Veterans, 1980

83. Wilson J: Conflict, stress, and growth: the effects of the Viet Nam War on psychosocial development among Viet Nam veterans, in Strangers At Home: Viet Nam Veterans Since the War. Edited by Figley CR, Leventman S. New York, Praeger Press, 1980

84. Van Putten T, Emory W: Traumatic neurosis in Viet Nam returnees. Arch Gen Psychiatry 29:695–698, 1973

85. Solomon G, Zarcone B, Yoorg R, et al: Three psychiatric casualties from Viet Nam. Arch Gen Psychiatry 25:522–524, 1971

86. Adebimpe V: Overview: white norms and psychiatric diagnosis of black patients. Am J Psychiatry 138:279–285, 1981

87. Parson E: The Kardiner-Ovesey fallacy: psychoanalytic formulation of the black personality revisited. Paper presented at the Third Annual Symposium on Selected Issues in Psychotherapy Highlighted by Minority Status. New York, Postgraduate Center for Mental Health, 1981

88. Carter J: Recognizing psychiatric symptoms in black Americans. Geriatrics 29:97–99, 1974

89. Kardiner A, Ovesey L: The Mark of Oppression. Cleveland, World Publishing Co, 1962

90. Halpern F: Survival: Black/White. New York, Pergamon Press, 1973

91. DeHoyos A, DeHoyos G: Symptomatology differentials between Negro and white schizophrenics. Int J Soc Psychiatry 11:245, 1965

92. Adebimpe V: Psychiatric symptoms in black patients, in Behavior Modification in Black Populations: Psychosocial Issues and Empirical Findings. Edited by Turner SM, Jones RT. New York, Plenum Press, 1982

93. Raskin A, Crook T, Herman K: Psychiatric history and symptom differences in black and white depressed patients. J Consult Clin Psychol 43:73–80, 1975

94. Hedlend J, Evenson R, Sletten I, et al: The computer and clinical prediction, in Technology in Mental Health Care Delivery Systems. Edited by Sidowski JB, Johnson J, Williams TA. Norwood, NJ, Ablex Publishing, 1980

95. Turner SM, Jones RT: Behavior Modification in Black Populations. New York, Plenum Press, 1982

96. Goldstein A: Structured Learning Therapy: Toward a Psychotherapy for the Poor. New York, Academic Press, 1973

97. Hollingshead A, Redlich F: Social Class and Mental Illness: A Community Study. New York, Wiley, 1958

98. Lorion R: Research on psychotherapy and behavior change with the disadvantaged: past, present, and future directions, in Handbook of Psychotherapy and Behavior Change: An Empirical Analysis, 2nd ed. Edited by Garfield S, Bergen A. New York, John Wiley & Sons, 1978

99. Sundberg N: Cross-cultural counseling and psychotherapy: a research overview, in Cross-Cultural Counseling and Psychotherapy. Edited by Marcella A, Pedersen P. New York, Basic Books, 1981

100. Acosta FX: Self-described for premature termination of psychotherapy by Mexican American and Anglo-American patients. Psychol Rep 47:435–443, 1980

101. Howard K, Orlinsky D: Psychotherapeutic processes. Annual Review of Psychology 23:615–668, 1972

102. Harrison I: Race as a counselor-client variable in counseling and psycho-

therapy: a review of the research. The Counseling Psychologist 5:124–133, 1975

103. Parloff M, Waskow I, Wolfe B: Research on therapist variables in relation to process and outcome, in Handbook of Psychotherapy and Behavior Change: An Empirical Analysis, 2nd ed. Edited by Garfield S, Bergen A. New York, John Wiley & Sons, 1978

104. Vail A: Factors influencing lower-class black patients remaining in treatment. J Consult Clin Psychol 46:341–349, 1978

105. Merluzzi T, Merluzzi B, Kaul T: Counselor race and power base: the effects on attitudes and behaviors. Journal of Counseling Psychology 24:430–436, 1977

106. Schmidt L, Strong S: Attractiveness and influence in counseling. Journal of Counseling Psychology 18:348–351, 1971

107. Speigel S: Expertness, similarity and perceived counselor competence. Journal of Counseling Psychology 23: 436–441, 1976

108. Acosta F, Yamamoto J, Evans L: Effective Psychotherapy for Low-Income and Minority Patients. New York, Plenum Press, 1982

109. Lewin K: Field Theory and Social Science. New York, Harper & Row, 1951

110. Lorion R: Patient and therapist variables in the treatment of low-income patients. Psychol Bull 81:344–354, 1974

111. Lorion R: Social class differences in treatment attitudes and expectations. Unpublished doctoral dissertation. New York, University of Rochester, 1972

112. Willie C, Kramer B, Brown D: Racism and Mental Health. Pittsburgh, University of Pittsburgh Press, 1973

113. Journard S: The Transparent Self. Princeton, NJ, Van Nostrand, 1964

114. Shorr J, Sobel P, Connella J: Imagery: Its Many Dimensions and Applications. New York, Plenum Press, 1980

115. Goldstein A: Psychotherapeutic Attraction. New York, Pergamon Press, 1971

19

Diagnosis and Treatment of Post-Traumatic Stress Disorder in Hispanic Viet Nam Veterans

Gregorio Piña, III, Ph.D.

19

In the 1980s Hispanic Americans will number 19,000,000. They are the second-largest ethnic minority in the United States (1). Hispanic veterans, descendants of Mexican-Americans, Puerto Ricans, Cubans, and Latin Americans, are an important veteran minority. Over 19 percent of Hispanic Americans in Viet Nam combat were wounded or killed (2), and traditionally Hispanics have been among the most decorated American combat soldiers (3).

Post-traumatic stress disorder in Viet Nam veterans has been described in detail (4–6). The disorder can vary in different cultures, and specific culturally determined treatment needs, if unmet, result in underutilization of services. Other related problems are overdiagnosing of psychopathology and premature termination of treatment by culturally insensitive professionals (7–10).

HISPANIC IDENTITY AS AMERICAN WARRIOR

Mucho antes de que llegaron los peregrinos a la Roca de Plymouth, mis nobles antepasados habian vivido aqui por generaciones. Teniamos sistemas de educacion, transportacion, arquitectura, communicaciones, astronomia, medicina, ciencias. . . . ¿Que pasa? O; No entienden. . . . Excuse me, you don't speak Spanish. I was saying that long before the Pilgrims landed at Plymouth Rock, my noble ancestors had been living here for generations. Our societies had systems of education, transportation, architecture, communication, astronomy, medicine, the sciences, taxes, religions, etc. But several factors, like conquerors and "Manifest Destiny," changed our history, languages, and governments and destroyed and broadened the roots of our identity.

My individual acculturation to "American" society began when I entered the first grade. The first English words I learned were "I pledge allegiance to the flag of the United States of America. . . ." Simultane-

391

ously, I learned and lived the pride that Hispanics have been the most decorated minority group warriors in the history of this country. This has been a double-edged sword for Hispanics, because our role as front line combatants has taken a disproportionate toll on our youth.

After World War II, we moved from agricultural valleys to the factories of cities. This was the chance to furnish our children with better opportunities. That was before Viet Nam. While we suffered disproportionate casualties in Viet Nam, we came back to fewer jobs and a realization that our youths' idealism, as well as their lives and limbs, had been ruthlessly used by those in power. Since the end of that war we have come to realize that it ate at the fabric of our individual identities.

As in previous wars, many Hispanic soldiers understood English poorly, some not at all. My speaking Spanish initially was not to mock you; it was to demonstrate the futile feeling of Viet Nam combat for many Hispanics. (based on reference 11)

FACTORS INFLUENCING HISPANIC IDENTITY AND POST-TRAUMATIC STRESS DISORDER

There has been an appropriate focus by psychodynamic theorists and clinicians on issues of identity when discussing PTSD in Viet Nam veterans. Ethnic identity involves a psychocultural dimension related to family and peer group socialization patterns, and to their interaction with past cultural traditions, immediate sociological factors, and larger social and political realities (12). In general, for Hispanics, the family system is of paramount importance. This includes the family of origin, family of procreation, extended family, and even close family friends. Saunders (13) and Madsen (14) indicate that many psychological problems are less severe in Mexican-American communities because of the emotional support provided by strong family structures. However, this hypothesis is also questioned in the literature (15).

With respect to identity formation and diagnosis and treatment, however, Hispanic culture (Mexican-American, Cuban, Puerto Rican, and Latin American) may be variously described as rigid, narrow, and defensive in one geographical area or flexible and incorporating in an adjoining neighborhood. Individuals may define a sense of self by maintaining barriers against potentially enriching experiences with other cultural groups. Among such individuals communication may appear clinically dysfunctional (11). In Hispanic veterans, then, PTSD may be masked and may masquerade as paranoia, machismo, a defensive posture, or a denial of symptoms.

Identity in Hispanics is further complicated by different types of acculturation (low, high, or multiacculturation). Participation in more than one culture—multiculturalism—or in widely different aspects of a sociocultural system, promotes personality flexibility, synthesis of experience, and subsequent expansion of one's behavioral repertoire (11). Language preference in psychotherapy, success in academia, and certain vocational choices are often related to being highly acculturated to the macrosociety. High acculturation permits traditional types of psychological interventions.

DeVos (12) describes a further effect of minority adaptation on identity maintenance. The minority individual may emphasize cognitive function, while abandoning his or her feelings about others. Ethnic identity can then be cast off or manipulated, depending on circumstances. This appears to resemble the psychoanalytic concept of splitting, although it can be carried out either consciously or unconsciously. The clinician's recognition of adaptation through identity denial not only assists with diagnosis, but also helps treatment when multiple patterns of acculturation and resultant defenses are present.

It is critical that the clinician who is not experienced with Hispanic culture understand the rich and extensive diversity which exists within each Hispanic culture (16). The common Spanish language causes the macrosociety to view these cultures as homogeneous. Failing to distinguish between different groups of Hispanics is analogous to ignorance of cultural differences between American blacks and Jews, British royalty and Irish farmers, or South African businessmen and Australian oilfield workers.

It is also important to distinguish between the influence of the culture of poverty and Hispanic culture on Viet Nam combatants. It is well known that in Viet Nam, as in previous wars, a disproportionate number of combatants came from economically disadvantaged groups (17). Hispanics were the second largest minority in Viet Nam. During the 1960s those who avoided the draft did so by going to college. In general, economically disadvantaged Hispanics have not done well in the educational system, and the college route of avoiding the military was therefore unavailable to most Hispanic youths.

THE DIAGNOSIS OF STRESS DISORDER
IN HISPANIC VETERANS

Many returning Hispanic veterans readjusted satisfactorily. Especially for the noncombatant, the readjustment to civilian life often proceeded smoothly. In this chapter, though, I shall discuss Hispanic Viet Nam combatants whose readjustment was stormy.

Often, like the individuals described by Benedek (18) and Milano

(19), Hispanic combat veterans had not noticed how far they had moved from their roots until they returned home with an altered personality. Milano described this process of personality change as "pronounced restructuring" of outlook following dramatic life experience.

The sociopolitical maturation of a soldier is accelerated by exposure to war and the subsequent transition to peace. This experience challenges the sense of self-continuity, and a painful struggle to find meaning and significance in one's life often ensues. Post–Viet Nam history in such cases may reveal chronic psychasthenia, depression, underachievement, and lack of progression toward major life goals.

The *Diagnostic and Statistical Manual of Mental Disorders, Third Edition* (20) lists criteria for the diagnosis of PTSD. Manifestation of symptoms is sometimes influenced by drug or alcohol abuse (18) or by pronounced identity change (4, 5, 19, 21). Either may increase the likelihood of misdiagnosis.

In response to the traumatic fear of annihilation an individual may have denied perceptions of immediate death and may have ignored the presence of danger. Psychic numbing may have developed. In cases where a veteran with PTSD is numb and disinterested, family members can be helpful in the clinical assessment. Interviewing close relatives not only allows discovery of specific symptoms (for example, a history of sleeping with weapons, nightmares, or problems with intimacy), but reinforces the healing potential of the family system.

The family physician is often helpful in evaluating and treating such symptoms as psychophysiological reactions, drug abuse, chronic anxiety, or depression. This is consistent with the observations of Karno and Edgerton (22), who write that Hispanics rely heavily on family physicians for help with emotional problems.

SOME PROFILES OF HISPANIC VIET NAM VETERANS

Viet Nam veterans are described elsewhere (23). Here the focus will be on variations specific to language, culture, and combat experience.

One type of Hispanic veteran was economically disadvantaged as a child, preferred Spanish, did poorly academically, dropped out of school, and was initially rejected from the military. This rejection led to significant concerns about manliness, or "machismo." After problems with the law—usually involving traffic violations, disorderly conduct, or public intoxication—the individual was reclassified "for the convenience of the government."

These men seem to have preferred being in the bush, not in the rear. They say they wanted to prove something, to find their niche, to show that they were not "rejects." Often they felt that this was their "once in a lifetime chance," the time to be "in uniform," to succeed in a task of manhood, a task of importance to the community. These individuals appear to have been willing to follow others blindly regarding free-fire zones, body counts, and extra duty. They boast of shunning the noncombat soldier.

Psychoneurological testing reveals a range of findings, such as aphasias and learning and language disabilities. There may be a significant pretrauma history of acting out and impulse control difficulties. A propensity to stay within traditional Hispanic culture may be evident. Anxiety is often found in these veterans, along with regressive use of Viet Nam behavior in postwar situations.

If a clinician unaware of PTSD made a previous diagnosis, it may be schizophrenia, sociopathy, or borderline personality disorder. For this type of Hispanic veteran, Viet Nam served to reinforce a previous identity as an inferior person. These men also suffer from a "profound shattering of images of self and humanity," as described by Blank (24). They give the impression that they have lost faith in the human capacity for goodness (24).

A second type of Hispanic veteran is the individual who as a youngster was average or better academically, finished high school, was then underemployed or unemployed, and entered the military to "pay his debt" to his country. These individuals also attempted to distinguish themselves in combat, conforming to the culturally reinforced view of heroic soldiering. Generally, their traumatic experiences have been dealt with by psychic numbing. Typical stress disorder breakthroughs have, however, made total denial impossible.

Some members of this second group have adopted the soldier identity and have proven vulnerable to agents who recruit soldiers of fortune or mercenaries. The political situation in Central America, their expertise in jungle guerrilla warfare, and their language capabilities make these veterans desirable recruits. If they are unemployed, they are even more receptive. Such a return to guerrilla warfare, like flashbacks and other forms of acute reliving of traumatic events, can be a symptom of PTSD.

There is a third group of Hispanic veterans. These men are neurologically sound and have a seemingly unremarkable pre–Viet Nam adjustment history. Issues of dependency, competition, and sexism were dealt with in culturally appropriate ways (16). They do develop PTSD, and their histories reveal the following contributing factors: a) trauma which takes on symbolic significance, b) subtle signs of weak personality structures as noted in careful reevaluation of adjustment to previous experiences, c) attempts at secondary gain, d) immaturity revealed by severe emotional conflicts at the time of traumatization, and e) ineffective efforts at treatment or support after trauma.

MACHISMO AND GUERRILLA WARFARE

Although, in general, predisposition is an important factor in PTSD, the brutality of guerrilla warfare dramatically elicits the most primitive aspects of machismo. Traumatic war experiences overwhelm individuals, who defend against fears of annihilation by splitting off emotions and memories. Thus, to accept the image of self as hunter and killer after the war becomes a therapeutic task.

Chronic exposure to dehumanization, killing, waste, and terrorism is incongruent with the traditions of Hispanic culture and the individual's previous identity. The therapist's task is to help the veteran accept and find meaning in the war experience. Survivor guilt, the need for expiation, and the need to mourn are often troubling. Some Hispanic veterans initially identified with the people of Southeast Asia, complicating their readjustment. The elusiveness of the enemy, the atrocities performed on our troops when captured, the isolation and danger of patrols, and the distrust of children and the elderly because of sabotage all brought about a type of prejudice against Asians, sometimes acted upon. This, too, complicates readjustment.

TREATMENT

Individuals relate to others on a continuum from the superficial to the intimate. The initial therapeutic goal is to develop a workable relationship. Within Hispanic cultures, relationships—especially between men —hold important meaning. Roll et al. (7) note that with Hispanics the therapeutic relationship can be intensely personalized, yet formal. The therapist must be aware of this and not react by pulling back.

Countertransference anxiety should be dealt with by proper consultation or supervision. In sum, the therapist must maintain the level of intimacy needed by the Hispanic veteran.

Initially the therapist's knowledge of Viet Nam and PTSD will assist in motivating Hispanic veterans to involve themselves in psychotherapy. However, knowledge that the veteran's suffering is understood, and emerging hope, may be followed by expressions of futility or depression. This reflects a resistance resulting in part from the need to block painful memories. The therapist needs to be aware of such defenses and interpret their use nonjudgmentally.

In PTSD, therapeutic warmth shows veterans that they are accepted and understood. This reinforces self-expression and guides resolution. Therapeutic confrontation with low-acculturated Hispanics can backfire because veterans can misperceive it as rejection or even as evidence of prejudice.

Hispanic veterans are often assisted by neutral questions regarding the chronological sequence of military events. Successful therapy requires dosing of probing comments. In contrast to typical psychotherapy, where the therapist maintains pressure for growth through silence, confrontation, and comment, with combat veterans it is sometimes necessary to reduce emotional pressure in order to reinforce effective ego functioning.

Treatment often involves clarifying previous emotional conflicts and models of the self which made the Hispanic veteran more vulnerable to the effects of trauma. In part because of evolving maturity in other areas, veterans are often ready in therapy to modify existing defense patterns. Reappraisal of trauma and its meaning is then possible.

Therapeutic trust must be reinforced before exploring traumatic events. While many Hispanic Viet Nam veterans speak of feeling "numb," the therapeutic relationship will reveal an intensity previously experienced in combat. This can approach symbiosis. Mutually interdependent combat relationships, established for survival purposes, served needs for nurturing (25). Seasoned therapists understand this level of intimacy. They also help the veteran explore memories which contain descriptions of "smelling gooks, death, the soil, etc." These reflect survival skills necessary in the war. Discussion of all this with the therapist helps the veteran approach and explore painful history.

Deaths of buddies take on special meaning in the transference relationship. Clarification of the "part self" (buddy) (25) that was killed is important because it can be experienced as a form of annihilation. Survival guilt is also relevant. The inability to mourn during combat, because of the requirements of survival, leave the veteran barren of feeling regarding the death of a buddy. Therefore, discussion of such events should be repeated as the veteran tolerates. For purposes of support, therapeutic clarification of the combat role and understanding of episodes of brutality by the veteran are important.

Building on all this, therapy can be directed toward mourning; this has been useful with Hispanic veterans. For veterans to learn to grieve, the therapist must explore with them the meaning of service and death in Viet Nam. Driven by idealism and culturally determined zeal to defend their country and the world from Communism, Hispanic veterans gradually awakened to the nightmare that the military goal in Viet Nam was ill-defined. Participation in Viet Nam also promised a better future at home. However, in the end Hispanic veterans felt disillusioned, doubted the value of Viet Nam service, questioned the sacrifice of their dead comrades, wished they had not killed, and felt less advantaged than many who had avoided service in the military. All of this must be explored in treatment. Hispanic Viet Nam survivors must also come to realize that their painful experiences have moral consequences, especially related to Hispanic ideals.

Distrust of the macrosociety and adaptation to mainstream America are complicated by the Viet Nam Hispanic experience. It is hard for veterans to understand the present, separate it from the past, fulfill personal ambitions, and focus individual strengths and idealism. The stagnation of personal, social, and employment development is likely to be accompanied by anger. Mapping out different life possibilities involving oneself and others is another therapeutic step.

HISPANIC FAMILY INVOLVEMENT

PTSD in Hispanic veterans is often manifested by marital, family, and interpersonal difficulties. The literature reveals family dysfunction and divorce in veterans suffering from stress, and therapists treating Hispanic veterans often see a need for marital therapy. Family oriented Hispanic culture further encourages such therapeutic interventions. In any event, a spouse or family interview to obtain historical data and provide orientation is useful.

Frequently in Hispanic families there is vacillation between emotional support and rebuke and criticism of the veteran, and even explosiveness toward him. Families are often aware that an unhappy member may strike out in a safe place. The family creates such an environment and the result is that the veteran relives the emotions of the combat situation within the family. This process, naively encouraged by loved ones, has left many Hispanic families scarred.

Veterans may encourage a spouse's denial of personal problems. Periods of increased marital discord may ensue, and in part owing to heightened emotions, symptoms are not resolved. A reinforcement of specific symptoms used to cope with stress may even occur.

Reliving of trauma or numbing may occur at such times, rebuke and criticism will be rampant in the family, and complaints regarding the veteran's poor adaptation are likely from family members. Interactional patterns may even reverse, with the veteran and spouse switching roles in the dyad.

Treating the Hispanic veteran alone has brought about transitory relief in some cases. However, the marriage relationship often reinforces the avoidance of intimacy and maintains pathogenic interpersonal behaviors. Family therapeutic interventions in these cases bring about clarifications concerning personal emotional dysfunctions, fears of abandonment, and the lack of models allowing long-term satisfactory relationships.

The process of treatment is straightforward. The spouse is formally invited to psychotherapy as ally, historian, and a possible agent of change. Fears of exposure and criticism are dealt with supportively and compassionately. The therapist offers a didactic description of the etiology and treatment of PTSD in Hispanic veterans. Treatment goals and duration are established. The spouse's presence promotes intimacy and a sharing of the burden of mourning. Hispanic veterans rarely relate wartime traumatic experiences to their spouses prior to treatment, so the therapeutic involvement of wives and significant others is crucial.

In treatment seemingly overwhelming challenges are divided into manageable, culturally relevant tasks. Culturally reinforced individual strengths are selectively supported. Therapy also involves catharsis. Ventilation of emotional pain has usually been discouraged in the Hispanic veteran's environment, where emotional control and superficial signs of courage are valued. The therapist facilitates the limited discussion of pain to permit all involved to get used to it, especially because the Hispanic veteran's suffering has unintentionally been reinforced by silence. The therapeutic goal is to facilitate the expression of grief, in circumscribed ways, in a culturally supportive framework.

SPECIAL ISSUES

Language

Especially with low-acculturated Hispanic veterans, language is an important issue. A Spanish-speaking professional facilitates the therapeutic process. When a Spanish-speaking therapist is not available, consultation by the therapist with an Hispanic colleague is helpful. If a language barrier is present, the therapist must keep sentences short and respectfully restrict interventions to areas where the therapist's language skills are adequate. Involvement with others in the veteran's family who speak English can be very useful.

Culturally Based Treatment

Each Hispanic culture has specific psychological treatment approaches for different problems, such as depression or anxiety. Therefore, culture-specific interventions may be appropriate at different times during treatment. A consultation between psychotherapist and cultural "healer" (such as a Curandero) may be useful.

TERMINATION

After exploration of the impact of Viet Nam trauma, termination begins. The therapist supports the veteran's attempt to incorporate the traumatic event and its aftermath into his cultural identity. Finding culturally approved aspects of painful experience and modifying identity appropriately is indicated. The Hispanic veteran is thus freed to recover from PTSD.

During the termination process current life stressors are confronted in new ways. The veteran also begins to consider the approaching loss of the therapist, which can trigger an exacerbation of old symptoms. Gradual working through of the separation reinforces previously developed techniques of modifying identity, adapting, and reducing the effects of stress (26). Therapist and patient also identify residual symptoms that the veteran will work on after termination.

In termination with Hispanic veterans the therapist continues to interpret the use of specific defenses and encourages further development of the observing ego. Planned follow-up is routine in these cases. This encourages the patient to establish further goals, which are culturally compatible. Thus, cultural cues reinforce ongoing psychological growth.

REFERENCES

1. Becerra RM, Greenblatt M: The mental-seeking behavior of Hispanic veterans. Compr Psychiatry 22:124–133, 1981

2. U.S. Department of Defense: Hispanics in America's Defense. Washington, DC, U.S. Government Printing Office, 1983

3. U.S. Department of Defense: Hispanic Heritage Week—Medal of Honor. Washington, DC, U.S. Government Printing Office, 1980

4. Figley CR (ed): Stress Disorders Among Viet Nam Veterans. New York, Brunner/Mazel, 1978

5. Figley CR, Leventman S: Strangers at Home. New York, Praeger Press, 1980

6. Wilson JP: Forgotten warrior project (mimeo). Cleveland State University, 1977

7. Roll S, Millen L, Martinez R: Common errors in psychotherapy with Chicanos: extrapolations from research and clinical experience. Psychotherapy: Theory, Research and Practice 17:158–168, 1980

8. Newton F: The Mexican American emic system of mental illness: an exploratory study. Spanish Speaking Mental Health Research Center Monograph Series 7:69–90, 1978

9. Padilla AM, Carlos ML, Keefe SE: Mental health service utilization by Mexican Americans. Spanish Speaking Mental Health Research Center Monograph Series 3:9–20, 1976

10. Martinez J (ed): Chicano Psychology. New York, Academic Press, 1977

11. Piña G: The historical identity of Mexican-American soldiers. (mimeo). Paper presented at the Second Training Conference, Operation Outreach. Pocano, Pa, Veterans Administration, 1981

12. DeVos GA: Ethnic adaptation and minority status. Journal of Cross-Cultural Psychology 2:101–124, 1980

13. Saunders L: Cultural Difference and Medical Care: The Case of the Spanish Speaking People of the Southwest. New York, Russell Sage Foundation, 1954

14. Madsen W: Value conflicts and folk psychiatry in South Texas, in Magic, Faith, and Healing. Edited by Kiev A. New York, The Free Press, 1964

15. Padilla AM, Ruiz RA, Alvarez R: Delivery of community mental health services to the Spanish-speaking/surnamed population. Spanish Speaking Mental Health Research Center Monograph Series 2:11–35, 1975

16. Gonzales J: The effects of language and culture on the assessment of psychopathology. Unpublished doctoral dissertation, University of Houston, 1976

17. Piña G: An investigation into the effects of language and acculturation in the assessment of psychopathology of Chicano neurotic males using the TAT. Unpublished doctoral dissertation, Washington, DC, The American University, 1978

18. Benedek T: Insight and Personality Adjustment: A Study of the Psychological Effects of War. New York, Ronald Press, 1946

19. Milano F: The politicization of the "deer hunters": power and authority perspectives of the Viet Nam veteran, in Strangers at Home. Edited by Figley CR, Leventman S. New York, Praeger Press, 1980

20. American Psychiatric Association: Diagnostic and Statistical Manual of Mental Disorders, Third Edition. Washington, DC, American Psychiatric Association, 1980

21. Zarcone VP Jr, Scott NR, Kauvar KB: Psychiatric problems of Viet Nam veterans: clinical study of hospital patients. Compr Psychiatry 18:41–53, 1977

22. Karno M, Edgerton RB: Perceptions of mental illness in a Mexican-American community. Arch Gen Psychiatry 20:233–238, 1969

23. Walker JI, Cavenar JO, Jr: Viet Nam veterans and their problems continue. J Nerv Ment Dis 170:174–180, 1982

24. Blank AS Jr: Stress of war: the example of Viet Nam, in Handbook of Stress: Theoretical and Clinical Aspects. Edited by Goldberger L, Breznitz S. New York, The Free Press, 1982

25. Brende JO: A psychodynamic view of character pathology in Viet Nam combat veterans. Bull Menninger Clin 47:193–216, 1983

26. Cameron R, Meichenbaum D: The nature of effective coping and the treatment of stress related problems: a cognitive behavioral perspective, in Handbook of Stress: Theoretical and Clinical Aspects. Edited by Goldberger L, Brenitz S. New York, The Free Press, 1982

20

Incarcerated Viet Nam Veterans

Bruce Pentland, M.P.A.
James Dwyer, M.S.W.

20

Even the best of men couldn't begin to realize what the war did to human beings. How it made good men bent and worse men blind.

—An Army Medic in Viet Nam

The effect of war on the warrior has been observed by artists through the ages. Ernest Hemingway's Krebs, in the story "Soldier's Home," is a World War I veteran who returns home to an experience of isolation and alienation. Krebs thinks that his salvation lies in escaping, in moving to another town.

Like Krebs, some Viet Nam veterans never really come home, but roam from one city to the next in search of a spiritual homecoming. Other Viet Nam veterans "come home" via criminal behavior and incarceration. The magnitude of this problem is unclear at this time, because studies that have been done up to now have not accurately measured this population, nor have they focused on specific experiences that lead some Viet Nam veterans into such a way of life

We will attempt to assess the magnitude and characteristics of this troubled group and describe an innovative project designed to assist incarcerated veterans. The Veterans in Prison Program (1) provides rehabilitative services to veterans, using several treatment approaches. An illustrative case study is also included.

As incarcerated Viet Nam veterans grow older, the opportunity for rehabilitation decreases; their pattern of antisocial action becomes more ingrained, and they see themselves as aliens existing outside "straight" society. Thus, timely and effective intervention that addresses criminal behavior as well as the Viet Nam experience is needed so that these veterans will not become career criminals who view incarceration as inevitable.

THE SCOPE OF THE PROBLEM

One popular stereotype holds that Viet Nam veterans have a significant chance of winding up in jail or prison. Articles continue to appear that suggest that as many as 50 percent of prison inmates are Viet Nam returnees. Reality is much less dramatic: current data indicate that Viet Nam veterans (those who actually saw service in Viet Nam) constitute five to 10 percent of the population of state prisons (2, 3). There are no accurate data for such men in federal prisons, local jails, or on parole or probation.

From the available data, incarcerated Viet Nam veterans do seem more disposed to violent crime than do incarcerated nonveterans. The overall picture indicates, however, that both groups suffer many of the same problems (such as alcohol and drug abuse) (Table 1). There is also a significant difference in the pattern of incarceration between Viet Nam veterans and their nonveteran counterparts; the veteran group is made up, for the most part, of men in their early to mid-thirties, many of whom are experiencing incarceration for the first time (2, 3). Most nonveterans were first incarcerated prior to reaching this age. We hypothesize that this pattern of incarceration indicates that many Viet Nam veterans in prison are there, at least in part, because of stressors related to the Viet Nam combat and homecoming experience. It is our observation that many of these veterans have not worked through these experiences, and until they do we believe that they will remain the "outlaw casualties" of that war. Our experience with the Veterans in Prison Program has taught us that many of these veterans can begin psychological rehabilitation while incarcerated, and that—if viable administrative controls are established—correction authorities will support such efforts.

THE NATURE OF THE PROBLEM

The overwhelming majority of Viet Nam veterans in prison have never been evaluated for post-traumatic stress disorder because this disorder was not considered relevant during their trials or encounters with law enforcement authorities. Our experience is that an understanding of PTSD is particularly important when working with veterans charged with and/or convicted of criminal offenses when the arrest occurred in the recent past. We must recognize that some incarcerated Viet Nam veterans were inducted or accepted into military service with preexisting behavioral problems, and in some in-

Table 1. Veterans and nonveterans in state prisons, by percentage in each group with specified characteristic and by age and sentence length, 1979.

Characteristic	Pre–Viet Nam veterans	Viet Nam veterans	Post–Viet Nam veterans	Nonveteran
Black	28	35	35	52
Hispanic	7	7	7	10
Not working at time of arrest	24	26	30	31
Convicted of violent crime	61	60	52	57
Regular heroin user	13	26	10	22
Heavy daily drinker	27	33	41	26
Less than honorable discharge	39	46	59	NA
Disabled	10	10	2	NA
Age (median years)	45.3	28.5	22.4	26.4
Maximum sentence (median years)	11.5	10.1	7.8	8.4

Reprinted from U.S. Department of Justice: Veterans in prison. Bureau of Statistics Bulletin, February 1981.

stances these individuals fall into the category of life-style or career criminals. Career criminals view incarceration as an occupational hazard. Youchelson and Samenow (4) have written about a treatment approach that can be utilized with this population. We would caution that this same approach is dysfunctional when applied to individuals with stress disorders, and that from our experience, relatively few Viet Nam veteran inmates, especially those who were more recently incarcerated, are in the career criminal category.

We have conceptualized three categories of behavior which lead to the incarceration of most veterans: 1) *conscious flashback behavior*, 2) *unconscious flashback behavior* (or the "*blind flashback*"), and 3) *action junkie behavior*.

Conscious Flashback Behavior

The most easily recognized category of behavior is that involving the conscious flashback (see Chapter 14). Veterans often can state that during the "crime" they were reliving a life-threatening Viet Nam experience, such as a combat situation, and behaved as one would when threatened with death. These veterans then regressed into action that was appropriate in Viet Nam: they sought to alter the ending of their past experience to make it "come out right."

Such behavior can be assaultive or in other ways violent. During the flashback, these veterans may shout at Vietcong or use language easily related to Viet Nam. They may later remember the original situation by discussing the flashback, but sometimes they may have no recall of the criminal event, or only limited recall. It may be possible for witnesses to provide the necessary data to indicate that a flashback did take place.

Unconscious Flashback Behavior

Unconscious flashback behavior has also been described as a "blind flashback" because of the absence of specific Viet Nam–related behaviors. It is therefore more difficult to assess. In most instances, veterans who display this behavior will not be able to provide the linkage of their current actions to past Viet Nam experiences, because they are consciously unaware of any such connection. They may also be quite resistant to the evidence gained in counseling which indicates that such a connection exists.

To complicate the situation further, since the event acted out may be a contrived condensation of a large number of experiences, it may be particularly hard to establish an understanding of the specific psychic motives for the behavior. We have also observed veterans who act out an emotion, or a set of emotions, that have been suppressed since Viet Nam. These emotions are associated with trauma of such intensity that the facts of the original incident(s) are all but lost in a state of deep repression, and all that remains is the emotional residue.

Action Junkie Behavior

The action junkie category (5) comprises the largest group of incarcerated veterans, and its members possess a wide range of personality styles and capacities for action. The critical feature of those in the action junkie group is that they seek out events or situations which are dangerous and risky seemingly for the pure "joy" of being in a threatening situation. They seek to recreate and reexperience the atmosphere of danger that was so prevalent in Viet Nam. It is not uncommon to hear veterans report that they never felt so high as when in combat; it was like being on a drug. Action junkies, because of some combination of a stress disorder and a personality predisposing to addiction and the need to act out, now try to involve themselves in situations where that same feeling of being high and in action can be duplicated.

In many cases, when an action junkie is incarcerated and the "high of action" is therefore impossible, he will begin to exhibit signs of stress disorder. It appears that the process of seeking out danger is a form of self-medication that defends the veteran against experiencing stress symptoms. At the same time he externalizes and seeks to master undigested memories of Viet Nam risks. We shall describe several action junkie behavior subtypes: revenge behavior, punishment behavior, and outlaw behavior.

Revenge Behavior. Revenge behavior is characterized by a desire on the part of veterans to extract some measure of "payment" from society for the wrongs suffered in Viet Nam and upon coming home.

These veterans see themselves as having been used and mistreated. They want to prove their abilities, for they perceive society as viewing them to be incapable.

These veterans are aware of these goals and direct their behavior toward reaching them. One man reported that when he arrived home, he found only minimum wage and minimum responsibility positions open to him. He responded by entering into a series of crimes that required a great deal of planning and courage ". . . to show [society] that I was capable of functioning at a much higher level than anyone was willing to recognize."

Punishment Behavior. This behavior is exhibited by veterans who seek to kill themselves (or otherwise be punished), though sometimes these men concurrently express the desire for help. When treating Viet Nam veterans in this group, it is crucial to remember that their behavior relates to acts they have committed in Viet Nam or feelings they have experienced about their participation in the war. These veterans might experience intrusive thoughts that cause them to fear that their behavior will endanger others. They may also struggle with war memories that can cause moral pain and guilt and lead to the wish for suicide. When these men commit criminal acts, they are usually of such a bizarre nature, or so poorly planned, that one cannot escape the conclusion that success was not the objective. Death is often the desired goal, although these veterans might be unable or unwilling to recognize this. They might also be blind to the fact that their actions are a cry for help.

Outlaw Behavior. A distinction must be made between career (or life-style) criminals and those demonstrating outlaw behavior. This distinction is most important for prison-based counselors, because it mandates different treatment (4). While outlaw behavior, in contrast to other Viet Nam–related categories described here, is marked by arrests and incarcerations prior to Viet Nam, or by frequent arrests since returning from Viet Nam, most of the offenses reflect poor impulse control. One is further impressed that this problem may have been exacerbated by the Viet Nam experience. Additionally, there is some clear capacity for maturation in the counseling setting; one finds that, unlike the career criminal, these individuals are not hard-core sociopaths.

Curiously, our experience indicates that it is with this group that counselors have the best chance of achieving rehabilitation. Members of this group have a strong need to conform and be a part of some type of "society." Timely counseling can help these individuals see that they have a "choice" with regard to life-style and actions and can therefore foster in these veterans a capacity to identify positively with society. This group responds very favorably when counseling incorporates the processing of V.A. claims, help with discharge upgrading, and other tangible "rewards."

BARRIERS TO TREATMENT

Before discussing treatment approaches, we must examine the barriers to treatment which exist in the prison setting. Counselors must recognize the pitfalls of peer sabotage, the difficulty of establishing a working relationship with the inmate/client, and the special problems of externalization in inmates and goal confusion in both inmates and counselors. No positive movement will occur if these barriers are not recognized.

Peer sabotage is an important treatment barrier. In prison, a hostile and structured caste system exists. Great value is placed on strength. Any sign of weakness can be used against an inmate. Thus, it is the responsibility of prison-based counselors to create programs that responsively work into traumatic areas.

A Viet Nam veteran who permitted himself abreaction in a rap group could place himself in a vulnerable position because he revealed the depth of his emotions. The inmate group must therefore develop sufficient trust and cohesion to allow members to express themselves and support each other without fear of reprisals.

Peer sabotage can also keep individuals from coming forward to seek counseling services because an "us (inmates) against them (society)" mentality pervades prison life. It can disrupt the development of a peer group because some inmates will seek to use the program for other forms of advantage, such as getting out of work assignments. Careful screening and tangible rewards for effective participation are techniques that have proven useful in dealing with peer sabotage.

The relationship between inmates/clients and counselors is a difficult treatment issue. The task of establishing a relationship is complicated by peer intimidation, threats of coercion, and more subtle forms of manipulation. Counselors must deal not only with unmotivated veterans, but also with direct hostility toward their goals and purpose.

Externalization refers to the tendency of veterans to place responsibility for their actions on outside forces. Many incarcerated veterans preface their individual histories with statements like, "All Viet Nam veterans. . . ," and go on to blame their current situations on the war. Counselors who are Viet Nam veterans are at an advantage in dealing with this attitude, but nevertheless the challenge to counselors is complex. It involves recognition of the tendency to externalize, as well as the sensitivity to recognize the very real effects of war experiences.

Prisons provide those who externalize with a compatible setting. Decision-making functions have been removed from the individual. Thus, assumption of individual responsibility must be encouraged. An effective prison program places emphasis on self-help, on building standards of individual responsibility, and on building standards of group responsibility, all in a setting where these pressures can be avoided.

In our experience, as these individuals accept responsibility for their thoughts, feelings, and actions, the Viet Nam experience is put into perspective. It is better understood and is not viewed as an all-powerful controlling force in their lives. The inmates/clients are able to focus on their own actions during Viet Nam and the distinctions between what war experiences they could and could not control. They can now get on with life without relating everything to Viet Nam and without the resulting sense of pervasive powerlessness.

Goal confusion is another barrier to treatment, one that is relevant to both inmates and counselors. It is imperative that before entering the prison setting counselors develop reasonable goals for the program (although in our experience these will likely be modified later).

The individual inmates may have a specific goal in mind as the result of becoming involved with a group of Viet Nam veterans, but some of these goals might be inappropriate or unattainable. Counselors must not only help inmates/clients define realistic treatment goals, but they must also be prepared to modify their own hopes for their veteran clients.

TREATMENT APPROACHES

The Veterans in Prison Program is broad-based and eclectic, and it emphasizes a self-help approach. As counselors in the program, we utilize relationship building and maintain a nonjudgmental, client-oriented attitude as we build insight. We employ techniques of reality therapy (6) and behavior modification.

Any successful treatment approach in prison depends heavily on engaging inmates in mutually supportive relationships. Reliability and straightforwardness in the counselors are essential, for inmates will search for signs of hypocrisy, insincerity, or inconsistency in the helping professionals. The counselor-inmate relationship, then, must be based on reliability (keeping scheduled appointments) and honesty.

It is most important that the counselor stay away from value issues and judgments. Eliminating value judgments from the counseling program sharpens recognition that the world is not just and that this lack of justice is a reality with which everyone, including inmates, must deal. Veterans/inmates must be challenged to look at their present situation, to recognize that they can make choices and exercise options.

The principles of reality therapy are important in this connection. In reality therapy, one supports the concepts of individual responsibility and choice and steers clear of viewing the client as a "victim." In many instances, a veteran's experiences, both prior to and in Viet Nam, cause him to adopt the self-image of the victim. He believes that Viet Nam proved that his actions are futile and that he has no "importance." Such a veteran will often express the idea that he is a tool to be used and then discarded.

Our counseling goal is to help veterans see their past lives as a problem to be managed. They must recognize that no matter how traumatic life has been, they should obtain their needs through actions acceptable to society. They must learn to deal with present needs as they resolve the thorniest issues of their past (Viet Nam and the homecoming and post–Viet Nam experiences). We use Viet Nam as a launching pad for developing more productive life-coping mechanisms. As inmates/veterans enjoy here-and-now success and better understanding of their past experiences, we find that they make better progress on the road home.

It has been impossible for many traumatized veterans to put the war behind them. We know they need a supportive environment that facilitates the working through of traumatic episodes. While traditional reality therapy ignores all historical input, we create an environment that allows veterans to discuss and digest their war experiences, to gain perspective by placing them in context.

We have indicated that the concept of self-help is an integral part of the treatment approach, and now we stress this again. Self-help groups in the prison setting encourage veterans to help each other. Group members do not passively wait for the counselor to provide all help, and we find this critical in the psychological growth of many inmates.

A most important part of our program involves behavior modification. As we have mentioned, the provision of immediate and tangible reward is most important. "Results" are rarely obtained as rapidly as the veteran desires, but the counselor can provide assistance with such issues as discharge upgrading, receipt of V.A. benefits, and help toward future employment. Although these may seem minor aids to the reader, they represent new and important experiences for the incarcerated veteran. Now, with the help and support of their counselors, veterans can experience the benefits of society, often for the first time.

This is instrumental in keeping inmates in the counseling group, for it gives them something palpable with which to confront peer sabotage. In most instances the process of obtaining such benefits is more important than the benefits themselves. It is a significant accomplishment for the veteran to participate in society, and the process provides the important lesson that society can aid the inmate. This lesson can be used by counselors when an inmate/veteran expresses the attitude that "society just doesn't work for me." We believe, then, that this form of activity represents a valuable behavior-shaping device. The change in inmate attitude also provides a foundation upon which further efforts at encouraging societally condoned "seeking behavior" can be based.

A CASE STUDY

Inmate Carl was a 30-year-old Viet Nam combat veteran. He was sentenced to a prison where a Veterans in Prison Program was in a formative stage. He had heard of this program through the inmate grapevine and sought out the counselor to ask why he would persist in coming to this particular prison, month after month, in the face of poor inmate response. Carl's initial comments were that the counselor must be crazy to keep wasting his time when there obviously wasn't any inmate interest. He said that if the counselor couldn't get you out of prison, there was nothing to be gained by participation in the program.

After several months, Carl began to spend more time with the counselor. He next brought a couple of other Viet Nam veterans with him to see this "fool." When he found that the counselor had also been in Viet Nam and was a combat veteran, his attitude changed markedly. He, and the two other inmates, formed a rap group.

With time, Carl opened up and told his story. He was from a town far from a large urban area. He enlisted after high school because he was convinced that it was his patriotic duty. While in Viet Nam he saw heavy combat, was once wounded, and was awarded numerous medals. He extended his enlistment for a second tour of duty, and upon his return home he received a traditional World War II homecoming. However, he had been changed because of his experiences, and was no longer sure that he had served his country well.

Carl was most confident that he himself had done an honorable job, but he had serious questions concerning the purpose of the war. Of greatest importance, he questioned the deaths of his comrades; he felt they had died for nothing. He stated that upon discharge he had really needed to sort things out for himself, and that the rousing "red, white, and blue John Wayne welcome home" he received had upset him.

He recalled that he had been called upon to address civic groups and high school students concerning the importance of serving one's country. He was treated as a powerful hero. He wanted to reveal his confusion and sadness, but when he tried to do this, no one wanted to listen. He was told that his war was over and he was home, and that it was important for him to serve as an example of strength to others.

As this situation continued, he began to drink in order to mute his unhappiness. As his drinking became more compulsive, he began to fight in bars. He became convinced that he was a coward because he couldn't talk to anyone about what he really felt unless he was drunk.

As his mental state deteriorated, his fights became more serious. He began to carry a weapon, and soon he was openly hostile to everyone, even when sober. He began to stay out late and engage in minor criminal behavior. He sought out dangerous situations. The local police and Carl's family and friends tried to ignore his behavior. Certainly, they did not understand his survivor guilt, his desire for punishment, or his cries for help. When he was picked up committing a crime, the victim did not press charges, and he did not receive the punishment he unconsciously sought. No one would "cooperate" with his unconscious need.

The culmination of this self-destructive behavior was a fight in which Carl nearly killed a man. He was arrested, tried, and convicted with hardly a mention of his Viet Nam service or experiences, and no mention of the pattern of his post–Viet Nam behavior.

It was well over one year from the time Carl first stuck his head into the counselor's office to the time he related his entire story. He felt, when we first began the rap group, that he was a very bad individual who had let everyone down with his actions upon returning home. This idea was persistent during most of the time it took him to relate his story. We worked on this idea about himself for an additional year and a half before he began to understand and accept just why and how he had sought punishment.

Eventually, Carl was able to gain some sympathy for his situation from the parole board, and based on a guarantee of counseling from a veterans program near his home, he was granted an early parole.

Furthermore, contact was maintained with his counselor through the mail, and reports indicate that his behavior continues to reflect an obvious optimism, a marked reduction in tension, and a dissolution of self-hate.

We understand that Carl is still concerned with his homecoming behavior and has not completely forgiven himself. In our view this is a good sign. We believe he now feels that he can function within a society, outside of prison, and that he is deserving of another chance. This, we feel, represents a balanced perspective.

SUMMARY

While the number of incarcerated Viet Nam veterans does not coincide with the popular stereotype, they do comprise a significant portion of the prison and jail population. These veterans can be helped by a counseling program that utilizes an eclectic approach and incorporates a self-help model. This program should be client-oriented and employ certain techniques of reality therapy and behavior modification. Although some serious barriers to treatment do exist in prisons, if these are recognized positive results are possible. It is essential that in establishing a Veterans in Prison Program the counselor be reliable, stable, consistent, and responsible.

Most Viet Nam veterans in prison are not career criminals but individuals who have been disillusioned and affected by Viet Nam experiences. In some cases these experiences have influenced an already existing inclination to criminal behavior, and in others we suspect that these veterans would not have come into conflict with the law had they not experienced Viet Nam and its aftermath.

Our experience is that even minimal attempts at "inreach" counseling help reduce recidivism. Existing resources within prisons, and in the community, can be utilized to provide many of these services. As we have done this work, we have come to feel more strongly a sense of moral obligation to these veterans. Many of these currently incarcerated individuals honorably served their country and were impeded in reintegrating into society by a lack of public support and understanding. We are convinced that the treatment program we have described allows incarcerated Viet Nam veterans to take the first steps on their individual journeys home, and that this model should be employed throughout the penal system.

REFERENCES

1. Pentland B, Scurfield R: Inreach counseling and advocacy with veterans in prison. Federal Probation 36:21–29, 1982

2. Pentland B, Rothman G: The incarcerated Viet Nam service veteran: stereotypes and realities. The Journal of Correctional Education 33:11, 1982

3. U.S. Department of Justice: Veterans in prison. Bureau of Statistics Bulletin, February 1981

4. Youhelson S, Samenow SE: The Criminal Personality, vol 1 & 2. New York, Jason Aronson, 1977

5. Wilson JP, Ziegenbaum SD: The Viet Nam veteran on trial: the relation of post traumatic stress disorder to criminal behavior. Unpublished Manuscript.

6. Glasser W: Reality Therapy: A New Approach to Psychiatry. New York, Harper & Row, 1965

21

Forensic Assessment of Post-Traumatic Stress Disorder in Viet Nam Veterans

John O. Lipkin, M.D.
Arthur S. Blank, Jr., M.D.
Raymond Monsour Scurfield, D.S.W.

21

Since the first use of post-traumatic stress disorder as a defense in a case involving a Viet Nam veteran in 1978, the criminal justice system has become increasingly attuned to the influence of unresolved PTSD in episodic criminal behavior. We estimate that through mid-1984, the question of PTSD has been a major element in several hundred cases nationwide. A special issue of *Behavioral Sciences and the Law* (Vol. 1, No. 3, 1983) reviewed a number of legal aspects of the application of this defense and can furnish the clinician with an overview.

In a number of cases, judges and juries have determined that, according to applicable law, behavioral outbursts resulting in criminal offenses have represented PTSD symptoms or have been caused by pressure from memories of combat trauma. These conditions were deemed sufficient to justify a determination of innocence by reason of temporary insanity or a mitigation of punishment following a determination of guilt. With and without such findings, courts have further decided to order specific treatment arrangements for certain defendants.

The criminal justice system can be expected to call upon clinicians to perform forensic evaluations in future cases. Such evaluations of Viet Nam veterans involved in criminal behavior pose an unusually complex challenge, with profound implications for the individual, the family, and the public safety.

In addition to the usual complexities of assessing the influence of any psychiatric disorder on criminal culpability, forensic assessment in these cases requires highly refined psychiatric history-taking and diag-

This chapter was originally published as "Post-Traumatic Stress Disorder in Vietnam Veterans: Assessment in a Forensic Setting," which appeared in *Behavioral Sciences and the Law* (1:51–67, 1983). Reprinted in revised form by permission of the Van Nostrand Reinhold Company.

nosis, as well as an understanding of the effects of past experience on present behavior and symptoms. Differentiation must be made between the impact on behavior of antisocial or impulsive character traits and combat experiences with resulting PTSD. For example, in these cases certain features are often found:

- General alienation,
- Reluctance to talk to a professional,
- Violent outbursts and assaults,
- Intolerance of authority, and
- Dysfunctional patterns of living, especially affecting employment and marriage stability.

All of these features may result from either character structure or stress disorder, and in the forensic situation the clinician is confronted with the task of determining which is causative.

In order to accomplish this task, the evaluator must be free of past professional biases about the effects of war trauma and must understand the evolution of the diagnosis of PTSD in American psychiatry. The evaluator must perform an unusually detailed psychiatric history covering the individual's entire life and must understand the individual's experiences in Viet Nam and afterwards. All of this is essential if the evaluator is to establish the presence or absence of trauma and its impact on the behavior at issue. This chapter will review these matters, cover key points in the conduct of the evaluation, and discuss the psychiatric contribution to the management of forensic cases.

Recognition of PTSD requires discovery of a stressor "that would evoke significant symptoms of distress in almost everyone" (1, p. 238). Rape, natural disaster, concentration camp or prisoner of war experiences, and combat are the most familiar events associated with the diagnosis. Yet it is our view that the peculiarly traumatizing circumstances of the Viet Nam experience must be explained at length to many clinicians; they have limited awareness of the unique circumstances of the war, and their clinical attitudes concerning diagnosis of combat veterans are biased by the two previous editions of the *Diagnostic and Statistical Manual of Mental Disorders* (2, 3) (*DSM-I* was in use from 1952 through 1968, when *DSM-II* was published.)

THE HISTORY OF THE PTSD DIAGNOSIS

As mobilization occurred for World War II, American psychiatry was hampered by a diagnostic nomenclature designed primarily for the patient population found in public mental hospitals. When civilians were screened for military service, it became obvious that only 10 percent of those rejected for psychiatric reasons could be diagnosed according to the standard nomenclature.

During the war, a variety of personality disturbances, psychosomatic problems, and psychological responses to combat were observed which were inadequately covered in the nomenclature. In response, military psychiatrists developed a more comprehensive system of classification. This was eventually adopted by the Armed Forces and the Veterans Administration. In 1948, a revised International Statistical Classification was adopted that closely resembled the model developed by the United States military. This process of review and revision of the diagnostic standards for psychiatry eventually led to the first edition of the American Psychiatric Association's *Diagnostic and Statistical Manual of Mental Disorders* (2, pp. vi–vii).

Although terms such as "shell shock" and "neurasthenia" were used as recently as World War II, *DSM-I*, in defining "gross stress reaction," indicated that

> The symptoms are the immediate means used by the individual in his struggle to adjust to an overwhelming situation. In the presence of good adaptive capacity, recession of symptoms generally occurs when situational stress diminishes. Persistent failure to resolve will indicate a more severe underlying disturbance and will be classified elsewhere. (2, p. 40)

The same manual indicated the following:

> Under conditions of greater than usual stress, a normal personality may utilize established patterns of reaction to deal with overwhelming fear. . . . The patterns of such reactions differ from those of neurosis or psychosis chiefly with respect to clinical history, reversibility of reaction, and its transient character. . . . It is also possible that the conditions may progress to one of the neurotic reactions. If the reaction persists, this term is to be regarded as a temporary diagnosis to be used only until a more definitive diagnosis is established. (2, p. 40).

Thus, psychiatrists were guided to the belief that any persistent reaction to combat stress must be classified as neurotic illness, psychotic illness, or personality disorder until the publication of *DSM-II* in 1968. Therefore, a strong bias that predisposing factors are responsible for chronic, as opposed to transient, stress reactions permeates the thinking of this period and continues to interfere with correct diagnosis by many of those who trained or practiced at that time.

In 1968, the year of the Tet offensive in Viet Nam, the previously used term "gross stress reaction" entirely disappeared from the no-menclature. It was replaced by "adjustment reaction of adult life." The only mention of combat in all of *DSM-II* is an example given to illustrate adjustment reaction of adult life. This example describes fear associated with military combat, "manifested by trembling, running and hiding" (3, p. 49). It is of further significance that this sole example of a stress reaction to combat evokes imagery of cowardice.

Since *DSM-II* was the official psychiatric nomenclature for much of the period of the Viet Nam War, it is not surprising to find that Viet Nam veterans were generally understood in psychological terms that failed to recognize the role of combat experience or trauma. Not surprisingly, clinical experience with Viet Nam veterans and their stress reactions influenced the development of *DSM-III*.

DSM-III and PTSD

DSM-III restored to psychiatric thinking the concept that individuals without predisposition to emotional disorder could experience a broad range of severe symptoms on the basis of overwhelming psychological trauma. The most striking feature of the PTSD diagnosis is its break with the traditional view that long-standing reactions to trauma must inevitably be the result of an underlying predisposition. Since this idea represents a major departure from certain traditional psychoanalytic concepts, and from the training experiences of a substantial majority of psychiatrists currently in practice, there has been substantial resistance to it among analysts and psychiatrists. Much less resistance has been noted in the fields of psychology and psychiatric social work.

Careful review of *DSM-III* provides a basic understanding of the elements of PTSD. We will now discuss the key issues and problems in conducting a thorough forensic assessment of Viet Nam veterans suspected of suffering from PTSD.

Post-traumatic stress disorder occurs as one outcome of exposure to extreme psychic stress. In our view, there is little or no evidence that predisposition is a primary factor in determining which individuals will develop PTSD. Thus, it is essential to begin a clinical evaluation on the assumption that normal individuals can and do develop PTSD, although the form and emergence of symptoms may be dynamically related to nonmilitary life experience.

Combat experience, like concentration camp experience, produces stress which cannot be fully comprehended by people who have not lived it. Furthermore, many features of the Viet Nam War contrast sharply with other wars in our history. Because these differences influence the clinical picture, some Viet Nam veterans with PTSD have symptoms and behavior patterns which seem unusual to the clinician inexperienced in dealing with this population.

THE NATURE OF THE VIET NAM WAR

Various writings provide information about the nature of the Viet Nam War. Lipkin et al. (4), Figley (5), Lifton (6), Santoli (7), and Hasford (8), among others, offer both objective and subjective descriptions of the war experience.

Attorneys and clinicians must recall that each period of the Viet Nam War was different, both in the war zone and in the United States. Civilian attitudes toward the war were often sharply divided, and community support for military service was often lacking. Viet Nam combatants were significantly younger than those in World War II and Korea. Instead of being assigned to units for the duration of the war, troops were sent to Viet Nam for 12 or 13 months. As a result, combat military units were made up of persons on different schedules, some new in Viet Nam and inexperienced, others "short" and superstitious or preoccupied about surviving another month, week, or day. Most men and women went to Viet Nam and returned from Viet Nam alone, often by plane. The transition from the combat zone to home town usually took less than 48 hours and included crossing many time zones by jet plane. Returning military personnel were sometimes dazed, exhausted, and bewildered by the rapid transition and by the hostile, critical, or disinterested responses of strangers, friends, and family. Upon return there was no social sanction for the tabooed behaviors that were demanded by military structure or required for survival in Viet Nam.

Finally, the nature of guerilla conflict forced many Viet Nam combatants to abandon long-held assumptions about women, children, and war. In the Viet Nam War, any American could be attacked in any part of the country, by any Vietnamese. A Vietnamese clerk in a U.S. Army office during the day might be an assassin at night. A crying child could be a deadly, explosive trap. Heat, humidity, jungle warfare, and the relentless unseen enemy made most jobs in Viet Nam dangerous, exhausting, and unpredictable. The political struggles surrounding the war influenced military strategy with bewildering effects for soldiers, who may have repeatedly captured and abandoned small bits of territory at devastating human cost.

MAKING AN ACCURATE DIAGNOSIS OF PTSD

In addition to the extraordinary multileveled complexity of the relevant traumas, the diagnosis of PTSD is made more difficult when the traumas occurred months or years before the examination. A variety of fixed behavioral patterns, defenses, and attitudes have been developed to secondarily deal with the traumatic aspects of experience. Also, some stress-related symptoms are not unique to PTSD. Therefore, there are relatively few cases without some significant symptoms which could fit into other diagnostic categories.

As an example, substance abuse was common among our forces in Viet Nam. Particularly after 1969, drugs were abused in an attempt to control fear, anxiety, rage, and exhaustion. Some combat veterans upon returning home experienced severe sleep disturbance related to their Viet Nam experience (nightmares and intrusive thoughts about combat). Some turned to alcohol and marijuana use as a means of controlling these symptoms. In some cases, this use occurred in those who had used a similar substance in Viet Nam. In other cases, there had not been previous alcohol or marijuana use. The chronological sequence of symptoms and behaviors and their relationship to each other and to traumatic events are of vital importance in understanding whether a specific psychiatric symptom is or is not a part of PTSD.

For a number of veterans, dramatic changes in life-style occurred following Viet Nam. Abrupt relocations and dramatic changes in occupation are listed in *DSM-III* under "associated features," but are not considered inclusionary criteria for a PTSD diagnosis. Research is needed to determine whether associated features listed in *DSM-III* such as anxiety, impulsive behavior, or depression should be considered core symptoms.

Work history may give clues about the presence of PTSD. Some Viet Nam veterans prefer jobs with little or no social contact or supervision, such as janitor, night watchman, gardener, etc. Others move impulsively from job to job, taking many different jobs each year. Skillful interviewing may reveal that discomfort with social interaction, intolerance of authority, or inability to keep commitments causes the veteran to abandon each job.

Another group who have PTSD appear much more successful. Such individuals invest so much time and energy in their jobs that they advance rapidly and become well paid. However, some of this group —which includes executives, clergy, lawyers, doctors, and nurses— work so compulsively that they have little meaningful interaction with friends and family. Fears of intimacy, guilt over survival, and attempts at restitution may underlie their overachievement.

A very negative attitude toward government, a suspiciousness of the motivations and honesty of various governmental officials and agencies, or similar phenomena may give clues to the presence of underlying PTSD, rather than indicating characterologic difficulties. This may also be the case for impulsive or acting out behaviors. However, most clinicians experienced with Viet Nam combat veterans have found that, in regard to impulse control, these veterans are more often over-controlled and preoccupied with a fear of losing control. Very few have a history of repeated loss of control (9).

Most clinicians who have worked extensively with combat veterans find that, while there may appear to have been a symptom-free period for a number of years following combat, careful examination reveals that there were "trouble signs" and subtle symptoms within the first two or three years after Viet Nam. Typically, upon closer inquiry, symptom-free veterans reveal that they have had substantial depression, sleep disturbance, confusion, lack of clarity about their values and purpose in life, and difficulty in staying with tasks or relationships in the years immediately after their war experiences.

Another example of such a history is that some veterans experienced nightmares or intrusive thoughts which on the surface did not have Viet Nam content. However, there was negative or life-threatening content and a feeling state identical to the feeling aroused during traumatic Viet Nam experiences. Still other combat veterans, like others who survive major psychological trauma, have years of symptom-free functioning before developing PTSD symptoms which clearly derive from war stressors.

Who Should Perform the Forensic Psychiatric Evaluation?

Ideally, the forensic evaluation should be done by a clinician with the following attributes:

- The ability to conduct a thorough psychiatric examination, following any standard outline. Physical, neurologic, and mental status examinations may be required, since the etiology of loss of control may require investigation.
- The willingness to obtain special examinations and consultations as needed. These additional sources of information may include laboratory tests, toxicological tests, electroencephalograms, psychological testing, or comments from family, former teachers, and others.
- Objectivity. It is essential that the examiner's attempt to perform a comprehensive evaluation not be biased by attitudes concerning culpability, Viet Nam veterans (either pro or con), or the Viet Nam War.

Chronicity, Repression and Denial, and the Forensic Assessment

The time which has elapsed between the Viet Nam War and the present makes the forensic evaluation particularly difficult. The presence of PTSD indicates that resolution has not been accomplished for some or all of that individual's experiences. In the absence of resolution the victim of massive psychological stress is likely to have developed an assortment of protective mechanisms or maladaptive behaviors. These may include repression and denial, suspiciousness and aggressiveness, apathy, withdrawal, and amnesia. When a Viet Nam veteran with PTSD commits a criminal act on the basis of a dissociative reaction, a flashback, or another element of the condition, he or she is particularly likely to have impaired access to the relevant material.

> *A former Army doctor, without prior criminal history, took a classroom of children hostage. The incident ended without injury. In jail, the veteran was evaluated repeatedly. Other than a history of migraine and evidence of chronic anxiety, depression, and irritability, little emerged during the course of two evaluations. During a third evaluation, in several sessions totaling 10 hours, it was found that the veteran had major classical amnesia concerning most of his duty at a field hospital in Viet Nam. This amnesia was partly penetrated by detailed, well-informed questioning. After several hours information was obtained concerning multiple mortar attacks, booby trap incidents, and an extraordinarily gruesome exposure to casualties at the field hospital. In about the eighth hour of interviewing, it was revealed that the doctor had shot and killed a North Vietnamese prisoner of war who was attempting to escape, a fact he had probably not discussed with anyone during the 12-year postwar interval.*

In connection with the general problem of obtaining a detailed combat history against a variety of obstacles, some examiners have found, as in this case, the use of audio tape recording helpful. This facilitates review of the sessions in fine detail and helps uncover of inconsistencies which may lead to important discoveries.

INTERFERENCES WITH DISCOVERY

Given the various peculiar circumstances of the Viet Nam War and the postwar social milieu, the clinician may unwittingly establish a context which decreases the chance that the veteran will be able to discuss relevant material. Sometimes even mildly stern, formal, or authoritarian behavior on the part of the examiner may be provocative, frightening, or antagonizing to a Viet Nam veteran. Such reactions can also be stimulated by an examiner's apparent lack of knowledge or interest in the importance of the Viet Nam experience to the veteran.

Such an atmosphere in an interview may stimulate the same defenses which led to the initial repression of military experience. Even in the absence of detectable authoritarian behavior or negative judgment about the veteran by the examiner, the image of the mental health professional as an authority figure may militate against revelation by the veteran. This is particularly so when the professional is employed by a governmental agency.

A strikingly inhibited lower-middle-class veteran with no record of previous criminal behavior attacked his girlfriend with a weapon for no apparent reason. He caused dramatic but non-life-threatening injuries. Despite persistent questioning over a period of several hours, he revealed very little about his Viet Nam history, until a combat veteran, who wasn't a mental health professional but who did have some counseling experience, was brought into the interviews. Almost immediately, the defendant began to reveal to the other combat veteran numerous important details of his experiences in Viet Nam.

THE MILITARY HISTORY

Standardized interview schedules concerning combat history in Viet Nam may be useful in this evaluation (10) (also see Chapter 13). Understanding the dynamics which bear upon the criminal episode depends on developing an accurate and richly detailed picture of the veteran in Viet Nam, as well as the effect of those experiences on the individual's life. The key elements of a thorough history of a Viet Nam veteran are discussed below.

A. *Character of Entry into the Military*

1. Psychosocial life context immediately prior to military entry, age, activities, etc.
2. Assessment of individual motivation for entry into the military, to include whether the veteran was drafted or enlisted, the reasons for enlistment, and the possibility of enlistment to avoid the draft or to avoid a civil court sentence.
3. Assessment of whether friends, siblings, and cousins were already in the military or in Viet Nam, and the impact of this on the veteran's decision to enter the military.
4. The family military history. This history may be extremely important, including combat history of father or uncles in Korea or World War II. In some cases, it has been noted that combat experiences of the father or other relative were hidden, that is, they had

never been discussed in detail with the Viet Nam veteran during his childhood and adolescence and served as an important family secret.

B. Basic Training and Events/Training and Experiences

It is important to assess the basic training experience, with inquiry as to how the veteran perceived it. Racial slurs may have diminished unit cohesion and identification with military leadership for minority group members.

The adequacy of training for functions to be performed in Viet Nam is important. Medics or nurses may have felt inadequately prepared for responsibilities they had in the war zone. For combat training, it is important to assess adequacy in light of the individual's actual combat experiences. This may provide essential information underlying the traumatic significance of Viet Nam experiences. Some veterans, such as combat engineers, had relatively little combat training beyond basic training and officially had noncombat duty in Viet Nam (building bridges, buildings, etc.). Some of these unprepared individuals, however, actually experienced a great deal of combat, which they found particularly traumatic.

C. Transport to and Arrival in Viet Nam

How did the veteran get to Viet Nam? Did the veteran go alone, with strangers, or with friends? Was there a positive send-off? Were family, neighbors, or others antagonistic or supportive?

The nature of arrival in Viet Nam is important as to 1) the degree of organization or disorganization which confronted the individual upon arriving; 2) the provision of jungle war training, or lack of it, in country during the first few weeks; and 3) the immediate circumstances of the individual's arrival at his or her unit in Viet Nam. The attitudes of members of the individual's unit toward replacements may also be significant. For example, an experienced person with six months in country may have taken a FNG ("fucking new guy") under his or her wing; conversely, FNGs may have been left to fend for themselves or may have been subject to ridicule.

D. Nature of Military Experience in Viet Nam

The specific details of the individual's tour of duty in the combat zone must be explored. It is helpful to review the basic facts of the tour chronologically, including units in which the veteran served, the nature of operations, the numbers killed and wounded, the coherence or lack of coherence of tactical and strategic objectives, the intensity of combat, and the presence of combat-free intervals. In addition, the quality of leadership and camaraderie throughout the tour needs to be assessed by specific questions about the abilities of the individual's immediate and more superior commanders.

It is often possible by asking basic questions about who did what, where, when, and why to develop important inferences about the quality of both leadership and unit morale. Use of marijuana, alcohol, amphetamines, opium, heroin, and other drugs must be evaluated, both as a group or unit phenomenon and in terms of the individual. Particularly in the post-1969 period, a number of units had widespread drug usage.

> *An individual was engaged in long-range reconnaissance. He and his buddies were regularly provided with combination barbiturate-amphetamine products by one of their commanders prior to going out on patrol. In addition, they purchased amphetamines locally and used both drugs regularly as part of their combat routine. Eliciting this particular history was of considerable importance in evaluating the individual's return to drug use some 14 years later.*

For apparent "noncombatants," it is equally critical to assess exposure to war trauma. Exposure to casualties was quite prevalent among medical personnel, including doctors, nurses, medics, and others on hospital duty. Such exposure also was common among chaplain's assistants and those on graves registration duty. Chronic traumatic states have been observed among all of these groups of veterans, including those involved in cleaning and preparing bodies for shipment to the United States. Some individuals obtained noncombat duties to avoid combat for a range of reasons, including fear of injury or death or opposition to the war. These veterans may have a particularly complex problem with survivor guilt.

In some cases the assumption that a veteran was a noncombatant is simply incorrect, and in many cases military records fail to report combat events which in fact occurred.

> *A veteran had an extensive and chronic history of postwar alcoholism with multiple admissions to a veterans hospital for delirium tremens and was diagnosed as having borderline personality disorder. His Viet Nam history had never been carefully explored, partly because he was allegedly engaged in noncombat duty on a riverboat. During the delirium tremens he made repeated references to destructive episodes, and on some occasions his hallucinations included Asians. A more complete psychiatric evaluation, which explored the military history, revealed that his boat was frequently attacked. On one such occasion he transmitted orders by radio to jets flying close*

support, which led to an air attack which he was told destroyed a village containing many Vietnamese.

Psychiatrists, other mental health personnel, all physicians, chaplains, and unit commanders frequently sent unwilling individuals back to combat and balanced the needs of individuals against the needs of combat units. This task, too, is associated with war trauma, guilt, anxiety, and rage.

E. Contact with the Vietnamese Civilian Population

There was a great range of contact between American troops and Vietnamese civilians. For some veterans there was little or no contact, for others substantial animosity developed. Other veterans made close positive relationships with the local population and learned its customs and culture. Many of these veterans established affect-laden relationships with Vietnamese children, women, or the elderly. For some veterans their first sexual experiences occurred in Viet Nam, often under unusually stressful conditions.

Finally, a number of veterans, particularly from minorities, identified with the local populace because of racist acts and attitudes they knew of toward Vietnamese and minority Americans. This was true even though many minority group members found a lack of racism in their combat units. They and others were still enraged by the racist attitudes which continued unabated outside of the combat unit and at home.

A soldier became involved with civilian support activities, providing food and other necessities to a Vietnamese orphanage. Later, several children from the orphanage were killed and wounded. This set the stage for the veteran's PTSD symptoms, which occurred many years later.

F. Other Items to Consider

Loss of buddies and the problem of survivor guilt are extremely important. Often the comradeship with one or a few others in Viet Nam was of an intensity that has not since been approached or matched. If close buddies were lost or wounded in combat, there may be guilt associated with the belief that the veteran was at least partly responsible: because the veteran went on R&R, because the injury or death occurred just after the veteran left his or her unit to return to the United States, or because he or she was at least partly responsible for the friend joining the service in the first place.

G. *Homecoming*

Completion of the military history requires a careful analysis of the homecoming and long-term postwar treatment opportunities. Many veterans returned to overtly hostile or nonsupportive friends, relatives, or communities. In the 1970s Viet Nam veterans experienced job discrimination, discrimination by some of the traditional service organizations in accepting them as members at the local level, and unspoken prohibitions against discussing their Viet Nam experiences.

Some women Viet Nam veterans suffered the additional stigma of being labeled homosexual or promiscuous. Ethnic minority veterans often faced racist practices at home, which increased their feelings of rage about their service in Viet Nam and the sacrifices they had made. Many combat veterans, as well as physicians, nurses, and other support unit veterans, experienced massive ambivalence about their Viet Nam service, which motivated them to avoid discussing Viet Nam.

In psychiatric examination of Viet Nam veterans, knowledge of military vocabulary or jargon may be essential in the discovery of vital material. Many examiners are not familiar with the jargon of Viet Nam, and a special effort must be made to understand the meaning of these terms. Reviewing notes or recorded interviews with a Viet Nam veteran familiar with the vocabulary may assist in discerning the meaning of events.

EMOTIONAL DYNAMICS IN INTERVIEWING COMBAT VETERANS

Chronic and delayed PTSD can be shaped in a complex and subtle way by the interplay of Viet Nam experience and preexisting values and concepts of self. Some veterans have enduring difficulties because their performance at some point during the combat tour was inconsistent with their expectations for themselves.

Great detail about the individual's experience must be obtained to accurately assess its psychological impact. This creates problems for many examiners, even if they are accustomed to evaluating individuals who have experienced trauma. Such detail may be painful, upsetting, and frightening to hear.

Dealing with emotionally laden material is potentially threatening to the combat veteran. This may reflect a fear of losing control or of reexperiencing the horrors of the revived trauma. In addition, the veteran may have had prior negative experiences in clinical situations, or with significant others, in trying to discuss combat trauma. Others have never before talked in detail about Viet Nam (10).

A veteran's recitation of personal Viet Nam history can be accompanied by intense and diffuse affect, such as rage or fear. This intensity, per se, may frighten or threaten examiners. If the feeling is experienced toward the examiner, both the veteran and the examiner may retreat from crucial data-gathering efforts.

These evaluations, when conducted in adequate depth, may blend into psychological treatment. The course of the evaluation may be guided by therapeutic considerations. A veteran may express rage at the nation, the government, or the public. These feelings must be understood and addressed by the examiner. The examiner should consider whether such rage is directed at persons or institutions that symbolically represent or actually caused trauma experienced by the veteran. As in all clinical settings, the clinician must not simply interpret what he or she hears literally or "objectively"; the clinician must empathize with the veteran and attempt to view what he or she hears from the veteran's unique point of view. This may be a painful task for a non-goer to Viet Nam.

ASSESSING CULPABILITY

Assessment of these cases for forensic purposes involves an integrated understanding of culpability, repetition, current patterns of behavior, and preexisting personality characteristics. An important task of the forensic examiner is noting psychological patterns and determining causal links between criminal behavior and combat experiences. First this is done without reference to culpability.

Premature consideration of culpability may obscure the task of observing how and to what extent the individual's criminal outburst is a symbolic repetition of war experiences, an expression of conflicts about such experiences, or an attempt at remembering deeply repressed experiences.

Following elucidation of the psychological links between present outbursts and combat experiences, an assessment is made of the individual's state of mind at the time of the criminal offense. This involves retrospective evaluation of the veteran's mental status in terms of dissociation, loss of contact with reality, and control over behavior.

Assessment of premilitary impulse control and criminal behavior before, during, and since the war is also pertinent.

The doctor described above who shot and killed an escaping prisoner of war had no history of premilitary criminal behavior. However, as an adolescent, he had been severely punished by his parents after a few episodes of fighting with family and friends. His medical activities involved a reaction formation to this very mild problem of impulse control and resultant guilt. This history predisposed to his extraordinarily intense guilt reaction after he killed the escaping prisoner in self-defense.

Examiners in forensic cases are usually called upon to comment either formally or informally on the matter of culpability in light of the individual's control over his or her behavior at the time of the criminal offense. In PTSD cases this is especially problematic, because a diagnosis of psychosis is usually critical in concluding there was an absence of self-control.

Whether as part of an insanity defense or of an evaluation establishing mitigating circumstances, the examiner must consider culpability from two particular perspectives. The criminal outburst might represent a flashback, a behavior that is psychologically linked to combat experiences. If it is determined that a flashback did occur, the content of the events reexperienced in this fashion should be carefully elicited and assessed. The objective is to determine the nature and force of emerging memories and the degree of challenge to the individual's defenses and controls. A second task is to assess the level of impulse control, as such, at the time of the offense. Once this is accomplished, it may be possible to estimate the degree to which the flashback undermined impulse control during the offense.

It should be noted that although PTSD flashbacks are common, those involving criminal behavior are rare. Furthermore, in our experience, the occurrence of criminal flashback behavior is not predictive of similar future episodes. Certainly, effective psychotherapeutic treatment for PTSD is helpful in enabling veterans to gain control over behavior associated with dissociation and flashbacks.

LEGAL DISPOSITION AND TREATMENT IMPLICATIONS

Because of the inherent treatability of PTSD, examiners asked to perform evaluations in PTSD cases should realize that they are involved in a treatment situation. Frequently, criminal outbursts are a manifestation of the veteran's attempt at retrieving and working through traumatic experiences which have not been resolved. Although it may be necessary for society to effect punishment or control a dangerous person, the evaluation of criminal behavior is an important step in beginning effective treatment.

Therapeutic considerations often influence legal proceedings. In some cases, the mental health examiner, the defendant, the defense attorney, and the prosecutor may agree on a legal arrangement which serves the needs of society and facilitates treatment for the veteran. This is frequently the case when by consensus an insanity defense and public exposure in a trial are avoided and treatment is made available. Thus, the strategic legal choice between an insanity defense and a guilty plea may be based on an understanding among all parties that PTSD is involved, that treatment is likely to be effective for the particular defendant, and that the veteran and society will be best served by a disposition which emphasizes treatment.

A further complexity is that some veterans with histories of rage have treatable PTSD, while others have less treatable, lifelong characterologic problems. Differentiation of veterans in these categories is essential. Finally, if the defense attorney and prosecutor turn out to be Viet Nam veterans, this may influence the disposition in a range of ways. Attention to this detail by the psychiatric consultant can be helpful.

A defendant had obviously committed a crime in the throes of a flashback, and an insanity defense would have been successful. The chief prosecutor was initially determined to exact extreme punishment, following the entering of a guilty plea. During the presentencing hearing, as detail after detail of the defendant's experience in Viet Nam emerged, along with an astonishing postwar history of misdiagnosis and improper treatment for PTSD, the prosecutor was deeply moved. He recalled his own Viet Nam combat experience. He revised his view of the case to the relief of his associates on the prosecution team, and after checking his reactions with them agreed with the judge's disposition, which emphasized treatment.

RESOURCES

The lack of expert resources is critical regarding the forensic evaluation of PTSD. Relatively few mental health professionals are able to perform the detailed examination that is necessary. Obtaining such evaluations from the private sector is financially prohibitive for most defendants. Federal and state facilities are limited in their ability to provide such services.

Frequently, adequate evaluation depends on funds from the court. Our current experience suggests that courts may be more generous than anticipated in making expert evaluation possible.

Defendants, attorneys, and examiners confronted with severe fiscal limitations are advised to consider the usefulness of reports from other Viet Nam veterans, from friends and family members, and from members of veterans service organizations. These may contribute significantly to the evaluation process and thus reduce the time and cost of the professional's evaluation.

VERIFICATION

Because of the increasing frequency of such cases, objective documentation of the military history is important. Official military personnel records obtainable from the St. Louis Records Center are often non-revealing: they provide names of the veteran's units and seldom give even basic data about where the units were. With enough time it is frequently possible to track down members of the defendant's unit or others familiar with combat operations in which the veteran participated. Judges frequently grant continuances for this purpose.

The Retired Officers Association has in some cases been a useful source of commanders who, because of professional and career interests, possess detailed recall, and sometimes objective records, of military operations and conditions. In the case of the doctor described above, two retired generals and a former infantryman were able to provide details concerning local conditions and events which occurred around the doctor's field hospital when he was there. These details helped overcome the defendant's amnesia and validated his history.

GENERAL ISSUES

After thorough evaluation, some cases will seem reasonably clear and simple. Unfortunately, others will be ambiguous. There is no fixed connection between psychological trauma and criminal behavior. The vast majority of combat veterans with PTSD never engage in either violence or criminal acts; some do. Whether a particular veteran with PTSD committed a particular crime partly or entirely because of the disorder is a determination which challenges the skill of the informed clinician.

We recommend that clinicians consider the following guidelines when trying to determine whether a connection exists:

1. Crimes related to PTSD usually reconstruct in some decipherable manner elements of traumatic situations. The evaluator must determine the presence of this isomorphism.
2. The presence of fugue states, dissociative reactions, and bewilderment supports the conclusion that criminal behavior reflects im-

pairment of the ability to control behavior.

3. Life events which force the individual to face unresolved wartime grief, guilt, or fear may stimulate otherwise unlikely behaviors and activities, including those necessary for survival in combat. For example, the birth or death of a child may evoke harshly repressed material and lead to survival behavior.

4. Careful clinical study should reveal understandable motives for the behavior. It is seldom the case, however, that an antagonistic or threatening clinician will uncover pertinent information. This may be particularly important in adversarial proceedings, where the prosecution examiner fails to elicit relevant material and expresses disbelief at the assessment of the defense examiner.

5. The most credible defense demonstrates a close relationship between the crime and a specific traumatic situation. In assessing such a case, details will emerge which will be convincing to open-minded clinicians, judges, and jurors.

6. Although many Viet Nam veterans with PTSD have improved over the years, some have not. Among those most troubled it is not surprising to find anxiety, depression, phobias, rage, substance abuse, divorce, unemployment, and suspiciousness. The presence of these signs, symptoms, and behaviors may mislead the objective clinician or provide data for the antagonistic clinician, resulting in misdiagnosis and pessimism regarding prognosis.

7. Some Viet Nam veterans in psychiatric hospitals suffer from forms of mental illness other than PTSD. However, since the first evaluations of Viet Nam veterans during the 1960s, clinicians have confused hallucinations with flashbacks, anhedonia with psychic numbing, and psychotic with nonpsychotic illness. Many clinical formulations before the publication of *DSM-III* in 1980 failed to diagnose cases of stress disorder or acknowledge the relevance of traumatic events.

8. Despite the most diligent efforts, there will be a group of forensic cases in which the relationship of existing PTSD to a criminal act remains unclear. In some of these cases, we believe that recent life events may have stimulated partial reliving of traumatic events or may have evoked behavior which was initially developed to deal with PTSD. Frequently, these responses include substance abuse, aggressive acts, or rage episodes. We recommend that, in the absence of a significant history of criminal behavior, emphasis be given to the causative role of PTSD. Such cases may be best managed by rehabilitation and probation rather than by simple punishment.

We do not assert that all criminal acts by combat veterans can be explained in whole or in part as sequelae of the psychological trauma of war. However, in cases where criminal behavior can be partially or entirely attributed to trauma, and where there is a possibility of meaningful treatment, we encourage judicious use of psychotherapy, along with probation or parole. If punishment is included, an element of restitution may be useful.

When PTSD is pertinent to crime, the carefully done clinical assessment and analysis of causality will be clear and parsimonious. When PTSD has been a critical issue, its discovery, treatment, and clinical course often clarify for both clinician and veteran many puzzling historical details of the period prior to the criminal offense.

REFERENCES

1. American Psychiatric Association: Diagnostic and Statistical Manual of Mental Disorders, Third Edition. Washington, DC, American Psychiatric Association, 1980

2. American Psychiatric Association: Diagnostic and Statistical Manual of Mental Disorders. Washington, DC, American Psychiatric Association, 1952

3. American Psychiatric Association: Diagnostic and Statistical Manual of Mental Disorders, Second Edition. Washington, DC, American Psychiatric Association, 1968

4. Lipkin J, Blank AS Jr, Parsons E, et al: Viet Nam veterans and posttraumatic stress disorder. Hosp Community Psychiatry 33:908–912, 1982

5. Figley CR (ed): Stress Disorders Among Viet Nam Veterans: Theory, Research, and Treatment Implications. New York, Brunner/Mazel, 1978

6. Lifton RJ: The Broken Connection. New York, Simon & Schuster, 1980

7. Santoli A: Everything We Had. New York, Random House, 1981

8. Hasford G: The Short-Timers. New York, Bantam Books, 1980

9. Scurfield R: Post-trauma stress assessment and treatment: overview and formulations, in Trauma and Its Wake, vol 1. Edited by Figley CR. New York, Brunner/Mazel, in press

10. Wilson J, Krauss G: The Viet Nam Era Stress Inventory. Cleveland OH, Cleveland State University, 1980

22

Conclusion: Stress and Recovery in Viet Nam Veterans

Stephen M. Sonnenberg, M.D.

22

In the last half-century, war has served American psychiatry as an unwanted stimulus to perfect our understanding of human behavior. Whether the concern was with the nature of aggression or the healing process among survivors, experiences at the front and in hospitals at home led mental health professionals to new insights. Knowledge expanded in the psychology, biology, and treatment of mental illness.

This volume has been a long time in coming, for it is now a decade since America's withdrawal from Viet Nam. Yet, sensitive and skilled diagnosis and treatment of post-traumatic stress disorder in Viet Nam veterans remains a challenge to the helping professions. For many veteran survivors the war rages on, and for many others life will never be the same.

It appears that during every period of peace certain central lessons of war are forgotten. In that connection, historians and political scientists might write of forgotten lessons of international experience. Mental health professionals might write of forgotten lessons concerning the psychological effects of war. These lessons include observations of the psychic trauma of combatants, civilians caught up in conflagration, and those who sit at home, wait, and watch.

The delay in recognizing the mental pain of Viet Nam veterans was a complicated psychosocial phenomenon in America. By the late 1960s the war was enormously controversial and profound divisions and confusion were dominant features of national life. By 1970 a majority of Americans opposed the Viet Nam War, and there was a repudiation of veterans as bearers of unwanted history.

In addition, the savagery of battle in Southeast Asia was viewed at closer range than were the events of previous wars, because technological advances in communication and transportation made possible detailed pictorial accounts of the war on the television screens of millions of American households. This daily experience did not inure viewers to the violence they witnessed. Rather, the human capacity for aggression was dramatically clear and led to an hypertrophied need to deny and repress what was observed.

Although the American Psychiatric Association had in its nomenclature the category of traumatic reaction to wartime experience following World War II and Korea, this clinical entity was absent from the official diagnostic literature during the era of Viet Nam. Some psychiatrists believe this is because PTSD can affect previously healthy individuals, and it therefore reminds mental health professionals of their own vulnerability to extreme stress. This blind spot in official psychiatric nomenclature was a part of the environment to which veterans returned.

Another reason for professional insensitivity to the needs of returning veterans is attributable to the psychiatric techniques used on the battlefields of Viet Nam. These modes of intervention stressed rapid reintegration and return to duty for those who showed signs of "battle fatigue." These successes of military psychiatrists suggested a very low rate of psychiatric casualty. At first, then, veterans who suffered were not well understood, for there was neither an expectation that they were ill nor a diagnostic category in which they could be placed. PTSD had to be rediscovered before those with the disorder could be evaluated and helped.

Many veterans, themselves suffering and recovering from the stress and trauma of war, worked in self-help settings. They approached the task of helping themselves and others with creativity and zeal. They grew psychologically and encouraged experienced psychotherapists to work with war survivors. This stimulated the first contemporary researchers in the field of PTSD and resulted in clarification of the effects of trauma. The contributions of Chaim Shatan, Robert Jay Lifton, and Mardi Horowitz are seminal works born of what became a movement.

These same veterans were to give rise to a second generation of thinkers, researchers, and healers who would refine the theoretical and clinical understanding of PTSD. Some of these veterans were already young mental health professionals when they served in Viet Nam, some were nurses or medics, some were Army or Marine foot soldiers or officers, and some served in the Air Force or Navy. Among those who were not already healing professionals, several earned advanced degrees in medicine, psychology, counseling, and social work.

Members of this group of trained practitioners maintained their interest in the suffering of their comrades. Many now work within the Veterans Administration, but others occupy a range of positions in the community of helping professionals. Wherever they went they explained to their colleagues the nature of PTSD and stimulated understanding, interest, and concern among many who did not serve in Viet Nam.

This is a unique psychiatric book. You, the reader, have been provided a scientific account of the psychological ravages of Viet Nam on the men and women who served there. But you have also heard the voices of these veterans—and those of the helping professionals they have directly touched—as they reverberate throughout this book. In that regard these pages are characterized by special sensitivity to the pain of those patients and clients whose stories are described. Similarly, those sections dealing with treatment reflect the wisdom of many who themselves have suffered the trauma and stress of war and have recovered. It is an axiom of psychiatry that many of its greatest discoveries began with the personal experiences and introspective efforts of the psychological scientist who proffers a new idea. Nowhere is that axiom more apparent than in this book.

You have just been exposed to a powerful account of the pain of Viet Nam veterans who suffer with PTSD, as well as the difficult challenge faced by the helping professionals who wish to provide assistance. You have learned of the anxiety, depression, and guilt with which so many survivors struggle. You have become aware of the role that traumatic past experiences play in the lives of these victims of stress, of the need to undo the past which unconsciously motivates so much of their behavior. You have read of nightmares and dramatic flashbacks. During the latter, you have learned, complicated behavior may symbolically repeat the past. You now know of the disruptions that PTSD causes in families and social systems.

You have read of the valiant efforts of veterans to help one another and of a range of creative therapies they developed. Some of these veterans are mental health professionals, and others are not. You have also become aware of interventions developed by nonveteran therapists, who were inspired by the commitment of those who survived the war.

You have been told of the role that social networks, peer support, somatic therapy, psychotherapy, and help from the Veterans Administration play in aiding veterans to integrate their experiences and resume an arduous process of maturation. The special problems of particular groups of veterans have been reviewed, and the need for outreach to forgotten populations has been discussed.

Some would like to believe that Viet Nam no longer affects the American people, but this seems to be mere wishful thinking. A generation of Americans were scarred by the Viet Nam War. If they themselves did not serve, it is likely that they experienced the loss of friends or family. And all of this took place in the context of a war which did violence to the ideals for which America stands.

Thus, you—the reader for whom this book has been written—are advised to explore additional contributions of other concerned individuals, contributions which describe the impact of Viet Nam from various other perspectives. These include political and diplomatic considerations, ecological effects, the impact on public mental and physical health, and the nature of a world led to view life with too little concern.

Out of the suffering of America's veterans and the people of Viet Nam, growth can occur and lessons can be learned. Psychiatrists and other mental health professionals can make important ongoing contributions to the national and international healing process that must continue. Mental health professionals have much to offer in the process of national appraisal that is a part of life in America. In this country there is the possibility of public debate and self-scrutiny. Americans have the opportunity to ask themselves how they interact with their government, refine and define their values, and shape their institutions.

In every society there is a pernicious danger that members of an underclass will be assigned the most unwanted burdens. This clearly happened when American boys were selectively drafted for service in Southeast Asia. Likewise, there is a tendency to scapegoat, to assign guilt to a pariah class. This certainly characterized the homecoming of those who served in Viet Nam. Psychiatrists and their professional colleagues are in a special position to provide leadership that interprets and clarifies the nature of this process.

There is still much to be learned concerning the trauma of war and the nature of PTSD, as well as the process of growth which can occur in recovering veterans. It is clear that the helping professions must play an active role if that knowledge is to develop and if more effective methods of therapy are to emerge. We are on a journey removed by a decade from Viet Nam, and it is all too easy to travel on without a sense of urgency. It is hoped that you, the reader, will recognize that our task is both urgent and imposing. It is hoped also that you will use the knowledge you have gained from reading this book to dedicate yourself to advancing your abilities to understand and assist those veterans who so desperately need your help.

Index

Index

DATE			
JUL 1 8 1988			
OCT 2 1 1989			
APR 0 9 2002			